FROM PARALYSIS TO FATIGUE

A History of Psychosomatic Illness in the Modern Era

Edward Shorter

THE FREE PRESS
A Division of Macmillan, Inc.
NEW YORK

Maxwell Macmillan Canada
TORONTO

Maxwell Macmillan International
NEW YORK OXFORD SINGAPORE SYDNEY

The Free Press
A Division of Macmillan, Inc.
866 Third Avenue, New York, N.Y. 10022

Maxwell Macmillan Canada, Inc.
1200 Eglinton Avenue East
Suite 200
Don Mills, Ontario M3C 3N1

Macmillan, Inc. is part of the Maxwell Communication Group of Companies.

First Free Press Paperback Edition 1993

Printed in the United States of America

printing number

1 2 3 4 5 6 7 8 9 10

Library of Congress Cataloging-in-Publication Data

Shorter, Edward.
    From paralysis to fatigue : a history of psychosomatic illness in the modern era / Edward Shorter.
        p.   cm.
    Includes bibliographical references and index.
    ISBN 0-02-928667-0
    1. Medicine, Psychosomatic—Social aspects—History.
2. Somatoform disorders—Social aspects—History.   3. Social medicine.   I. Title.
    [DNLM: 1. Fatigue—psychology.   2. Paralysis—psychology.
3. Psychophysiologic Disorders.   4. Psychosomatic Medicine—history.   5. Social Environment.   WM 90 S559f]
RC49.S435   1992
616'.001'9—dc20
DNLM/DLC
for Library of Congress   91-24912
                                                                            CIP

To my parents,
Joan and Lazar Shorter,
in gratitude

Contents

Preface   *ix*

1. Doctors and Patients at the Outset   *1*

   Psychogenic Symptoms   *2*
   The Symptom Pool   *5*
   An Eighteenth-Century Symptom Census   *10*
   The Doctors' Story Begins   *12*
   Three Eighteenth-Century Views of Mind-Body Relations   *14*
   Irritation and the Reflex Arc   *20*

2. Spinal Irritation   *25*

   The Diagnosis Crystallizes   *26*
   Spinal Irritation Appears in the Patients' World   *29*
   Center and Periphery   *33*

3. Reflex Theory and the History of Internal Sensation   *40*

   Applying Reflex Doctrine to Patients   *41*
   The Triumph of Reflex Theory   *45*
   Reflexes from the Sex Organs   *48*
   The Medicalizing of Women's Internal Sensations   *51*
   The Last Gasp of Reflex Theory: The Nose   *64*

4. Gynecological Surgery and the Desire
   for an Operation   *69*

   The Pelvic Organs as a Supposed Cause of Insanity   *69*
   Gynecological Surgery to Cure Nervous and Mental Illness   *73*
   Gynecology in the Hands of Psychiatrists   *79*
   Clitoridectomy   *81*
   The Desire for Surgery as a Psychosomatic Symptom   *86*
   Sexual Surgery on Males   *92*

Contents

5. Motor Hysteria   95

  Hysterical Fits   96
  The Rise of Hysterical Paralysis   102
  A Picture of Paralysis   108
  Triggering Paralysis   112
  Male Hysteria   117
  The Family Psychodrama   120
  The Doctors' Dislike of Hysterical Paralysis   125

6. Dissociation   129

  Spontaneous Somnambulism and Catalepsy   130
  The First Wave of Hypnosis   134
  Hypnotic Catalepsy   136
  Induced Somnambulism   146
  The Second Wave of Hypnosis   150
  "Permanently Benumbed" and the Climate of Suggestion   155
  Multiple Personality Disorder   159

7. Charcot's Hysteria   166

  Charcot's Life   167
  Charcot's Doctrine of Hysteria   175
  The Hospital as Circus   181
  The Diffusion of "la Grande Hystérie"   186
  A Turn Toward the Psychological?   193
  The Disappearance of Charcot's Hysteria   196

8. The Doctors Change Paradigms:
   Central Nervous Disease   201

  The Destruction of the Reflex Paradigm   202
  *The Rise of Central Nervous Theories of Psychosis
     and Neurosis*   208
  Nerve Doctors for Nervous Diseases   213
  Neurasthenia   220

9. Doctors, Patients, and the Psychological Paradigm   233

  Forerunners of the Psychological Paradigm   233
  The Psychological Paradigm Becomes a Major Competitor   239
  Patients' Medical Therapy Is Physicians' Psychotherapy   245

Contents

The Psychoanalysts Hijack Psychotherapy | 253
Patients Reject the Psychological Paradigm | 261

10. The Patients' Paradigm Changes | 267

The Decline of Motor Hysteria | 267
The Paradigm Shift on Harley Street | 273
Chronic Fatigue | 277
Psychogenic Pain | 285

11. Somatization at the End of the Twentieth Century | 295

A New Sensitivity to Pain | 295
Fatigue | 300
Fixed Illness Belief | 301
The Epidemic of Chronic Fatigue | 307
The Media and the Loss of Medical Authority | 314
Somatization and Postmodern Life | 320

Notes | 325
Index | 411

vii

Preface

The history of psychosomatic illness in the modern era is a complex and sometimes tangled tale. The present work provides the essential narrative of the story, beginning with such notions as hysteria in the eighteenth century, and continuing into our own time with such contemporary disorders as chronic fatigue syndrome. It is a history of shifting maladies as experienced by patients and perceived by doctors, an account of how historical eras shape their own symptoms of illness. (A future work will focus on the social and biological themes in psychosomatic illness, seen in historical perspective.)

It should be emphasized at the beginning that from the patient's viewpoint psychosomatic problems qualify as genuine diseases. There is nothing imaginary or simulated about the patient's perception of his or her illness. Although the symptom may be psychogenic, the pain or the grinding fatigue is very real. The patient cannot abolish the symptoms by obeying the simple injunction to "pull up your socks," for what he or she experiences is caused by the action of the unconscious mind, over which he or she by definition has no rational control. Thus this book does not view patients with "somatoform" symptoms as bizarre objects but as individuals who enjoy the dignity that all disease confers; our task is rather to understand why the kinds of psychosomatic symptoms that patients perceive change so much over the ages.

Because I am a historian, the interplay between culture and the problems of the individual interests me. Here the unconscious mind intervenes. In psychosomatic illness the body's response to stress or unhappiness is orchestrated by the unconscious. The unconscious mind, just like the conscious, is influenced by the surrounding culture, which has models of what it considers to be legitimate and illegitimate symptoms. Legitimate symptoms are ascribed to an underlying organic disease for which the patient could not possibly be blamed. Illegitimate ones, by contrast, may be thought due to playacting or silliness. By defining certain symptoms as illegitimate, a culture strongly encourages patients not to develop them or to risk being thought "undeserving" individuals with no real medical problems. Accordingly there is great pressure on the unconscious mind to produce only legitimate symptoms.

This cultural pressure is the crux of the book. The unconscious mind desires to be taken seriously and not be ridiculed. It will therefore strive to present symptoms that always seem, to the surrounding culture, legitimate evidence of organic disease. This striving introduces a historical dimension. As the culture changes its mind about what is legitimate disease and what is not, the pattern of psychosomatic illness changes. For example, a sudden increase in the number of young women who are unable to get out of bed because their legs are "paralyzed" may tell us something about how the surrounding culture views women and how it expects them to perform their roles.

Psychosomatic illness is any illness in which physical symptoms, produced by the action of the unconscious mind, are defined by the individual as evidence of organic disease and for which medical help is sought. This process of somatization comes in two forms. In one no physical lesion of any kind exists and the symptoms are literally psychogenic; that is to say, they arise in the mind. In the second an organic lesion does exist, but the patient's response to it—his or her illness behavior—is exaggerated or inappropriate. Culture intervenes in both forms, legislating what is legitimate, and mandating what constitutes an appropriate response to disease. Our late-twentieth-century culture, for example, which values individual dynamism, regards physical paralysis and sudden "coma" (both common before 1900) as inappropriate responses.

Psychosomatic illnesses have always existed, because psychogenesis— the conversion of stress or psychological problems into physical symptoms—is one of nature's basic mechanisms in mobilizing the body to cope with mental distress. People have always tried to achieve some kind of plausible interpretation of their physical sensations. They cast these sensations on the model of well-defined medical symptoms available in a kind of "symptom pool." Only when an individual's act of making sense amplifies the sensations, or attributes them to disease when none exists, does psychosomatic illness come into play.

The two actors in this psychodrama of making sense of one's sensations are, and always have been, doctors and patients. The interaction between doctors and patients determines how psychosomatic symptoms change over the years. Doctors' notions of what constitutes "genuine" organicity may alter, perhaps as a result of increased scientific knowledge or of new cultural preconceptions. Although patients' notions of disease tend to follow doctors' ideas—a kind of obedience that has started to break down at the end of the twentieth century—patients may also change their notions of the legitimacy of symptoms for reasons that have little to do with medicine. The point remains, however, that the relationship between doctors and patients is reciprocal: As the ideas of either party about what constitutes legitimate organic disease change, the other member of the duo will respond. Thus the history of psychosomatic illness is one of ever-changing steps in a pas de deux between doctor and patient.

This book begins with the late-eighteenth-century status quo and brings the story up to the present. The nature of psychosomatic symptoms changed relatively little before the second half of the eighteenth century. Premodern patients responded not to an official medical culture but to a fairly constant and unchanging body of unofficial medical folklore that was probably a thousand years old. Before 1750 doctors, too, believed in a relatively unchanging core of "humoral" medical doctrines, the basic components of which reached back to the ancient Greeks. Then, after the mid-eighteenth century, the presentation of psychosomatic illness began to vary—changes reflected in the following chapters.

Finishing in the present exposes one to all the risks of writing contemporary history, in which the underlying factors do not stand out from the superficial detail with the clarity lent by remoter times. Still, as a historian, I am attracted by the idea (however illusory and deceptive it might be) of using the past to illuminate today's problems. So striking is the impact of culture on psychosomatic illness, that both doctors and patients today might learn something by seeing medical symptoms, which are considered intensely personal and idiosyncratic, in light of the past.

Some thanks are in order. I owe much to the inventiveness and energy of my library assistant Kaia Toop, and I am happy to acknowledge here the help she has given me over the years. I have been privileged to work in the Science and Medicine Library of the University of Toronto. My friend Walter Vandereycken, M.D., read critically an earlier draft. Joyce Seltzer at The Free Press has been a wonderful editor, and Susan Llewellyn a superb copy editor. I should also like to thank my dear wife, Anne Marie Shorter, M.D., who read each chapter of the manuscript and offered helpful comments. Grants from the Connaught Fund of the University of Toronto and the Social Science and Humanities Research Council of Canada helped support some of the research. Of the many archives and libraries in Europe and England in which I have worked, I must single out the Institut für Geschichte der Medizin in Vienna as a reminder that intense scholarly effort is not incompatible with a setting of warmth and hospitality.

CHAPTER

1

Doctors and Patients
at the Outset

The descent from mind to body is a tricky one. How does the mind interpret the signals the body gives off? A young executive feels a stomachache before an important presentation. There is nothing physically wrong with her stomach. In the absence of any physical lesion, her mind perceives pain coming from the stomach. That pain is psychogenic, unlike the pain of a gastric ulcer, which is somatogenic. (*Somatogenic* means there is something physically wrong with the body, and damaged nerve endings are causing the pain.)

Do psychogenic symptoms have a history of their own? Have they perhaps always been more or less the same, as coughing up sputum, if one has pneumonia, has historically been invariant? One factor that confers a history is the doctor's attitude. Patients want to please doctors, in the sense that they do not want the doctor to laugh at them and dismiss their plight as imaginary. Thus they strive to produce symptoms the doctor will recognize. As doctors' own ideas about what constitutes "real" disease change from time to time due to theory and practice, the symptoms that patients present will change as well. These medical changes give the story of psychosomatic illness its dynamic: the medical "shaping" of symptoms.

Not until the eighteenth century, with the advent of new theories about "nervous disease," does such shaping begin to change. Patients start the narrative by breaking with an age-old pattern of traditional psychosomatic symptoms. And the doctors' part of the story commences just as some important scientific advances occur. But these discoveries about the nervous system led to some unscientific theories about how nervous disease arises—

1

theories that would suggest to patients a new pattern of psychosomatic symptoms. The symptom shift thus begins with the rise of such "nervous" symptoms. A set of symptoms, such as hysterical paralysis, arose which was quite specific to the late eighteenth and nineteenth centuries. These symptoms would in the twentieth give way to quite different symptoms—those of chronic fatigue, pain, and allergy sensitivity.

Psychogenic Symptoms

By definition psychogenic physical symptoms arise in the mind, in contrast to somatogenic symptoms, which come from organic disease. To the patient, however, both kinds of symptoms *seem* the same: Both appear to result from real bodily disease. There is very little cultural shaping of the symptoms of organic disease, and people presumably turned yellow with liver failure in the fourteenth century just as they do in the twentieth (liver disease causes jaundice, giving a yellowish cast to the skin). Although the mind may still edit somatogenic symptoms, they are mainly shaped by organic disease. But the shaping of psychogenic symptoms is left to the fantasy of the unconscious.

Nevertheless, the unconscious is not entirely abandoned to its own resources. The surrounding culture provides our unconscious minds with templates, or models, of illness. If our unconscious decides, for example, that we are to be in pain, it determines how pain will be dealt with: perhaps with the stoic jaw clenching of Anglo-Saxon cultures or with the tying about one's head of a kerchief, as in Italy. These are examples of culturally determined templates the unconscious uses to instruct itself.

All these templates, or different ways of presenting illness, constitute a symptom pool—the culture's collective memory of how to behave when ill. For Western society since the Middle Ages, the number of potential symptoms in this pool has been relatively unchanging. Symptoms of headache, tiredness, and a twitching left leg are some of its contents, which have been available for centuries. Some symptoms from other cultures—such as "koro," a perception among South Asian and Chinese males that the penis is retreating inside the abdomen—do not form part of this pool.[1] The symptom pool of the Occident has always harbored certain standard items. Until the middle of the twentieth century, people knew about the contents of this pool from popular culture, an oral tradition that communicated from generation to generation whatever individuals told each other about aches, pains, and other bodily woes. Today the media more than any other conduit tell us about the symptom pool.

The contents of this particular symptom pool are psychogenic, in that all may be caused by the action of the mind. (Turning yellow is not part of the psychosomatic symptom pool.) But headache, tiredness, and a twitching left leg may be caused by organic disease as well, and someone has to decide whether they are psychogenic or somatogenic. Perhaps it is the individual, him- or herself, in deciding whether to seek out the doctor for a particular symptom. Perhaps it is the doctor, in deciding whether to operate or to counsel the patient. In historical studies informed retrospection tries to decide. Yet the decision must be made, or the notion of a well-circumscribed psychogenic symptom pool is meaningless.

In some historical periods certain items in the pool are frequently drawn on, in others scarcely at all. How does the culture of a given period decide which symptoms to select? It depends on representations of what is thought to be legitimate organic disease. No patient wants to select illegitimate symptoms, to become a laughingstock or be dismissed as hysterical. Thus any given period will have a predominant notion of what it considers real disease.

Robert Musil makes this point, in a slightly different context, in his novel about Viennese life at the turn of the century, *The Man Without Qualities*. Ulrich, the chief protagonist, is thinking about photographs of beautiful women from decades past, and as he tries to achieve some kind of rapport with the faces in the photographs he notices "a whole number of small features which actually constituted the face, and yet which seemed very improbable. All societies have always had every kind of face. But the standards of the day single out one particular face as the dominant one, the essence of happiness and beauty, while all other faces attempt to imitate it."[2] So it is with symptoms. Our bodies send us the most disparate variety of signals about physical sensations. Under some circumstances, we interpret these signals as evidence of disease, but the symptoms into which our minds cast this disease are just as determined by fashion as was the fashionable face of fin-de-siècle Vienna.

These symptoms fall into four general categories: sensory symptoms, such as prickly skin or tiredness; motor symptoms, such as paralysis; symptoms of the autonomic nervous system, such as a churning bowel; and symptoms of psychogenic pain.

Sensory and motor symptoms, the first two groups, belong to the body's somatosensory nervous system. This is a nervous system with its own privileged pathways. Certain parts of the spinal cord are reserved for it, as are certain areas of the brain. If a young man suddenly developed a loss of feeling in half of his body (and had no organic disease), he would

3

have a psychosomatic sensory symptom. A young woman who awakened one morning unable to walk because of a paralysis of her legs (and had no neurological illness) would belong in the motor category.

A third group of symptoms are autonomic, meaning they are controlled by the autonomic nervous system, which regulates the action of internal organs and the diameter of blood vessels. Thus diarrhea, blushing, a racing pulse, and all kinds of internal sensations come into this category.

Finally, there is psychogenic pain, which means pain that the patient perceives as real but that is not caused by an organic lesion in the body. The pain arises in the mind. If I get a headache as I sit at my word processor thinking how to make this clear, I am suffering a psychogenic headache.

Of course all these symptoms could result from organic diseases too, which is precisely the point. In somatization the unconscious mind chooses symptoms that will be taken as evidence of real, physical disease and that will win the patient an appropriate response.[3] Thus most of the symptoms in these four compartments of the symptom pool have always been known to Western society, although they have occurred at different times with different frequencies: Society does not invent symptoms; it retrieves them from the symptom pool.

One objection comes immediately to mind. With the exception of those in the last chapter, the patients described in this book are all dead. Is it certain that their symptoms were not caused by an organic disease? Retrospectively, it is not. There is only the presumption of psychogenesis, based on (a) the history of the illness, such as paralysis after seeing a frog on the road, and (b) the response to what was essentially placebo therapy, such as hydrotherapy or administration of a laxative. These two circumstances give certain symptom patterns a flavor of psychogenesis.

An elderly neurologist in Marseilles told me about young Italian female patients, usually from southern Italy, who would be brought to his clinic—much more prestigious than the Italian clinics—in an ambulance, convulsing and thrashing in fits. "It would take four men to hold them down," he said. He cured them with sugar pills. He opened his desk drawer to show the three colors of pills he gave, some "stronger" than others. Of course the patients thought they were powerful medicine.

Were these young women epileptic?

"No, hysterical," he said. "You can smell this quality of hysteria." He gestured expansively to his nose. "*Ça sent de l'hystérie.*"

Whatever the cultural reasons for the illness behavior of these southern Italian women—and one may presume many such reasons on the part of powerless young women in a patriarchal society—they probably did not have epilepsy. So it is with many of the men and women in this book: They probably did not have an organic illness, although we cannot be sure.

The Symptom Pool

The pool of psychosomatic symptoms, physical symptoms caused by the action of the mind, has a history. Of the various types of psychosomatic symptoms, those attributable to the motor side of the nervous system are the most colorful. Reaching back into antiquity, they include sudden loss of the power of speech (hysterical aphonia);[4] the inability, all at once, to open the eyelids; contractions, incapable of relaxation, of the elbows, wrists and fingers; and failure to get out of bed one morning because the lower limbs are paralyzed. Historically, the commonest of the motor symptoms have been fits, or pseudoepileptic fainting and writhing about. In fits, motor activity is apparently out of control, the limbs twitching histrionically, the eyes turned back in the head, the affected individuals (they do not become "patients" until they see a doctor) often screaming, cursing, and attempting to bite those nearby.[5]

In the domain of pseudoepilepsy there is truly nothing new under the sun. According to a note in the November 7, 1711, *Spectator*: "Mr. Freeman had no sooner taken coach, but his lady was taken with a terrible fit of the vapours, which, 'tis feared, will make her miscarry, if not endanger her life." "After many revolutions in [Mrs. Freeman's] temper of raging, swooning, railing, fainting, pitying herself and reviling her husband, upon an accidental coming in of a neighbouring lady . . . she had nothing left for it but to fall in a fit." Mrs. Freeman was quite accustomed to throwing teacups into the fire and berating the menfolk surrounding her. Whatever the true cause of her unbridled behavior ("this fashionable reigning distemper"), it is unlikely that she had epilepsy.[6]

Far from London in rustic Edale, Dr. James Clegg went to visit his mother on September 14, 1730: "She was seized whilst I was there with a most violent hysteric fit exactly at the time the moon came to the full. I lodged there that night."[7] Again, Dr. Clegg's mother probably did not have epileptic attacks at full moon, though we cannot know for sure. There was Mrs. King, thirty years old, of Northfleet and a patient of John Woodward, a distinguished London physician. In the spring of 1705 "a great grief" affected her, whereupon "she fell into a most violent griping pain of her stomach. In a quarter of an hour she perceived a tingling, and afterwards a deadness of her left hand, which gradually ascending up her arm, took her head, when she lost all sense, and became finally cold, stiff, and was thought dead." Mrs. King had a long and complicated medical history: "She had once a fit upon a fright, in which she lay as dead for three or four hours." Further: "Upon grief she has had frequently risings in her throat and chokings. A fright affects her back instantly with pain. . . . It also brings on a flight vertigo and pulsation in her back and head, as also palpitation of the heart with a flushing and heat of her head and face."[8] Thus a whole riot of bodily symptoms could accompany an attack of fits, for somatizing patients often experienced all major varieties of psychosomatic symptoms simultaneously.

Mrs. King's case merely hints at another kind of motor symptom: *globus hystericus*, the sensation of a ball rising from the depths of the abdomen and lodging in the throat, whereupon an attack of fits begins. In 1713 a Mrs. Cornforth described to Doctor Woodward what she experienced in such a fit: "First her legs became feeble, so that they would not bear her weight and she could not possibly stand up." Then back pain commenced: "Immediately her heart begins to throb and palpitate, the throbs pointing at, and forcing [radiating] towards the part of the back so pained; they also force to her arms, neck, and head at the same instant, and the pulsations, in all, keep time exactly with the heart and back." She feels nauseated, and then "she sensibly perceives something fluid ascend from the place pained in her back up into her shoulders, the scapulae, arms, neck, and head." At this point Mrs. Cornforth describes much "throbbing" and writhing in her upper body and internal organs. Finally "she feels something descending down her back to her stomach, and the fit is instantly at an end."[9]

"Vapours, otherwise called hysterick fits and improperly, fits of the mother," said London physician John Purcell in 1702, "is a distemper which more generally afflicts humankind than any other whatsoever." Its symptoms? "First they feel a heaviness upon their breast, a grumbling in their belly, they belch up, and sometimes vomit. . . . They have a difficulty in breathing and think they feel something that comes up into their throat which is ready to choke them; they struggle, cry out, make odd and inarticulate sounds or mutterings; they perceive a swimming in their heads, a dimness comes over their eyes; they turn pale, are scarce able to stand; their pulse is weak, they shut their eyes, fall down and remain senseless for some time."[10] These are typical accounts of fits, which dominate the motor hysteria scene until well into the nineteenth century.

The motor symptom of inability to walk owing to supposed paralysis of the lower limbs reaches far back into time as well. Occurring chiefly in young women, these psychogenic paralyses would become virtually epidemic in the nineteenth century. But they were not unknown in the seventeenth century, when sufferers sought relief at such watering places as Bath. Thus in 1682 Mrs. Budghill of Exeter, "a comely young gentle-woman" of twenty-five, came to Dr. Robert Pierce, "all parts enfeebled and benumbed, but especially the lower parts, so that she could neither stand nor go, and the sense of feeling was depraved in all parts." Multiple sclerosis? A spinal tumor? She was "first put into the Queens-Bath, after-wards in the King's; and after a whiles bathing was pumped [given an enema]," and given various medications, so that she "at length very well recovered the perfect use of, and sense in, all her limbs."[11] Accordingly Mrs. Budghill's paralysis was probably psychogenic.

The evidence given at canonization hearings for possible saints, reflects the whole range of premodern forms of hysteria. Thus at the hearings for François de Sales, bishop of Geneva, who died in 1622, much testi-mony was accumulated of miracles performed in the countryside around Annecy in the 1650s in the deceased bishop's name. Thirty-four of the miracle cures in adults concerned paralyzed and crippled limbs. For ex-ample, after a series of maladies, in 1658 the gentleman Roget de la Bisolière found himself "paralyzed in all limbs, particularly below the waist, and since about two months I had also lost the sense of feeling." After praying to François via the intermediary of the Virgin, the man "felt an extraordinary power in all his joints" and was able to walk again easily. In 1639 Jeanne-Marie de Viry, "having been paralyzed for twelve years," was able to walk again after praying at the bishop's tomb. There were many similar cases.[12] Thus there is little new in the realms of hyster-ical paralysis and paresis.

On the sensory side, seventeenth-century witches represent a familiar historical example of anesthesias, the absence of feeling in the skin. Sometimes women accused of witchcraft were alleged to have induced anesthesia in their victims, sometimes themselves to be anesthetic, the anesthesia discovered only during the investigation. Lisa Tutken of the village of Sydinghusen in Germany, for example, was arrested in 1631 because of "black magic" and was thereupon interrogated. Undressed before the examining judge, "a stigma is discovered on her right shoulder-blade, as though [the devil] had seized her with three fingers; when the needle is stuck in deeply, she feels nothing."[13] This woman evidently suggested herself into an actual sensory deficit, on the basis of the general

7

belief that individuals such as herself must be anesthetic. Her form of symptom must have been well established in the symptom pool of early modern society.

Psychogenic pain poses more of a problem for historians because one is usually unable to rule out organic sources of pain in a given person. Yet in some cases the pattern is so striking that a physical disease is unlikely to have been the cause. Here, for example, is Martha Greswold, a twenty-three-year-old gentlewoman who was brought to Bath in May 1663, "so weak as not able to use hand nor foot, nor so much as to lift her hand to her head, but was carried from place to place, and lifted into and out of her bed." The striking aspect in this case, however, is not her weakness, which could have been caused by many different diseases, but the pattern of her pains. She had already had an attack of joint pain at thirteen. Now, "after taking cold, this wandering arthritic pain took first one knee, after a while the other, and so leaped from joint to joint till it had gone over all her limbs." There was an even-more-pronounced psychiatric element: "Her head was concerned in her general weakness; she apprehended everything that was said to her, but remembered little or nothing." A final argument against the organicity of her pain is that Doctor Pierce's therapy cured her. A vigorous round of enemas, laxatives, and bathing improved her so that seven weeks later she was able to ride homeward (a two-day journey on horseback). She then remained well for ten years—her husband dying in the interval—until clinical signs of gout (nodes at the joints and so forth) became apparent.[14] Even if Mrs. Greswold had already experienced early symptoms of gout in 1663, her total debility still represented a form of somatization.

The fourth compartment in the symptom pool is the body's internal organs, regulated by the autonomic nervous system. The unconscious mind is able to achieve what the conscious mind cannot: manipulation of the smooth muscle of the esophagus, stomach, and intestines. (It is extremely difficult deliberately to make one's esophagus swallow smoothly or one's bowels function.) Many disorders involving the bowels, for example, are psychogenic and have been familiar to doctors and patients since time out of mind. In 1816 Dr. G.L.V. Hohnstock of the village of Silkerode in central Germany described a kind of bowel-obsessed patient, chronically plagued by constipation, diarrhea, and abdominal pain. In the course of the patient's story, we reach the point where he has finally achieved an "opening," a bowel movement.

Often as a result of the relief he now feels, he falls into ecstasy. Now he directs his attention very specifically to his B.M.'s because he knows

8

what agony and anxiety constipation have caused him. Whenever the subject comes around to constipation socially, he perceives again these hypochondriacal complaints. He is happy to spend long sessions upon the toilet. To extend his stay he lays in a supply of books. Also he takes purgatives to combat constipation, and any doctor can insinuate himself with [the patient] who is willing to prescribe them. . . . The hypochondriac now believes that life is impossible without laxatives, and if none are available, he gives himself enemas. He also pays quite exact notice to his stool and its composition, keeps a diary of it in which he records daily with great exactness the quantity and quality of the excrement.[15]

It is evident from this description that the bowels of Dr. Hohnstock's patient were influenced by the action of his mind.[16]

Dr. Hohnstock's patient is also of interest for several other reasons. He perceived a good deal of abdominal pain, which may have arisen from the disordered action of the gastrointestinal tract. This would be an example of what is now called irritable bowel syndrome. (Although the problem seems ultimately to be psychogenic, its immediate impact is a real disruption of function.) Then there was the man's own analysis of his problems, his illness attribution, for Doctor Hohnstock's patient was hypochondriacal.

Hypochondria is a separate dimension of psychosomatic illness, more a state of mind than a physical symptom as such. It is found in three different contexts.[17] First, hypochondria means a preoccupation with bodily symptoms, amplifying or misinterpreting what one is actually perceiving.[18] Permitting oneself to become chronically debilitated and bedridden by a strained back, for example, represents the amplification of a symptom. Second, there is unreasonable fear about disease, a phobia of catching tuberculosis from door handles (as at the turn of the century) or of contracting AIDS from one's waiter in a restaurant (as many fear today). Such phobias play a role in understanding societal responses to illness, but most psychosomatic patients do not merely fear disease: They are already highly symptomatic. Third, there is misguided disease conviction—attributing one's symptoms to a certain disease, such as colitis among the upper crust of late-nineteenth-century France or chronic fatigue syndrome today. In the past, patients with irritable colons have imagined that their bowels had impassable strictures in them. Other patients might believe that their insides have "turned to water" or no longer even exist. These are both frankly delusional extensions of the same theme of fixed false beliefs about the body's internal state. Among premedical examples of such fixed attributions were witchcraft and demonic possession.[19] Medicalized versions of such attributions begin with "animal magnetism" and "catalepsy" in the last quarter of the eighteenth century.

The larger point is that patients' representations of disease help form the contents of the symptom pool. What people thought they had plays an important role in the history of psychosomatic illness, the more so because these attributions are especially vulnerable to medical "shaping."

An Eighteenth-Century Symptom Census

The historical story lies, in fact, just as much in changing attributions as it does in changing symptom patterns. Both must be considered in assessing the pattern of psychosomatic illness in a given period. One asks, for example, if the background hum of normal, day-to-day discomfort actually changes over the years? What symptoms does one experience in any given day, without their necessarily being defined as major illness for which medical help is sought? This question is impossible to answer for any historic population as a whole, for records usually have not survived of what individuals experienced on a day-to-day basis. Yet for small, literate elites in the eighteenth century and after, there are such records, in the form of diaries and letters.

Some eighteenth-century English data suggest that this "background hum" of bodily perceptions that are not necessarily defined as disease may change little historically. The diaries and letters of seven eighteenth-century figures—three men and four women chosen more or less randomly from the large corpus of memoir and diary literature—were sampled in order to answer the questions: What patterns of somatization occurred in the daily flow of ordinary life? To what kinds of bodily symptoms were these individuals most sensitive?[20] To some extent, these "respondents" were noting organically caused symptoms, such as infections or arthritis, as well as somatization. Yet enough complaints of apparently psychological origin emerge to convey a sense of garden-variety somatization at the outset of our story.

Dudley Ryder, for example, a political figure who by 1754 had become lord chief justice of the king's bench and privy councillor, was a young man in his mid-twenties preoccupied with his health. His diary entries for 1715 and 1716 offer a tale of somatic woe. January 21, 1716, saw the first mention of shoulder pain; a day later the pain had spread to his neck and the other shoulder. He drank a bottle of ale to "sweat" the pain out, but by the following day it had spread to his thighs. By March 1 the pain, previously in his shoulders and thighs, was in his foot. On March 15 he entered into a contract with the mistress of a bathhouse for a year.

> The reason of my design [to go often] is that I think it will strengthen my body, purge it of ill humours, fence me against cold, prevent convulsions which I have sometimes been afraid of by reason of those sudden startings which I have sometimes. I have heard also it is good against the stone and gravel, which I have been afraid of upon the account of those sharp pains I have about my belly. . . . It will also cure the laxity of the nerves which is the occasion of what they call the vapours.

Two weeks later he came home from a walk and began to feel uneasy, having a sore throat, elevated pulse, and hot hands. Two weeks later his hands had grown even hotter. By May 6 arm pains had begun. A week later he was cupped (underwent bloodletting) to stop the arm pains. By mid-July his family was losing patience with this sensitive young man. "[His cousin Marshall] thinks that my case [of rheumatism] is as much hysteric as rheumatic if not more." All the while, heavy thoughts lay on his mind, and indeed he exhibited some evidence of depression: "There was one thing troubled me extremely . . . and that was the apprehension I was under that I was not capable of getting my wife with child if I had one. I find myself not very powerful in that way and it makes me very uneasy to think my wife should have reason to complain." On and on went the record of "swooning," "giddiness," and "melancholy." Ryder lived another forty years.

By contrast the duchess of Northumberland, forty-four as we encounter her in 1760, complained more of fatigue and gout. May 6, 1760: "Tired to death." September 8, 1762: "I was very ill." July 1, 1771: "Being too lame on my arrival in England to pay my duty to their Majesties in public . . ." May 20, 1772: "I forgot my gout and got out and walked part of the way." Of course she may have had gout, but her entire circle of young upper-middle-class society women believed themselves gouty as well, and it is likely that most did not have organic disease of the joints.

Bridget Byng, healthy enough to outlive her husband, John—the fifth Lord Torrington—by ten years, was continually ill throughout the 1780s and early 1790s. Early in June 1781, when she must have been in her late thirties or early forties,[21] she said she was unable to walk far without pain. Two weeks later husband John wrote, "As Mrs. B. was not well, I stayed at home after my walk." Six days thereafter she was "tolerably well, tho she has been much fatigued with the rumble to Gloucester." In August of the following year John fulminated not only against his wife but her whole set: "All my ladies were so fatigued by the toil of the day, that they hurried home to bed; a most precious, nervous set, encouraging each other in sickness and fancies; never drinking one glass of wine but by the advice of the doctor. The maids, in imitation of their mistresses, fall sick likewise, and complain bitterly of their bad health!!" By 1794 little had changed. September 15: "Mrs. B from illness quickly retired to bed."

It is clear that this well-to-do coterie suffered from quotidian psychosomatic illnesses not entirely unlike those of today.

Some statistical analysis can be made of the references in these letters and diaries. Of a total of 243 somatic complaints, almost half are the hypochondriacal mopings of Dudley Ryder. The other six individuals, although symptomatic from time to time, were not high symptom reporters. If one assigns these 243 symptoms to major categories, pain is the major single complaint (21 percent of the total). Only 12 of the 243 symptoms concern the motor side of the nervous system, and the incidence of classic hysteria in day-to-day life must surely have been low (although spectacular when it occurred in the form of sudden blindness, deafness, paralysis, and so forth). Thirty-five complaints were attributable to the routine somatic symptoms of anxiety and depression (sweating and fast pulse in anxiety, tiredness, lack of appetite, and insomnia and the like in depression). And 42 notices appeared of some other variety of sensory complaint. The remaining symptoms were too varied to outline in this manner. In sum, the volume of perceived aches, pains, and weariness has probably changed little historically. What changes is people's readiness to seek medical help for these symptoms, to define them as disease, and to give them fixed attributions.

The Doctors' Story Begins

From the outset it must be emphasized how unreliable medical diagnoses have been historically. One may go badly awry in thinking that the diagnostic label pinned on the patient necessarily reflects the reality of his or her illness. The many young women with multiple sclerosis who received the diagnosis "hysteria" are a perfect case in point.

The difficulty of breaking through the diagnosis to the reality of the illness was a problem not just in the eighteenth century but throughout. By the late nineteenth century, for example, medical diagnostics had greatly improved. Yet doctors still had great difficulty untangling the psychogenic from the neurogenic, as we see in the example of neurosyphilis ("tabes," "progressive paralysis," "general paralysis of the insane"). Here is Josef P., a senior official in Austria's internal revenue service, who in 1893 at age thirty-five presented to his family doctor with symptoms of "nerve pain over his entire body, attacks of dizziness, headaches and colics." He also displayed some behavioral abnormalities, "yelling and screaming so that the neighbors yards away could hear, slamming doors so that the house shook, and seeming more confused from month to month." Over the months to come Josef P. consulted three of Vienna's most eminent neuropsychiatrists, Richard von Krafft-Ebing, Julius Wagner-Jauregg and Moritz Benedikt. Each had an international reputation and had written books about psychiatry and neurology. So what disease did Josef P. have?

Professor Benedikt said that he had "hysteria virilis." Professor Wagner-Jauregg diagnosed "polyneuritis." And Professor Krafft-Ebing believed that he had "progressive paralysis," the nineteenth-century term for neurosyphilis. Thus on the basis of the same data three eminent professors had arrived at three entirely different diagnoses.[22] Although Krafft-Ebing's diagnosis was the correct one—the patient would die insane and paralyzed in an asylum—we see what difficulties would be encountered by a historian who wanted to write a history of "hysteria" or "polyneuritis" on the basis of diagnostic terms alone. If one wants to press through to the historic reality of patients and their illnesses, it is unwise to satisfy oneself solely with diagnoses. A reasonably full record of the course of the illness is needed. However, medical diagnostics play a role in shaping illnesses and cannot be ignored.

A history of psychosomatic illness has little reason to dwell on medical theories before 1800, for two reasons. One is that most patients did not come into contact with physicians but rather with midwives, herbalists, and other such paramedical figures. Although patients' views might have been influenced by these professionals, little medical shaping of their symptoms occurred. The second is that traditional doctors did almost nothing by way of clinical examination or investigation, and accordingly were far less capable of differentiating somatogenic from psychogenic illness than even the Viennese professors of a later era.

Was a lesion present or not? Before 1800 physicians were usually unable to give a reliable answer. These doctors suspected, of course, the existence of symptoms without diseases, as doctors since the ancients have always done. But the eighteenth-century categories for pigeonholing such problems—"hysteric and hypochondriac affections" and "the vapours"—were so shot through with obviously physical disease that the average physician's competence at separating organic from psychosomatic must have been tenuous at best. It is striking in the literature on hysteria to see how many patients have a fever (meaning they have an infectious disease), and how many die soon after the diagnosis is made.

To illustrate this point: Mary Prettyman, twenty-three and "of tender habit" (delicate) was a patient of John Andree's early in the eighteenth century in the London infirmary. "About ten weeks ago [she] was taken with a great working in her bowels, swelling at stomach, after that grew hot and feverish, then had a tremor all over, and fell into a fit, crying and laughing alternatively, which lasted about three hours." These symptoms persisted about two weeks. "This case is properly hysterick," noted Doctor Andree, attributing her problems to a missed period. We ask retrospectively, if Miss Prettyman was experiencing fits of psychological origin. The answer is probably that she had some kind of febrile delirium from an infection.[23] In other words, most medical accounts written before the beginning of careful clinical investigation of patients in the nineteenth century run the risk of conflating the organic and the psychological. As a result we learn little about the actual occurrence of somatization from earlier medical reports.

Three Eighteenth-Century Views of Mind-Body Relations

For some purposes the quality of the diagnosis is irrelevant. When, for example, we discuss medical theories as an independent influence in the shaping of patients' symptoms, it does not matter whether the doctors' diagnoses were correct or not. What counts is the physician's expectation of disease presentation, however ill founded in reality his expectation might be. Because it is this expectation that helps to determine what the patient brings to the doctor, in the hope of having his or her ailment diagnosed as legitimately medical, it is necessary to sketch the main eighteenth-century views of how body and mind influence each other and then see how the advance of basic medical science contributed to shifting these views. In this shift lay the basis of nineteenth-century "reflex" theory, a major moment in the history of psychosomatic illness.

Before the revolution in the neurosciences that occurred late in the eighteenth century, traditional medical views of mind-body relations could be divided into three groups: humoral theories, "master organ" theories, and theories stressing the role of nerves.

Humoral theory, the doctrine that the body was composed of four humors, had the most distinguished ancestry of the three. These humors then determined temperaments, and specific kinds of disease were associated with each temperament. Given that disease resulted from an imbalance of the humors and temperaments, medical therapy should be directed toward getting them into balance again. As Edward Baynard, a society doctor who divided his time between Preston and Bath, poeticized in 1719:

> For in ten words the whole art [of medicine] is comprised,
> For some of the ten are always advised:
> Piss, spew and spit,
> Perspiration and sweat
> Purge, bleed and blister,
> Issues and clyster.
> These few evacuations
> Cure all the doctor's patients
> If rightly applied
> By a wise physic guide.[24]

Baynard gives us here a thumbnail sketch of traditional humoral therapeutics: Get those humors right by giving drugs that cause the patient to salivate, sweat, urinate, or evacuate his bowels (a clyster is an enema). He also alludes to a refinement of humoral therapy called "counter irritation," creating skin lesions in order to draw up those poisons from below. Caustic material (an "issue"), for example, might be bound to the skin in order to encourage the formation of pus. All this polypharmacy was directed toward getting out the bad humors and righting the good.

Humoral diagnosis and therapeutics retained their millennia-old grip on many physicians right until the middle of the nineteenth century. For example, in 1836 a professor of psychiatry in Würzburg, Johannes Friedreich, could explain various mental illnesses in terms of notions about the humors and temperaments that had gone comfortably unchallenged for hundreds of years: Depression was caused by the melancholy temperament (once associated with the humor black bile), mania by the choleric temperament (yellow bile), psychosis (*Narrheit*) by the sanguine temperament (blood), and dementia by the phlegmatic temperament (phlegm). Treatment of mental illness could therefore be aimed at the internal organs, which were responsible for the humoral balance acting upon the brain.[25] In its ability to explain how the parts of the body communicated with one another in health and disease, humoralism had great apparent power and gave ground only slowly to its competitors.

A second group of eighteenth-century theories explaining how the body influenced the brain invoked specific internal organs, and made these organs a kind of master control that guided the brain. Theories inculpating the uterus as the master organ, in women at least, are ancient.[26] John Sadler, a physician in Norwich, having "consulted with Galen and Hippocrates for my proceeding," concluded in 1636 that, "among all diseases incident to the body, I found none more frequent, none more perilous that those which arise from the ill affected womb: for through the evil quality thereof, the heart, the liver, and the brain are affected." Therefore a typical affliction of women, resulting in symptoms that would later be labeled "nervous," was "suffocation of the mother [uterus]." Sadler explained it was not that the uterus itself was strangled, "but that it causes the woman to be choked. It is a retraction of the womb towards the diaphragm and stomach, which presses and crushes up the same," resulting in suffocating and fainting. A synonym in Sadler's work and others' for "suffocation of the mother" was "the hysterical passion." The womb was its seat.[27]

The great English physiologist William Harvey wrote in 1651 in his work *Anatomical Exercises on the Generation of Animals*: "For the uterus is a most important organ, and brings the whole body to sympathize with it. . . . When the uterus either rises up or falls down, or is in any way put out of place or is seized with spasm—how dreadful, then, are the mental aberrations, the delirium, the melancholy, the paroxysms of frenzy, as if the affected person were under the dominion of spells, and all arising from unnatural states of the uterus."[28]

These uterine-centered views were widely accepted by the population as a whole, male and female. Midwife Jane Sharp was certainly a partisan of them, as she wrote in her midwives' guide in 1671, "Amongst all diseases, those that are called hysteric passions or strangling of the womb are held to be the most grievous. Surrounding and falling sickness [dizziness and fits] are from hence, by the consent the womb hath with the heart and brain, and sometimes this comes to pass by stopping of the terms [menses], which load the heart, the brain and womb with evil humours." It was sympathy between brain and womb that, in Mrs. Sharp's view (which she believed was that of Hippocrates as well), caused ill humors from the uterus to produce headaches. Worse: "Some are frantick [insane], others so silent they cannot speak. Some have dimness of sight, dullness of hearing, noise in their ears, strange passions and convulsions."[29]

For centuries people had believed that one could treat the uterus by subjecting it to noxious odors, burning a foul-smelling herb called asafetida, for example, to procure an abortion as the woman crouched over the

16

smoke, or burning feathers under her nose to cure hysteria. As William Roots, on staff at St. Thomas's Hospital in London, explained to the medical students in 1836: "My impression is that one of the beneficial results of these foetid substances in hysterical conditions is the peculiar effect that they produce on the mind, through the medium of the olfactory nerves. You all know that nothing is more common, when a woman is hysterical, than to see her relieved for a time by the burning of feathers under her nose. It would be difficult perhaps to find anything much more digusting than that."[30] Uterine theories, in other words, made the patients of St. Thomas's responsive to this particular placebo therapy.

Even after the uterus had passed from fashion as "master switch," an association between uterus and hysteria remained in the popular mind. Both were believed somehow linked to perverted sexual desire. In 1894 Robert Sommer, a psychiatrist at the University of Würzburg, urged his colleagues to avoid the term hysteria in dealing with patients, "who almost without exception think of something sexual. If a doctor, for example, gives a mother the happy news that the prognosis of her seven-year-old daughter is favorable because her convulsions are merely 'hysterical' in nature, the mother will be silently indignant—or sometimes very loudly as well—at the presumption that her little sweetheart is already ruined sexually."[31] Thus we are dealing with a culture already highly inclined to believe in fabulous notions about the sex organs, providing a fertile soil for further medical suggestion.

One final point about the physicians who considered the uterus a master organ: Many of them were particularly interested in nervous disease. This is important, for uterine theorists provided direct continuity between age-old inculpations of women's reproductive organs and nineteenth-century "reflex" views. In England such otherwise progressive obstetricians as Edinburgh's John Aitken continued late in the eighteenth century to indict the pelvic organs in "furor uterinus, or nymphomania, an itching sensation about the os externum [vaginal cervix]," whose symptoms were, "lasciviousness, micturition, and convulsive motions."[32] Dublin obstetrician Edward Foster defined furor uterinus as "a vehement desire of venery, attended with melancholy or mania." Among its causes were suppressed menstruation; among its remedies emmenagogues (drugs to induce menstruation) and "acrid pessaries."[33]

Nor was this incrimination of the uterus in psychiatric ailments some specifically British quirk. Only those vapors that cause hysteria come from the uterus, not all vapors, conceded Edme-Pierre Cauvot de Beauchêne, later a consulting physician to Louis XVIII. How were the victims of this "hysteric nervous illness" to be recognized? "Some women fall to the ground in convulsions and screaming, others are silent. Some fall into an alarming faint which manifests itself under the false guise of a peaceful sleep. The convulsions and fainting spells then may give way to laughter without apparent cause, or in other patients perhaps to unmotivated tears."[34] Jean-Baptiste Louyer-Villermay, a Paris physician and author of a widely read work on hysteria, considered the uterus fundamental. After presenting evidence on the different clinical courses of hysteria and hypochondria, he concluded, "All this proves that in hysteria, the uterus is the affected organ and that it plays the principal role."[35]

What other organs controlled the mind, producing hysterical symptoms? A second major candidate alongside the uterus, particularly in France, was the digestive tract. Continental medical writers were especially interested in the stomach. They held it to be the seat of the emotions and considered that various psychiatric disorders originated from the stomach and its nerve plexuses.[36] In 1774 the Erlangen professor Jacob Friedrich Isenflamm, for instance, produced a murky tract on the cranial nerves and the stomach as keys to the nervous system.[37] In a series of papers in 1796 and 1797, Pierre Jean Georges Cabanis, a Paris academic and hospital administrator, spotlighted "the immediate action of the stomach upon the brain." At fault, he believed, was "the improper distribution of energy [la mauvaise distribution des forces] which is common to all nervous diseases and is specially evident in those having as their site the stomach and the diaphragm."[38] Several years later the noted Paris anatomist Marie François Xavier Bichat implicated the ganglia of the autonomic nervous system, the gastrointestinal tract, and the brain in a quite elegant model of nervous disease. Whereas paralysis, hemiplegia, infantile convulsions, and the like had their seat in the head, other disorders such as hysteria, hypochondria, and melancholia had their seat in the belly, perhaps in association with the nervous "ganglia." Bichat thought this made sense empirically because visceral pain had (and has) a different quality than does somatosensory pain. Furthermore, "I think it very probable . . . that the sympathies [among these organs] play a real role in hysteria, in certain kinds of epilepsy where the fits begin with a painful sensation in the epigastrium, and in the whole group of so-called nervous affections, which the laity conflate under the name 'vapours.'"[39] The result of all this peripheral localization theory—notions that attribute psychic states to the action of body parts other than the brain—was to pave the way for the systematic treatment of such mental disorders as hysteria by treating the periphery of the body.

Some authors asserted that the nerves control the mind. We have been discussing prescientific views of mind-body pathology in the eighteenth and early nineteenth centuries, views held by authors who either wrote before the explosion of mid-eighteenth-century empirical research into neurophysiology, or whose work was little affected by it. As a part of such prescientific views, other writers stressed the nervous system itself. The belief that the nerves must somehow influence such nervous phenomena as epilepsy reaches far back into the history of medicine.[40] It received a new impetus at the beginning of the eighteenth century from the theories of Friedrich Hoffmann, who in 1693 accepted an appointment as professor of medicine in the newly founded university of Halle. Hoffmann, like a number of his early-eighteenth-century counterparts, set out to construct a system to account for the body's functioning in health and disease. These systems were all more or less castles in the clouds, built abstractly from "first principles" and lacking (aside from anatomical dissection) any empirical basis. Hoffmann's system, articulated in numerous publications from 1718 onward, hypothesized a "nervous ether" radiating out from the brain and setting the rest of the body mechanically in motion. Illness occurred when contractions (arising perhaps from the stomach) closed down the pathway of this fluid. Hoffmann believed that such contractions preferentially affected the spinal column.[41] Hoffmann's system was thus of particular interest because it called attention to the nervous system, especially the spine.

After Hoffmann, many eighteenth-century writers focused explicitly on the nerves in "vapours," "spleen," "hyp" (hypochondria), and the like. "These hysterical affections as well as hypochondriacal sometimes begin in the brain, where the spirits are first irritated and impelled into inordinate motions," wrote London physician Richard Blackmore in 1725. "Thence the tempest drives through the nerves down to the lower parts, and carries great disorder and confusion wherever it comes." He believed that his ideas "will facilitate our conceptions [of] how hysteric fits are produced in the head."[42] The great Italian pathologist at the University of Padua, Giovanni Battista Morgagni, was quite contemptuous of "the old exploded and long rejected error" that the uterus ascended in the body. For Morgagni, in hysterical and hypochondriacal illness, "the chief disorder is in the nervous system, as it is called."[43] This tradition of doctrinaire and a priori theorizing reached a provisional high point when in 1777 the Edinburgh professor of medicine William Cullen added the disease class of neuroses, ailments of the nervous system, to a celebrated nosology, or classification of diseases, which he had first published in 1769.[44] With Cullen's work, the nervous system was drawn firmly into theoretical view.

19

How did the nerves work? Among abstract theorizers of the nervous system, the doctrine of "sympathy" had particular resonance. It was particularly on sympathy that later writers about spinal irritation and reflex neurosis would draw with gusto. Many of the above-mentioned authorities had invoked sympathy among the organs as the explanation of how body systems communicate with one another. Indeed, the doctrine of "sympathy" goes right back to Galen in the second century after Christ.[45] And practice-oriented physicians often noted that the organs were in communication. For example, the obstetrician William Giffard observed early in the eighteenth century that administration of an enema to a mother in labor seemed to quicken the action of the uterus: "A clyster not only makes more room, by freeing the rectum from the excrements contained in it, but very much forwards the delivery, by putting the muscles and uterus in motion by its irritation."[46] But as to how this intercommunication between body systems worked, theorists had not really got beyond some unspecified mechanism of sympathy, which regulated the message traffic, causing the breasts to swell as the uterus enlarged in pregnancy, or the bladder to give off a "large flow of pale colourless fluid" after an epileptic or hysterical fit.[47] It remained for the eighteenth-century neurophysiologists to give new impetus to this familiar notion of sympathy.

Irritation and the Reflex Arc

Simultaneous with arid theorizing, practical research on the nerves and their illnesses was going on across a wide range of basic medical sciences. Some of this work amounted simply to sniffing out anecdotes in support of preconceived notions; other work led to a virtual scientific revolution that destroyed humoralism. The result of all this research activity was, by 1800, to cast the spotlight on two particular phenomena of great importance to nervous disease: (1) a specific kind of pathology called "irritation," and (2) a proposed mechanism to explain disease, called "the reflex arc."

What exactly happened to the body in nervous disease? After Hoffmann, the nervous system would become the preferential territory in searching for causes of hysteria and hypochondria. This story began with the work of the Swiss physiologist Albrecht von Haller, who in 1736 accepted a post at the newly established university at Göttingen. Having earlier studied with Hermann Boerhaave in Leiden, Haller was pricked by the budding Enlightenment spirit of empiricism. He actually did experiments with muscle fibers rather than merely theorizing about them, and thus gave an empirical basis, in his great work published between 1757 and 1766, to the ancient doctrine of irritability. He had observed that muscle fibers shorten briefly as they contract, thereby showing themselves to be irritable. As Charles Singer and E. Ashworth Underwood put it, "The characteristic of irritability is that a very slight stimulus produces a movement altogether out of proportion to itself, and that [the muscle] would continue to do this repeatedly so long as the fibre remains alive."[48] This doctrine represented a major accomplishment of empirical research, one of the first of modern times. It suggested a concrete, physical mechanism of what exactly was wrong with the nervous system: It was too irritable.

The next chapter in the story, alas, represents a mere caricature of research and medical advance—the writings of the Scottish physician John Brown. Brown had studied with William Cullen and hoped to wrench himself from poverty by building a great system, similar to those of Hoffmann and others. Clearly borrowing from Haller's notion of irritation, though without acknowledging it or doing any research on the subject, Brown postulated in 1780 that all the tissues of the body were "excitable." Disease occurred when tissues were too little excited (asthenic) or overexcited (sthenic).[49] All this "Brunonian" (from Brown) theory, a house of cards having little to do with Haller's work, could be forgotten had it not had such an enormous impact on theorizing about nervous disease, especially on the Continent.[50] Now physicians would be asking not whether the humors were out of balance but whether the nervous system had become too "excited." And because excited is close to irritable or irritated, they might also ask whether nervous disease was not a result of irritation.

Irritation acquired a kind of spurious legitimacy because for a period of time it was conflated with inflammation.[51] Inflammation represents a real disease process in which the affected part is hot, turgid, red, and painful and exhibits loss of function. Irritation has only the last in common with inflammation: There is some functional deficit but no lesion, no evident pathological change. Such authorities as François Joseph Victor Broussais in Paris, inventor in the years after 1808 of yet another medical system in which patients were bled, used terms like *inflammation* and *irritation* almost interchangeably, suggesting that one was just a subtype of the other.[52] Such sloppy usage helped elevate irritation to the dignity of a genuine pathological entity.

At the end of the eighteenth century, the doctrine of irritation began to be applied clinically, to the spine as well as to other parts of the body. In

21

1800, for example, another Scotsman, the Glasgow surgeon John Burns, explained how sympathy could carry disease processes in the body far from their original sites. Burns switched back and forth in his account between the terms *inflammation* (which he generally used when clear pathological changes were at work, but sometimes when they were not) and *irritation* (which he apparently regarded as a kind of global term for disorder). In Burns's view, whenever irritation or inflammation appeared, some kind of local treatment was necessary.

The significant difference between irritation and inflammation was that the presence of irritation had to be hypothesized on the basis of other symptoms, such as unusual behavior on the patient's part or symptoms far distant from the irritated site. Inflammation was obvious at the site. Thus the assumption of irritation gave license for a series of invasive, meddlesome, and unnecessary interventions that presupposed the presence of disease where none actually existed. Burns had suggested treating inflammation of the spine, for example, by putting an "issue," or caustic compress, on the skin of the back in order to excite pus and pull the irritation away from the affected parts below.[53] By 1800 we are thus close to the doctrine of spinal irritation and its treatment.

A second scientific narrative from the late eighteenth century traces the course of the reflex arc in the nervous system. Just as inflammation is a genuine natural phenomenon, so do reflex arcs exist. In the knee-jerk patellar reflex, for example, a sensory signal from the kneecap produces a reflex twitch of the quadriceps muscle, which extends the knee joint. Defects in the twitch point to genuine organic disease of the nervous system. Although previous writers such as René Descartes had speculated about reflexes, it was Edinburgh physiologist Robert Whytt's animal experiments in the 1750s that demonstrated that the spinal cord (rather than the various ganglia of the abdomen) formed the center of the body's nervous communication. However the signals might arrive and depart, the spinal cord reflected them. Hence it is fair to say that Whytt established the reflex action of the spinal cord.[54]

But, in addition to experimenting on research animals, Whytt was also a clinician. In his seminal work on nervous diseases, published in 1765, he linked these hard scientific findings to more abstract musings about how sympathy produced hysteria, hypochondria, and other nervous conditions—an association that lent his speculative views on illness in humans a scientific basis they did not in reality possess. Whytt thought nervous disorders in general were caused by "a too great delicacy and sensibility of the whole nervous system," as well as by the deficient function of certain body organs. The behavior of pregnant women, for example, showed that the irritated nerves of the uterus could produce "those symptoms commonly called nervous or hysteric." Or obstructed menses could sympathetically affect the stomach, whose many nervous connections might then, again by means of sympathy, produce hysterical symptoms elsewhere in the body. "That pains in the head often proceed from a sympathy with the stomach is rendered probable by the violent vomiting which sometimes accompanies the *clavus hystericus* [a headache that felt as though a nail were being driven into the head], and by observing that people much troubled with wind in their stomach and flying pains in their head are not so often affected with these pains when they are free from the flatulence." The basis of nervous disease, in other words, was a physical affliction of the nerves (though Whytt allowed for a certain influence of "passions of mind"), and nervous symptoms could be abolished by the standard medical treatments of the day.[55] For establishing scientifically the centrality of the spinal cord in reflex action, and culturally, as the author of the first major work on nervous diseases defined as such, Whytt emerges as a crucial figure in the story. Yet if Whytt had not existed it would have been necessary to invent him, for the whole idea of nervous illness lay in the Zeitgeist, specifically in previous scientific writing and nonscientific speculation about the nerves.

Up to this point, no one knew how the many nerves running in and out of the spinal cord on both its front (anterior) and back (posterior) sides shared the responsibility for sensation and motor action. In 1784 Georg Prochaska, one of the many talented Viennese doctors from the Czech province of Moravia, suggested, on the basis of frog experiments, that distinct sensory nerves carried the signals inbound to the cord, and distinct motor nerves carried them outbound from the cord.[56] It remained for the English physiologist Charles Bell to establish in 1811 that the anterior spinal roots had motor functions (the motor nerves carried the outbound nerve impulse from those roots), and eleven years later for the Frenchman François Magendie to demonstrate that the posterior spinal roots had sensory functions.[57] Therewith the anatomy of the reflex arc had been completely described. An apparent scientific basis for the concept of reflex neurosis had been laid.

Distinctive to the late eighteenth century was the clinical establishment of nervous illness, a concept that had two sources: the abstract theoretical speculations about the nervous system in the sterile tradition of school medicine running from Friedrich Hoffmann down through William Cullen, and the empirical research tradition established by Albrecht von Haller and Robert Whytt. In the 1760s and after in Britain and on the Continent, works proliferated on diseases of the nerves, diseases we would

23

recognize as mainly psychiatric in nature. In 1763 Pierre Pomme of Montpellier explained that vapors were, as he thought, caused by dried-up nerves. Among the symptoms of the vapors: pounding headaches (*le clou hystérique*), "sadness, melancholy and discouragement which poison every pleasure," bad teeth, bowel noise, leg cramps, periodic paroxysms, fainting, fits, and so on.[58] Pomme's work was typical of the genre explaining hysterical paralyses and the like as a physical derangement of the nerves.

Inevitably, supply rose to meet demand. Patients began presenting themselves to doctors with nervous illnesses rather than with the hyp. In 1783 a learned society in Utrecht sponsored a prize competition for essays on "the causes of the increasing nervous disease in our land." The Amsterdam physician Jan Petersen Michell indicted "overworked minds," "neglected physical activity," too many parties, too much "reading of novels that depict romantic activity," and the like.[59] We are, in other words, at the interface of science and society, where basic scientific advances became cast in terms comfortable to the prejudices of doctors and patients. As early as the 1770s hysterical and hypochondriacal patients started appearing in doctors' offices claiming that their nerves felt very tense. They were probably echoing some popular understanding of Haller's doctrine of muscle tensing and irritability, and now were avid to hear from the doctor a confirmation of this "quite unusual tensing" ("*ganz besondere Anspannung*"), as Erlangen's Jacob Isenflamm put it. Isenflamm indeed found it quite exasperating to convince patients on the basis of his own experiments that a physical tensing of the nerves was impossible.[60]

But it was at the very epicenter of somatization, the spa at Bath, that the impact of newly discovered nervous disease on patients' symptoms showed most visibly. In 1786 James Makittrick Adair, a Scotsman who had some time earlier come to Bath to practice medicine, indicted Whytt's book as the cause of the modern plague:

> Upwards of thirty years ago, a treatise on nervous diseases was published by my quondam learned and ingenious preceptor Dr. Whytt. Before the publication of this book, people of fashion had not the least idea that they had nerves. But a fashionable apothecary [general practitioner] of my acquaintance, having cast his eye over the book, and having been often puzzled by the enquiries of his patients concerning the nature and causes of their complaints [began telling them], "Madam, you are nervous."[61] The medical shaping of symptoms had begun.

24

CHAPTER

2

Spinal Irritation

The modern medical shaping of psychosomatic symptoms did not really begin with eighteenth-century diagnoses of hysterical and hypochondriacal disorders. These terms were far too general to suggest any specific disease presentation. Also, hysterical disorders in the eighteenth century were mainly fits, and fits had been around for hundreds of years, a product of popular belief in demonic possession unrelated to medical views. The shaping of somatization begins with the diagnosis of spinal irritation in the 1820s.[1] This pseudodisease, which flourished in medical diagnostics until the 1870s and beyond, offered the first modern instance of a cultural shaping of patients' symptoms, in this case with the doctor acting as the agent of the culture.

On the patient's part, spinal irritation meant a sensitivity to sensation in the general area of the back ("the spine"), as well as the belief that far-distant peripheral symptoms were caused by an invisible but nonetheless real disease of the spinal cord. On the doctor's part, spinal irritation represented the belief that a local irritation of the cord was responsible for the patient's other symptoms via reflected action.

There were certainly legitimate medical reasons in those years to look for spinal disease[2]: Tuberculous osteitis ("spinal TB"), or bone infection, in the vertebral column and in other bones was, for example, quite common. But here one would expect objective findings of fever and inflammation, abscesses that could be palpated; bladder and bowels would have ceased to work; the vertebrae might collapse. In irritation, by contrast, there were no local symptoms except subjective tenderness or pain. Moreover, spinal TB was seen in both sexes, whereas spinal irritation was a disease almost exclusive to young women. Spinal irritation was a particularly appropriate diagnosis for an era in which young women were

25

seen as waiting passively for marriage and for the events of life to sweep them along, because it called for the patients to lie flat on their backs for months.

The Diagnosis Crystallizes

In the years before 1820 all the components of the diagnosis were already in the air: the concept of irritation, a new awareness of the nervous system, local treatment of the back and spine, and the doctrines of sympathy and reflex, which would assign to remote parts of the body the consequences of local disease.[3] It simply required someone to pluck them from the air and bolt them into place in the form of a specific disease.

The diagnosis of spinal irritation first took form not among the professors of medicine but among provincial English surgeons and apothecaries. For example, in a letter "On Irritation of the Spinal Nerves" to a medical journal in 1821, R. P. Player, a surgeon in Malmsbury, called attention to a kind of spinal disease marked by "the occurrence of pain in distant parts." On examination, as the doctor pressed on the tips of the vertebrae, patients reported pain. "But in many instances patients are surprised at the discovery of tenderness in a part, of whose implication in disease they had not the least suspicion."[4] In other words the patients' backs were perfectly fine until called to their attention by Player's physical examination. About a year later Player published a further account of this "preternatural tenderness," not just of individual vertebrae but of the entire spinal column, treatment of which could cure "cases of goutty affection of the stomach itself," as well as "diseases in general." For local treatment (meaning treatment of the skin directly over the spine), Player recommended cupping with large cupping glasses, bleeding, and blistering.[5] Player's two articles illustrate an early congealing of the diagnosis of spinal irritation.

In 1826 Benjamin Travers, senior surgeon at St. Thomas's Hospital in London, gave a boost to the notion that local irritation could be "reflected" to the whole system, although he did not dwell on the spine in particular.[6] Two years later John Abercrombie, an Edinburgh surgeon and general practitioner who was the king's personal physician in Scotland and whose main interest was neurological lesions, alluded rather skeptically to "certain obscure and anomalous affections which . . . present many of the characters of disease of the spinal cord, though their termination in general is more favorable." "The affections occur almost entirely in women, chiefly those of the higher ranks, and are generally extremely tedious and untractable." They left as suddenly as they had come, he said.[7] By the time of Abercrombie's writing, therefore, the diagnosis was certainly abroad in the profession.

In the same year, 1828, Thomas Brown, senior physician at the Royal Infirmary of Glasgow, wrote the first major account of spinal irritation: "I allude chiefly to those morbid affections of the spinal nerves so often met with in young females." Indeed, he deemed it a disease peculiar to females, of whom he had seen many in the Glasgow Lock Hospital for venereal diseases, in the infirmary, and in his private practice. "I find some difficulty in giving a name to this disease," he wrote, "but as it consists perhaps in a state of increased irritability in some of the spinal nerves, we may name it SPINAL IRRITATION."

How did Brown diagnose spinal irritation? It presented as a peripheral pain somewhere in the body, such as beneath the breast or near the sternum, in addition to tender spots on the spine of which the patient had not been aware until the examination. Pressing on the spine then elicited the peripheral pain, "thus distinctly proving the connexion between the two." The disease had two forms: one in which only a single spinal nerve seemed to be affected, and this was seen in men too; and "those in which there is a more general and constitutional irritability, in which the irritation is apt to affect different parts of the spine in succession." This kind was associated with "the peculiar action of the uterine system," and was said to "occasion a whole train of singular symptoms." Some of Doctor Brown's patients would temporarily go blind. One vomited all that she ate. Another, a young woman of seventeen, had a paralyzed left arm and could swallow only liquids. He cured her with a large blister on her neck (using a substance like acetic acid to raise a large fluid blister on the skin).[8] One appreciates the beauty of such a diagnosis: There need be nothing wrong with the spine at all. Merely attributing symptoms to it would justify treatment, and the more convincing and resolute the treatment, the greater the success in cases of psychosomatic illness. The ensuing orgy of blistering, leeching, and cupping of the spine probably represents the first (unwitting) use of placebo therapy in modern surgery.

After the official birth of spinal irritation in 1828, the diagnosis grew rapidly in popularity. It was initially picked up by provincial Anglo-American physicians, rather than by hospital consultants in the medical capitals. Thus a surgeon in Leeds, Thomas Pridgin Teale, wrote the first book on the subject in 1829. Teale said:

The lower extremities become the seat of various morbid sensations, spasms, tremors, et cetera, for the most part resembling those which have been described in the upper limbs. The patients also complain of a sense of insecurity or instability in walking; their knees totter and feel scarcely able to support the weight of the body. . . . This irritation, or subacute inflammatory state [meaning no inflammation was demonstrated] of the spinal marrow is not necessarily connected with any deformity of the spine or disease in the vertebrae.

The success of bed rest and "local depletion" (cupping and the like) in Doctor Teale's hands is an indication that his patients probably did not have an organic disease of the spine.[9] In his account the evocation of organicity relies on such code words as *subclinical inflammation* to suggest the hidden presence of real inflammation, a recognized disease with pathological findings, rather than using irritation, in which there was no pathology.[10] (This occurs again, much later, with "myalgic encephalomyelitis" and "chronic fatigue immune deficiency syndrome.") Also, the descriptions of these young female patients staggering and falling about constitute early references to what will be a rising theme in the story: hysterical paralysis.

In the usual pattern of dissemination of innovation in medicine, ideas pass from the professors of medicine and consultants at the center to small-town practitioners at the periphery. The dissemination of spinal irritation was quite the reverse, flowing from the periphery to the center. In 1830 T. N. Smart, a medical practitioner in Cranborne, Dorset, reported the case of a woman of twenty-three who, after having various bodily pains, "soon became stiff-necked and the motion of the jaw impaired . . . she is subject to hysteric fits; menstruation generally painful." Four days later: "The muscles of the neck and jaws are rigid; not able to open the mouth wider than will admit the thin end of a spoon; saliva dribbling; voice inarticulate; deglutition [swallowing] painful," pain everywhere. Smart found, "on examination of the spine, *tenderness between the shoulders.*" Diagnosing hysteria and spinal irritation, he blistered and bled her, and she speedily recovered. This case helped convince him that "uterine sympathy" had been overrated and that the key to understanding hysteria and tetanus was the spine.[11]

In Ireland, too, spinal irritation was reported not from the Dublin consultants but from small towners, brothers named Griffin, the more famous of whom, William, had collected his observations on the disorder while practicing in the village of Pallaskenry.[12] From the United States in 1832, which then counted very much as the medical periphery, came a report from young Dr. Isaac Parrish, who had just received his M.D. from the University of Pennsylvania and had interned at the Philadelphia Alms House Infirmary. Among his patients with spinal irritation were:

- Mary Ann Ledden, nineteen and "of delicate nervous temperament," who had come into the hospital with pain all over her lower limbs that seemed to have no organic cause. "At the time I saw her she was confined to the bed, being unable to move her lower limbs without experiencing acute pain. On examining the spinal column, I found most acute tenderness on pressure over the lower dorsal vertebrae [at the level of the shoulder blades]." He first cupped her, then blistered her, and in a few days she was well again.
- Mary Hall, twenty-three, had experienced a partial paralysis of the lower limbs for about a year. Because she had stopped menstruating at the time she came into the Alms House, her problems were deemed uterine. Then a few months later she "was attacked with an unusually violent paroxysm of mania, for which she was sent to the cells; she was alternately singing, talking, and laughing in a most boisterous manner; her lower extremities were powerless." Leeching and cupping her back and neck repeatedly produced a recovery, evidence in Dr. Parrish's mind that her diagnosis had really been spinal irritation.[13]

After the early 1830s reports of spinal irritation became quite frequent. Such fashionable London consultants as Evans Riadore, who had an office at 73 Harley Street and staff appointments at several London hospitals, began to produce tomes on the disorder, ensuring that it would be seen among upper-middle-class as well as poor and peripheral patients.[14] In 1854 Robert Bentley Todd, a London consultant with a vast private practice, said that uterine-caused hysteria could result in irritable spine, thus linking mind, spine, and pelvis in a circle of pathology.[15]

The diagnosis also began to be reported outside the Anglo-Saxon world. On October 4, 1844 a small-town practitioner in Switzerland noted in his diary: "I went over to Mattweil [village] for a consultation, where there was supposed to be a twenty-year-old girl of very fragile constitution who suffered from somnambulistic [hypnotic] phenomena. Such phenomena consist quite simply of excess nervous irritation and nervous activity [*excessive Nervenreizung und Nerventhätigkeit*] and have their seat and origin in the spine."[16] Thus spinal irritation had been well launched in the world of medical practice.

Spinal Irritation Appears in the Patients' World

Although the diagnosis was a medical figment, either a false explanation of real, organically caused symptoms or a code word for psychosomatic symptoms, patients nonetheless developed symptoms of spinal irritation. Or else they embraced the diagnosis for whatever symptoms they had. On February 8, 1825, Dr. John Simpson of the textile town of Bradford noted in his journal, "I called to see Dorinda Simpson who is at present at Leeds under Mr. Hey's care for a disease of the spine. I was happy to find her much better. Diseases of the spine have increased considerably of late years, and principally among females." Doctor Simpson attributed it to corset-wearing. He continued, "Spinal affections are most common in large towns and more frequent amongst the better ranks of society."[17] Already in the early 1820s young women were picking up on the growing climate of medical suggestion about the spine.

Spinal irritation was a disease attribution remarkably easy to implant by suggestion in the patient's mind. A vigorous physical examination of the hitherto asymptomatic spinal column would suffice. In 1849 Walter Johnson, a consultant at Guy's Hospital in London, explained how his colleagues proceeded with their young female patients:

> The method of examination at present generally pursued is the following. The examiner stands behind the patient, and, commencing just below the neck, makes firm pressure with his knuckles successively on each projecting ridge, or spinous process as it is called, that stands out from the spinal column. Less usually he tries the effect of scalding the patient by a sponge dipped in hot water. In the course of his investigations it frequently happens that as soon as he presses or scalds one particular ridge or vertebra, he perceives his patient wince or give some evidence of pain. "Aha!" says the physician, "there it is."

The physician might stop there if he believed that particular vertebra to be the seat of "a local circumscribed inflammation or irritation of a corresponding point in the spinal marrow." "Sometimes however," Doctor Johnson continued,

> he is baffled, but then instead of yielding the point, he will begin to punch or hammer the vertebrae, as he before pressed them. In this way it very rarely happens but that he at last succeeds in finding some sensitive spot, which he can assume to be the seat of the disease. He now feels it a clear duty to apply leeches to the culprit vertebra, or mercurial inunction, or a blister, or an issue or seton [a few silk threads inserted into a surgical incision in the skin, to excite pus], and strictly enjoins perfect quiet and the recumbent position.

But in addition to having confirmed his own fantastical diagnosis, the physician has also implanted the disease attribution in the patient's head.

She becomes focused on her spine. Doctor Johnson continued, "Attracting the patient's chief attention and filling her head with the fear that some disease exists in that situation [the spine], greatly misleads the practitioner." Some other physician, let us say, has now taken charge of this case, and "his attention is wholly arrested by the pain in the back, which leads him to apprehend inflammation or ulceration of some of the joints in the spinal column." Fearing something like spinal tuberculosis, the new doctor "impresses on his patient the necessity of a rigid maintenance of the horizontal position. Obeying this recommendation, which accords with her own instinct, the unfortunate maiden stretches herself supine upon the bed or sofa, and vegetates many a weary month in slothful languor."[18]

Thus we encounter the early Victorian spectacle of many young middle-class women spending years on the couch. Benjamin Brodie was a distinguished London surgeon, a consultant at St. George's Hospital and disbeliever in the diagnosis of spinal irritation, which he considered a form of "local hysteria," originating not in the uterus but the nervous system and corresponding to what later generations of doctors called psychogenic regional pain.[19] Brodie described patients who not only felt this back pain subjectively but permitted themselves to become "paralyzed" by it:

> Hysterical affections, in which the symptoms are referred to the spine, are of very frequent occurrence. Such cases are, in many instances, mistaken for those of ulceration of the intervertebral cartilages and bodies of the vertebrae; and in consequence of this unfortunate impression on the minds of the medical attendants, I have known not a few but very numerous instances of young ladies being condemned to the horizontal posture, and even to the torture of caustic issues and setons, for several successive years. . . .
>
> In these cases the patient complains of pain and tenderness of the back. . . . The pain in the back is seldom confined to a single spot, but it extends to different regions of the spine, and it not unfrequently shifts its place from one part to another. The tenderness of the spine is peculiar. The morbid sensibility is chiefly in the skin, and the patient for the most part flinches more when the skin is even slightly pinched than when pressure is made on the vertebrae themselves. The pain is in the majority of cases more severe than in those of real vertebral diseases.

Brodie said these shifting skin sensations might induce further complications in the young patients, including "a sense of weakness in the lower limbs, so that they are scarcely capable of supporting the weight of the body, and even actual paralysis."[20] Thus a diagnosis that was itself the product of medical imagination sufficed to induce in patients further products of suggestion.

Another London surgeon, Frederic Skey of St. Bartholomew's Hospital, looked back in 1855 upon past decades of spinal illness. He mentioned the ease with which hysteria patients could reproduce the symptoms of true neurological affections, leading to misdiagnoses and inappropriate treatment:

> There is no locality more fruitful of this error than that of the spine. Within twenty years of the present time, our sea-bathing places of resort were crowded by hundreds of young women who were confined to the horizontal or semirecumbent posture for years, were excluded from society, debarred their education, restricted in their natural food, and compelled to adopt the miserable substitute of a medicated diet for years, simply because a hot sponge created a sensation of uneasiness, or, if you prefer it, of pain, at a given vertebra. . . . Now true disease of the spinal column is very rare in any class of society; but these cases were one and all cases of hysteria—cases of impaired health in young women, varying in age from seventeen to twenty-five. . . . Diseases of the spine were the rage and fashion of the day.[21]

Spinal concerns also spread among women because of doctors' use, when in a hurry or otherwise puzzled, of irritation as a wastebasket diagnosis with which to fob off patients. In 1871 the celebrated Boston physician Oliver Wendell Holmes, Sr., told the graduating medical class of Bellevue Hospital College in New York: "Some shrewd old doctors have a few phrases always on hand for patients who will insist on knowing the pathology of their complaints without the slightest capacity of understanding the scientific explanation. I have known the term 'spinal irritation' to serve well on such occasions."[22]

Spinal irritation continued to roll through the lives of patients in the nineteenth century, a magical explanation to which one could cling for symptoms that seemed otherwise bewildering or difficult to face. Among patients at the medical "center," the big cities of England and Western Europe, the heyday of spinal irritation was the 1840s, but at the periphery of North America and Eastern Europe it lingered longer. As late as 1906 an anonymous medical correspondent of the *Boston Medical and Surgical Journal* (later the *New England Journal of Medicine*) praised a sanatorium at Monte Verità, a chic artists' colony in southern Switzerland: "You cannot conceive of a place better fitted for jingling nerves and irritable spines."[23] The Viennese neurologist and psychiatrist Moritz Benedikt recalled a Hungarian countess who had been referred to him with vertebral pain and a diagnosis of spondylitis (inflammation of a vertebra):

> She had been flat out for months atop an ice pack and the very afternoon that I saw her she was to be fitted for a heavy corset. I thought the diagnosis was suspicious, and I succeeded through the application of a metallic magnet in making the pain disappear. [Patients attributed great powers to magnets.] Thus I realized that the pain was hysterical in nature. This was exactly the season for ice-skating in Vienna, and I asked her if she liked to skate. She said yes, and on that very same day she used ice-skates rather than the ice pack.[24]

This Hungarian countess owed her symptoms, as well as her fixed belief in the diagnosis of "spondylitis," to suggestion, either on the part of her friends, the press, or previous medical attendants. The point is that in the patient's world, symptoms attributable to spinal irritation once seemed very real.

Center and Periphery

If diagnoses lingered longer in popular memory in some countries than others, it was partly because of leads and lags in the development of medicine and science. Until the 1930s, London, Paris, Vienna, and the German university towns counted as the center, where knowledge drove ahead rapidly on a roadbed of new discoveries. Italy, Eastern Europe, the Iberian Peninsula, and North America, on the other hand, were the periphery, whose doctors would come to the center for postgraduate education and whose wealthy patients would seek out its professors for consultations. In the rise and fall of a nondisease such as spinal irritation, one discerns—unlike the usual pattern—the center embracing the idea more slowly and letting it fall more quickly. The periphery derived the notion from scientific ideas that were in the air in the 1820s.

Spinal irritation had a long and healthy life in the United States. In 1938 William Macartney would be able to look back on a career of medical practice in which he and his colleagues had constantly to wrestle with symptoms without lesions. What did they tell the patients?

> Change of life and the menopause can ring the changes and give us pause [relief from enquiries] as well. This will be a satisfactory diagno-

33

sis in any obscure trouble in the fair or fairer sex between the ages of thirty and ninety-six, after which senility may be cautiously substituted. . . . Poor circulation and creeping paralysis should receive due consideration and there is something peculiarly suggestive and appropriate about the latter. Spinal irritation was once in excellent standing but is no longer used by the elite owing to the dictates of fashion.[25]

Thus in the real world of medical practice, in the 1920s and 1930s American family doctors were still weighing the diagnosis.

Few documents could testify more eloquently to the retarded state of American medical practice around the turn of the century than the work of William Alexander Hammond, former surgeon general of the United States Army and cofounder of the New York Post-Graduate Medical School. In a book, *Spinal Irritation,* published in 1886, he prided himself on having discovered the disease in 1870 in the United States, although he did concede the existence of several "elaborate treatises" in Europe. In 1,000 cases of spinal irritation seen by him, "sexual excess" had been the cause of 180, masturbation of another 57, and so on. Hammond concluded, "In general terms, it may be said that any cause capable of reducing the powers of the system may produce spinal irritation."[26] In 1908 surgeon Ap Morgan Vance of Louisville, Kentucky, using an implicit model of spinal irritation, described how he treated his young hysteria patients. One of them, an eighteen-year-old girl, developed a hysterical, or false, pregnancy two years after having had a "paralysis":

Her abdomen was enormously swollen and she was wearing a "Mother Hubbard." I looked her over and found that she had simply a tremendous distention of the intestines [probably from air swallowing]. I examined her back and found a tender spot about opposite the tops of the scapulae [shoulder blades]. I applied the cautery again that afternoon, the abdominal swelling was absolutely gone within a few hours and she was able to dress in her usual clothes, including a corset!

Thus, in a standard treatment for spinal irritation, he had cauterized her back with a hot iron. Vance pointed out:

Something must be done as a rule to impress the patient with the fact that the doctor is "boss.". . . The best method of impressing the patient is the "white-hot iron," best applied along the spine, though hot water douching, fly-blistering [raising a vesicle with "Spanish fly"], good spanking, sometimes even a good "cussing" will often serve the purpose.[27]

34

The judgment of North America as a medical backwater is probably not an unfair appraisal of the world of Doctor Hammond and Doctor Vance.

The diagnosis spinal irritation would become popular in Germany only after 1840, "introduced" by the brilliant thirty-year-old surgeon and neuroanatomist Benedict Stilling of Cassel. Stilling doubted that the frequency of the condition was any greater among women than men.[28] Later in 1840 Moritz Romberg of Berlin laid his seal of approval on spinal irritation in an authoritative textbook.[29] In France, Charles-Prosper Ollivier (called Ollivier d'Angers) described the diagnosis in 1838.[30] In 1863 August Axenfeld, a distinguished Parisian internist and physician of Beaujon Hospital, wrote a textbook on nervous disease that widely publicized the condition, invoking spinal congestion as its cause and advocating bleeding as the therapy.[31]

In terms of the sociology of ideas, it is of interest that Stilling, Romberg, and Axenfeld were all Jewish, at a time when few Jews were in medicine. Axenfeld had been born in Odessa. Neither Stilling nor Axenfeld received a university post, in Stilling's case definitely owing to anti-Semitism. (Axenfeld died at fifty-one, his last years clouded by an unspecified brain disease, which may explain his lack of academic advancement.) Romberg, though just promoted to professor in 1838, was not at a hospital clinic in Berlin at the time he wrote the book but had a private practice. Hence these promoters of spinal irritation to their fellow physicians counted professionally as rather marginal men.

Even after its introduction, spinal irritation made few inroads in the German and French medical establishments. In France this is probably because Jean-Martin Charcot, an advocate of organic brain disease of hereditary origin as an explanation of patients' symptoms, never took to the notion.[32] As for Central Europe, only a couple of authorities ever expressed much enthusiasm about spinal irritation after the 1850s. But they were very enthusiastic: Wilhelm Erb, the well-known Heidelberg neurologist, and Richard von Krafft-Ebing, the Viennese professor of psychiatry. Erb's opinions were in no way marginal, and it is actually quite astonishing that a man of his reputation would have clung so late to this figment. Krafft-Ebing's opinions on the other hand became somewhat discounted after the publication in 1886 of *Psychopathia Sexualis,* which caused him to appear in his colleagues' eyes as something of a pornographer.[33] Aside from them, there were in Germany and France no other major supporters of spinal irritation whose opinions counted in neuropathology.

It was in the spas of France and Central Europe that the idea of spinal irritation did ring a bell. Although Europeans had sought out mineral springs ever since the Middle Ages, the spas (so named after the Belgian watering place Spa) experienced a great new boom in the nineteenth century. This came partly as a result of the railroad, which made these towns much easier to reach, and partly because a newly wealthy middle class cherished the notion of a privileged, vacationlike "cure," in which they would rub shoulders only with social equals and dally in conversation in tree-shaded spa parks, all the while sipping "healing" mineral water rather than experiencing "heroic" cupping, leeching, purging, and the like.[34] Beach resorts and mountain resorts also became included in the notion of "spa," offering "healing" seawater and mountain air. Before the 1880s these spas provided almost exclusively hydrotherapy, both internally in glasses of tepid water drunk ritualistically at 7:00 and 11:00 A.M., and externally in the form of bathing, showers, and the like. What more ideal therapy for spinal irritation could one imagine than jets of water directed against the spine? Thus spa physicians greeted spinal irritation joyously as a diagnosis.

At the spa, women seem to have been a particular therapeutic target. Perhaps this is because they had more time to travel than their businessmen-husbands, perhaps because they were less forthright in asserting, No thank you, my spine is *not* tender at that spot. Here, for example, is a female patient whom Louis Verhaeghe, a spa physician at the Belgian channel resort of Ostende, described in 1850: "a member of high society, twenty-four years old and of delicate constitution, who had suffered greatly from scrofula [tuberculosis of the lymph nodes] in her youth, marrying at twenty-two. Two deliveries in rapid succession and prolonged breastfeeding weakened her greatly." Her doctors had diagnosed spinal irritation and sent her to Ostende.

> Pain around her three upper thoracic vertebrae radiated with feelings of prickliness [*fourmillement*] to her upper limbs and her lower limbs down to the sole of her feet. Pressure on these vertebrae immediately caused pain radiating into her abdomen and arms. This patient came to Ostende only after the repeated failure of a series of medications. She improved considerably in one season of bathing, but two more seasons were required to restore her completely.[35]

Clearly spinal irritation was good for Doctor Verhaeghe's business.

At the well-known spa of Plombières in eastern France, spinal irritation was a big drawing card. Spa doctor Sébastien-Didier Lhéritier said in 1854: "We see a large number of patients, especially females, who complain of pain at some point along the spinal column but who are afebrile [meaning not tuberculous]," nor did they bear any other sign of organic disease:

> The pain generally coincides with a multitude of neuralgic or hysterical symptoms, sometimes for example tearing stomach pain, sudden fainting fits [*lassitudes spontanées*] and feelings of numbness in the limbs, or other times with a sensation of constriction about the chest, changes in their voice. . . . These patients have nothing other than spinal irritation.[36]

The Germans and Austrians took the lead in differentiating spas on the basis of which mix of particles in the spring water would best suit which particular disease. In this hiccup of pseudoscience, originated by the Viennese hydrotherapist Wilhelm Winternitz, some spas were deemed best suited for gynecological complaints, others for heart disease, still others for nervous complaints. Thus in his 1882 handbook on balneotherapy Georg Thilenius, the spa physician in Bad Soden, counseled victims of spinal irritation and spinal neurasthenia to seek out Schlangenbad in Hesse, Wildbad in Württemberg, Ragaz in Switzerland, and Gastein in Austria. (For patients with poliomyelitis and the like, the waters of Rehme, Nauheim, and Soden were more appropriate.)[37]

German spas in particular experienced a proliferation of private nervous clinics and sanatoria where somatizing patients, under more direct medical supervision than that available in the bathhouse of a crowded spa, could receive "individualized" physical and dietetic therapy.[38] Spinal irritation was aptly fashioned for such close attentiveness to somatizers: Virtually any therapy save massage would serve, and the patient's stay would last as long as the symptoms did or until the money ran out.[39] Even in 1900, long after spinal irritation had faded as a respectable academic diagnosis, we find the physicians of these private nervous clinics beguiling their patients with it. Hermann Determann, who owned a veritable empire of clinics in Sankt Blasien in the Black Forest and in San Remo, Italy, had this analysis of spinal irritation: "Seen mainly in anemic women, it is characterized first by annoying and often very painful sensations, especially burning, in the spinal column. . . . In addition may be listed the phenomena of heightened muscular excitability (restlessness, a drawing sense, shaking, twitching) and finally the phenomena of localized or general motor weakness which may reach extreme expressions [that is, paralysis]." What could be done for these unfortunates? Doctor Determann recommended "calming procedures" with lukewarm baths. "Damp cold" could also be effective.[40] In these private clinics, therefore, spinal irritation served the doctors' need to remain competitive vis-à-vis other clinics by medicalizing under this label the patients' ill-defined subjective sensations, and the patients' need to have their apparently organic symptoms taken seriously, which they accomplished by paying the clinics' high fees.

Spinal irritation was such a face-saving fig leaf for hysterical paresis and paralysis that it is almost a shame the diagnosis was discredited. Patients certainly found it more comforting to think their spines were irritated than that their problems were psychological. Yet its discrediting drives home a final reminder about center-periphery differences: It was first discarded in London, Paris, and the German university towns, and only last in the periphery. By 1851 Moritz Romberg, now professor of pathology at the University of Berlin and the most influential figure in neuropathology in Central Europe, had cooled on spinal irritation, regretting the frequency with which the diagnosis was made. He criticized a general tendency to see nervous symptoms simply as the result of pathological and chemical disorders elsewhere in the body, rather than stemming from intrinsic disease of the nervous system itself.

Deplorable enough in the universities, this trend is completely out of control in the everyday practice of medicine. Practitioners have been chasing after the will-o-the-wisp of spinal irritation, which appeases their relentless desire to be able to explain everything. Therewith the entire domain of neuropathology is reduced to a region [the spinal column] that may be palpated with the tips of one's fingers.[41]

Many other voices spoke out against spinal irritation in the 1860s and 1870s, and the diagnosis slid from view in academic medicine on the Continent.

Did spinal irritation go out of style because of better science or more acute clinical observation? Unfortunately, the eclipse of this nondisease was little related to the progress of medical science, for what replaced it in the middle of the nineteenth century was another doctrine that was even more outrageously unscientific: reflex neurosis, the view that not just an irritated spine caused disease at far-distant spots, but that any irritated organ could cause irritation in any other organ in the body, including the brain. The eclipse of spinal irritation thus resulted from a further maniacal plunge into error, taken in the name of science. It seemed inadequate to physicians to make merely the spine the seat of reflex changes that could affect the entire body. It appeared much more logical to incriminate every organ in the body, because, empirically, interconnections among the organs—among heart, kidneys, and lungs for example—were quite clear. What doctors thought of as better science and closer observation was really just the heaping of pseudoneurophysiology on a cultural base in which women seemed the more passive gender. Hence it made intrinsic sense that they would be more obedient to the commands of their internal organs.

CHAPTER

3

Reflex Theory
and the History
of Internal Sensation

From the doctrine of spinal irritation, it was a short step to an assertion that every organ in the body could reflexly influence every other organ. This was reflex theory: the view that nervous connections running via the spine regulated all bodily organs, including the brain, quite independently of human will. And if an organ could exercise its influence at far-distant sites, then disease at these sites could be treated by treating that organ. It was this simple logic that gave reflex theory its breathtaking capacity to inspire meddlesomeness among doctors, and to suggest patients into preoccupations with fashionable organs that in reality had nothing to do with their symptoms.

In particular, reflex theory provided the justification for massive medical intervention in the female organs of reproduction. In these events the uterus, which had briefly been displaced by the spine as the source of irritation, rushed back into full view as the target organ for treatment in nervousness. As the uterus regained its centrality, many women in turn became riveted by internal sensations from the abdomen and attributed various symptoms to supposed pelvic disease. Reflex theory, which linked the uterus to the brain, thus represented a conjunction of medical theories that reduced women to the status of automata regulated by their uteri, and cultural prejudices that saw women as womb-centered and more passive than men.

Applying Reflex Doctrine to Patients

In the 1830s Marshall Hall was the first physician to bolt into a thera-peutic program the concepts of irritation, reflex, and local therapy then flying through the air. Hall thus counts as the founder of reflex theory. But he was immersed in a medical culture that believed that the uterus spread its disorders throughout the body via the mechanism of "sympa-thy."[1] Hall was merely the first to dress up the metaphor of sympathy with a theory. Born in 1790, the son of a Nottingham industrialist, Hall completed his medical studies in 1812 in Edinburgh. After a three-year scientific tour of Continental universities, he returned to Nottingham in 1815 to practice medicine. There he acquired an extended gynecological practice, and in 1827, at thirty-seven, he published his first book on women's diseases.[2] At that time Hall moved to London and, at his Gros-venor Street address, soon developed a large gynecological practice among the upper classes, thereby immersing himself in all the chic jargon of the day about irritation and nerves.

In the early 1830s Hall's interests shifted to the scientific study of the nervous system. Here he made an important contribution to knowledge, from 1832 onward seeing the "reflex arc," as he baptized it, as part and parcel of a whole separate spinal nervous system in the body. He thought that this system was autonomous of the brain, though influenced by it, and that it controlled the activities of all body organs. Some of Hall's ideas about the autonomy and workings of this spinal nervous system later turned out to be false, but he nonetheless established the spine as the central control board of a vast network of reflex actions governing the body as a whole.

What was less scientific in Hall's work—and based more on the fash-ionable pseudoneurophysiology of the day—was his assumption that spi-nal centers were responsible for nervous symptoms. There was no sys-tematic scientific evidence for this, only guilt by association, such as attributing vomiting in women generally to irritation of the uterine nerves, on the grounds that some women vomit frequently in early preg-nancy. A typical passage from Hall: "Many of the symptoms and diseases of pregnancy are excito-motory [his neologism for spinal] in their nature. Vomiting is caused by irritation of the uterine excitor nerves. The ner-vous cough of pregnancy is pure reflex. I have known a patient suffer from spasmodic asthma during pregnancy and at no other time. The cramps of pregnancy are reflex and spinal."[3] Hall's overpowering vanity made him the more unamenable to correcting his abstract ideas in light of empirical experience.[4] Indeed, his vanity and contentious personality

41

made him an object of hatred among London's medical establishment, and he never received a distinguished hospital appointment (comparable to a professorship in Germany).

The parallels between Hall and Jean-Martin Charcot, the famous late-nineteenth-century French neurologist, are interesting. Both men made fundamental scientific contributions that induced in them a sense of infallibility. Both had extensive experience with upper-middle-class women, Charcot in his private consulting practice in the Boulevard St. Germain in Paris, Hall in his society practice in London. Both acquired fixed and decidedly unempirical ideas about nervous disease in women, to which they then clung with an incorrigible tenacity. Finally, both were profoundly influential. Evans Riadore gave Hall credit for discovering the mechanism of the "laws of sympathy."[5] An enthusiastic review in 1846 of one of Hall's books in the *Lancet,* the British medical weekly, called Hall "the Euclid of the nervous system."[6]

Most subsequent writing on reflex neuroses and the like after the late 1830s would acknowledge Hall as the pioneer of the concept.[7] In 1835 Benjamin Travers, senior surgeon at St. Thomas's Hospital in London, was already explaining, with bows to Charles Bell and Marshall Hall, how "reflected irritation" radiates around the body via the route of sympathy.[8] And Travers's colleague Benjamin Brodie opined that "an impression made on one part of the body will often produce a nervous affection elsewhere, at a distance from the original seat of the disease."

In support of this theory of remote action Brodie said:

> The late Dr. Wollaston was accustomed to relate the following history. He ate some ice cream after dinner, which his stomach seemed to be incapable of digesting. Some time afterwards, when he had left the dinner-table to go to the drawing-room, he found himself lame from a violent pain in one ankle. Suddenly he became sick; the ice cream was rejected from the stomach; and this was followed by an instantaneous relief of the pain in the foot.[9]

Although Brodie did not cite Hall nor mention the doctrine of reflex action, this was the doctrine in practice. By 1842 a sufficient number of authors had specifically invoked reflex theory for overviews of the literature to begin to appear.[10] Doctors were now discovering "reflex points" in the spine where once only vague irritation had prevailed.[11]

The decisive point in reflex theory's incrimination of the uterus came in 1846, with the second installment of the great Berlin neurologist Moritz Romberg's work on nervous diseases, begun in 1840. If one had to name the three most influential neurologists of the nineteenth century, Romberg would probably be one of them, in addition to Charcot and Karl Westphal. Romberg's authority gave reflex theory a boost that would carry it for the next half century. In 1845, at age fifty, Romberg received the chair of special pathology at the University of Berlin, "special" in this case meaning neuropathology. His views on the uterus as the cause of hysteria, a "reflex neurosis," would evolve somewhat over the next few years (until the final version of his textbook was published in 1857), but the gist is that hysteria—understood as convulsions, the ascending ball that lodges in the throat, paralysis, and so forth—was caused by irritation in the genital organs. While in theory both men and women could get it, women became symptomatic more commonly than men because their uteri were in a condition of permanent irritation. Male genitals, by contrast, were only occasionally irritated. Peak moments of irritation in women, such as the menses, would produce attacks of hysteria, but even between attacks the nervous system was in a state of irritable weakness (*reizbare Schwäche*). The attacks spread themselves via the sympathetic ganglia of the abdomen more so than via the spine. One would accordingly treat hysteria by (1) removing the reflex irritation from the uterine system with local treatment; (2) generally reducing the reflex excitability of the nervous system with baths and such; and (3) strengthening the patient's will to resist her bodily impulses.[12] Romberg had thus sketched out a theoretical justification for vaginal douching and pelvic surgery, for spa going, and for strengthening women's "will" not to masturbate. All three themes would have great medical resonance during the nineteenth century.

One more point about Romberg: Not only did he indict the uterus in women's nervous diseases, he invoked the ovaries as well. Foreshadowing Charcot, he said that the doctor could provoke a hysterical fit by pressing on the ovaries through the anterior abdominal wall.[13] The ovaries? Where had this subject come from?

We must go back a step or two. For the first incrimination of the ovaries as a cause of women's nervous symptoms we return to a twenty-eight-year-old physician at the York County Hospital in England named Thomas Laycock, who in 1840 wrote *A Treatise on the Nervous Diseases of Women*. Laycock had been born of good family in the town of Willerby in Yorkshire, apprenticed as a surgeon, then studied at University College, London, and in 1833 in Paris under the great surgeons at La Pitié. He graduated in medicine in 1839 from Göttingen.[14] Having studied the reflex ideas of such writers as Georg Prochaska in Vienna, Laycock acquired the view that reflex irritation emanated not from the uterus but the ovaries. He believed, not entirely wrongly, that the ovaries drove the uterus, the latter being more or less an appendage of the former. Laycock also said that reflex signals did not stop at the top of the spinal cord, as Marshall Hall had thought, but continued on to the brain. All this he expressed in the murky pseudoneuroanatomy of the day ("neuroanemic diseases" were thought to migrate from one end of the cord to another, and so forth), the main implication being that treatment of "ovarian hysteria" should be directed at the female pelvis.[15]

Romberg cited Laycock's work in his 1846 text. But it was through the celebrity of Romberg's own views that the notion of ovarian hysteria seized wide numbers of colleagues. In 1846, after reading Romberg's work, Charles Schützenberger, professor of medicine at Strasbourg, first indicted the uterus as the reflex cause of hysteria, then later that year the ovaries. As evidence of the ovaries' pathogenic qualities, Schützenberger adduced the case of Élise Richert, a servant of seventeen. A year and a half previously she had started fainting, ten months after her menarche had begun. By November 1844 the fits had become frequent, the timing not linked to the menses. Admitted to hospital, she complained of a rising *boule* (lump ascending to throat) before the attacks, followed by fainting and fits lasting from a few minutes to a half hour. At examination there was no sign of hyperesthesia (skin pain or prickly sensation), but light palpation "in the area of the ovary" did produce "a very lively reaction [*sensibilité*]," with pain radiating to the epigastrium followed by fits in the form of "rigidity of the truncal muscles, convulsive movements of the diaphragm, epiglottal spasms, loss of consciousness and convulsions lasting about ten minutes."

One sees how the reflex paradigm claimed empirical confirmation. Here was proof that the area of the ovaries was pathogenic. Moreover, Mlle. Richert had not yet ceased to give lessons. She had been discharged from hospital in November 1845. Four months later she had a fright as her period was beginning. The flow stopped at once, followed by lower abdominal pain and a sensation of globus. A month later the pain had progressed to full fits and daily fainting. She was readmitted. Now pressure on a very painful right ovarian region produced fits. "We are able to evoke these symptoms at will by pressing on the ovary, just as one may automatically produce coughing by tickling the nasal mucosa." They leeched and blistered her, the symptoms vanished, and she was discharged in May not to be heard from again.[16] Thus did ovarian hysteria make its way out into the world.

The Triumph of Reflex Theory

Between 1850 and 1900 reflex theory became one of the dominant medical models of nervous disease. Reflex theory modified the way many doctors treated their patients, particularly patients in whom hysteria had been diagnosed. It is really because of hysteria, or psychosomatic symptoms, that this triumph of reflex theory is germane to our story, for patients would present to doctors the kinds of symptoms called for by the reflex model. When one remembers that reflex theory predicted motor symptoms, and that in the reflex arc an inbound sensory signal produced an outbound muscular response, in the form of twitches or paralysis, it seems likely that a theory calling for motor hysteria might have contributed to some of the new forms of this kind of hysteria.

To understand how an abstract medical theory about neurophysiology could have influenced the real world of patients' behavior so profoundly, one must remember how alluring both doctors and their patients found this theory. For patients it provided a mooring of certainty in the face of the body's bewildering signals: it was just those pesky pelvic reflexes again. For doctors reflexes provided a general explanation of how disease in one part of the body affected other parts: Nervous signals from any irritated organ could travel up and down the spinal cord to any other target organ in the body. In women, the uterus and ovaries were thought the organs most susceptible to irritation, thus the organs that drove forward disease processes elsewhere. But reflexes could also spread to the brain, offering explanations of nervous and psychiatric symptoms in men and women generally, but particularly in women because of the permanent state of irritability of the female pelvis.

Although in Central Europe it had been Romberg who focused reflex theory on the pelvis, in the French and Anglo-Saxon worlds the elevation of reflex theory to a general explanation of many kinds of symptoms—not just nervous—was the work of Charles-Édouard Brown-Séquard. Brown-Séquard, one of the strangest intellectual hybrids of the nineteenth century, laid the basis for the total-body-reflex theories of the years after 1860. His father was the Philadelphian Edward Brown, his mother a Frenchwoman named Séquard. Brown-Séquard was born in Paris in 1818, got his M.D. there in 1840, and plunged into experimental work on human physiology. After holding various medical appointments in England and the United States, in 1869 he became a professor of medicine in Paris and in 1878 Claude Bernard's successor in the chair of experimental medicine at the Collège de France. In addition to a long list of other scientific accomplishments, Brown-Séquard contributed in 1889 to founding the discipline of endocrinology, in the form of his enthusiasm for injections into humans of extracts of dog and guinea-pig testes.[17]

Brown-Séquard was also interested in reflexes. Although the notion that any organ in the body could affect any other organ via irritation lay implicit in pre-1850 reflex theory, Brown-Séquard argued that in disease the nerves gave off secretions (which they did not normally do) and that these secretions traveled in the blood to affect distant organs. He laid these views out in a widely read series of articles in the *Lancet* in 1858. For example, the secretions from the nerves of an irritated anus were thought to produce a change in gastric secretion, so "that digestion becomes almost impossible." Hence hemorrhoids would cause an upset stomach. Or "reflex irritation starting from the stomach" could produce croup. Especially subject to irritation, as we have seen, were the contents of the pelvis. "Diseases of the genito-urinary organs can be the cause of paraplegia," he wrote, noting as well that the bowels had been implicated in paralysis.[18]

Of course these reflexes could travel to the brain. "[In] an *immense* number of recorded cases, insanity in its various forms, epilepsy, chorea, catalepsy, extasis, hydrophobia, hysteria, and all the varieties of nervous complaints may be the result of a simple and often slightly felt irritation of some centripetal nerve." Of particular interest were the therapeutic implications of this total-body-reflex doctrine: "When we wish to produce a modification in the condition of any organ, we must apply the means of irritation [to the body parts] which have the most evident nervous relation with it." To influence the uterus, one would therefore treat the breasts, and vice versa.[19]

Here at last was "science." Brown-Séquard's writings had a great influence upon transforming reflex theory from an antique-sounding invocation of "sympathy" to a doctrine that looked and felt scientific. One critical practitioner, looking back at the turn of the century, wrote: "The reflex theory dates back many years. Early in this century, and perhaps still earlier, it was offered as an explanation for certain neurotic phenomena, but its prominence in the medical mind of today is due to the lectures of Brown-Séquard on the physiology and pathology of the nervous centers, delivered in London in 1858."[20]

In every Western country, diagnosis and therapy based on total body reflexes became entrenched between 1860 and 1900. A few examples, all taken from mainline medicine, may at least illustrate this vast subject. Someone like Erwin Kehrer of Heidelberg, an obstetrician like his famous father Ferdinand Adolph Kehrer, believed implicitly in reflex neurosis. In an extensive tract on relations between the colon and the genitals published in 1905, Kehrer argued that "dropped organs," such as the stomach falling down in the abdomen or the kidneys slipping out of place, could create an instability in the central nervous system that reflexly would cause hysteria. The therapy: an abdominal operation to "prop up" those falling organs.[21] Falling-organ arguments figured prominently in academic medicine before World War II, and would vanish only after X-ray demonstrations showed that a wide range of positions for stomach, kidney, et cetera was within normal limits.

Although Vienna's Alfred Adler is usually associated with depth psychology, his theory of "organ inferiority" stated that a genetically based inadequacy of such organs as the bladder would reflexly cause hysteria, as well as eliciting "the jerking of the feet, inability to urinate in the presence of others, dysuria . . . involuntary evacuation of the bowels" and so forth. The mechanism of these derangements was not psychodynamic but physical, inherent in the reflex structure of the nervous system. For example, Adler attributed various deficiencies in the reflexes of his diabetic patients to inherited organ inferiority:

> Margit B.; constipation extending to her earliest childhood, defects of speech, attacks of singultus [hiccup] in puberty, hysterical anxiety. No palatal reflex and a very weak pharyngeal reflex. The father died of diabetes. A brother suffered up to his twelfth year from incontinentia alvi [fecal incontinence], a sister had hysterical attacks of unconsciousness. Here also we find the connection between reflex anomalies and diabetes, neurosis and infantile defects . . . among the individual members of the family.[22]

This was straightforward reflex theory among the Viennese psychologizers, with a dash of pseudogenetics thrown in.

What reflex therapies were regarded chic in pre–World War I Paris? Pulling on the tongue to stimulate the heart ("Laborde's method"), dilating the urethra to diminish the symptoms of *tabes dorsalis* ("Denslow's method"), cauterizing the skin to cure ulcers, and cauterizing the mucosa of the nose to cure everything imaginable. "Such is the current state of reflex therapy," the author concluded who cited the above examples:

> What has been done to date is quite small in comparison with the work that lies ahead, but these findings are quite solid and nothing is capable of overturning what had been intuition among scholars across many lands and times. Moreover, we have been able to transform the old theory of sympathy and to derive from it practical applications of capital importance, of certain efficacy and without side-effects.[23]

Clearly, in Paris reflex theory was imagined to represent a splendid scientific advance.

But the most fertile soil of all for such theories was the Anglo-Saxon world. It seemed perfectly reasonable to Leonard Williams, author in 1906 of an advice manual to English physicians, that peripheral irritation should cause distant neuralgias. What organs were suspect in a neurotic female? "The teeth, the tonsils, the ears, or the eyes." Eyestrain, for example, might cause distant disturbances in the nervous system. Any peripheral disorder could elicit migraine, he said. Accordingly, migrainous females should be checked by a gynecologist. Whereas the ovaries and uterus produced a vertical headache, constipation and diabetes produced a frontal one by dilating the cerebral blood vessels. Hence purgatives were good for headaches at the front of the head. "In very persistent headaches which resist all treatment, it is well to try the effect of a blister on the nape of the neck." He also urged the use of savin ointment (a caustic, from the savin plant) to keep the blister open.[24] Such was the practice of medicine in 1906.

The United States, which until World War II offered a secure home for much that was medically goofy, embraced total body reflex notions wholeheartedly. Dr. J. M. Hooper of Sulphur Springs, Texas, reported in 1884 a case of "reflex paralysis" in a girl of thirteen. He found her "sitting in a chair, with her hands and feet cold and the tongue twisted in the shape of a corkscrew to the left and protruding from the mouth. She was unable to articulate distinctly, the pupils were somewhat dilated." Dr. Hooper gave her calomel (mercury) and castor oil to make her bowels move and applied a mustard plaster to her spine. She had a bowel movement two days later at noon, whereupon "the paralysis [of the tongue] gave way."[25] For Doctor Hooper and his patients, in other words, "paralysis of the tongue" was a real disease caused by reflex action from a constipated colon or an irritated spine; and appropriate treatment would cure these bothersome reflexes that darted all over the body. Such cases could be multiplied manyfold in the three decades before World War I. A "corkscrew" tongue had become legitimate. Reflex theory had become a major moment in the practice of medicine, figuring in the messages doctors conveyed to patients about what constituted legitimate symptoms.

Reflexes from the Sex Organs

Yet a majority of those cases would concern not the stomach or the tongue but the organs of reproduction. Of the vast pelvic literature, only a small portion concerned the ovaries, and by now the reader has sampled its flavor sufficiently to make extensive quotation from it superfluous.[26]

Before World War I the organ held responsible for the greatest amount of reflex pathology was the uterus, not the healthy uterus of the ancients that bumped about the abdomen causing suffocations here and vapors there, but the diseased uterus. A whole school of German ophthalmologists, for example, inculpated the uterus in diseases of the eye. In 1877 Richard Förster, professor of ophthalmology at the University of Breslau, theorized that disturbances of the uterine nerves reflexly affected several of the cranial nerves, which in turn caused eyestrain. He coined the term *kopiopia hysterica,* meaning eyestrain of uterine origin.

> These patients are usually very garrulous and speak constantly of their pains, often in exaggerated terms. . . . One patient had to close her eyes every time she went through a door, because otherwise the drafts caused her eye pain. Another patient said her eyes could not stand it if someone stood too close to her while speaking, a third said that reading gave her abdominal pain, a fourth claimed that after reading for a while the black letters started to seem green, the paper red and so forth.[27]

Doctor Förster's patients apparently colluded with him in this diagnosis of hysterical eyestrain, for they perceived symptoms in the abdomen and elsewhere as they read, which they then reported to him.

The distinguished Strasbourg professor Hermann Wolfgang Freund worked out a system whereby the uterus influenced not just the eye but the thyroid, heart, skin, ear, and stomach.[28] Pierre Berthier, a French psychiatrist and champion of reflex theory, elaborated a plan in which the uterus reflexly controlled the entire body. He found it remarkable that this organ could influence the rest of the body more strongly than an amputation of an arm or a thigh. The key to this great power lay in a special spinal center that controlled the reflex activity of the uterus.[29] Along with many of his contemporaries, Berthier believed in special spinal centers of uterine and ovarian control. All these pseudoneurophysiological speculations about the spine would start to be abandoned after experimental demonstrations in 1874 by Friedrich Leopold Goltz and others that the internal organs could work even independently of the spine (that is, after the cord had been transsected in experimental animals).[30]

Probably the largest body of uterine reflex theory came from Anglo-Saxon gynecologists, who were intent on linking uterine disease to nervous disorder. From the 1860s to the 1890s, the list of British gynecologists who believed the uterus caused nervousness, reads like an honor roll of the profession: Fleetwood Churchill, professor of obstetrics in Dublin; Arthur Edis, obstetric physician at Middlesex Hospital in London; Alfred Galabin, obstetric physician at Guy's Hospital; and Henry Macnaughton-Jones, who taught obstetrics and gynecology first at Queen's University in Cork, later becoming a prominent Harley Street gynecologist in London.[31] A similar list could be compiled for the stars of American gynecology in these years, but the point has been made.[32] Several entire generations of men whose professional concern was with women's pelvic organs believed those organs toxic to the emotional health of their patients.

These ideas were not merely theoretical but applied on a daily basis in the practice of medicine. Here for example is Dr. Jean Sarradon, a twenty-seven-year old small-town physician in Gallargues, France, who, around 1907, saw a young woman from Aiguesvives who complained of vaginal discharge (leukorrhea, or *pertes blanches*) and *crises nerveuses*. Now twenty-eight, she had had a postpartum infection about four years previously. "From that moment on, her previously well-balanced personality became capricious. She often feels nervous." Two years after giving birth she experienced a classic attack of hysteria. Now she was having "crises" two or three times a week. Dr. Sarradon cured her by irrigating her uterine cavity and cauterizing her cervix.[33]

At the other end of the world, figuratively speaking, was Dr. Mary Putnam Jacobi, a prominent physician in New York with a special interest in the health care of women. Doctor Jacobi was also a believer in reflex theory. In the late 1880s she treated an

> unmarried woman, a teacher—subject for several years to attacks of transient amblyopia [dimness of vision without a detectable organic cause in the eye] coming on many times a day and lasting from a few seconds to a minute or two. . . . During a year before consultation the patient was also subject to nervous attacks, in which consciousness seemed to be, not abolished, but perverted for a while. The condition is imperfectly described by the patient, who can only say that "everything seems strange."

Doctor Jacobi examined the patient and found a prolapsed uterus, which means the uterus was sliding down the vagina, the cervix rubbing against the labia minora. Doctor Jacobi supported the uterus with a cup pessary "and the cerebral attacks immediately and permanently disappeared." Doctor Jacobi's analysis of the causes fitted firmly within the reflex tradition of pseudoneurophysiology: "Impressions have been generated on a diseased endometrium, or among pelvic nerves which, though not giving rise to local pain, may when transmitted to the sensory centres of the cortex so overexcite them that they inhibit the remaining cortical areas."[34] Several female physicians aligned themselves against reflex theory, yet adherence to it was not solely a phenomenon of maleness.

Nor were all the patients who suffered reflex irritation from their genitals women. Men's reproductive organs could be irritated too, though the number of male patients in the literature is far fewer than of female.[35] In 1890 the Swiss internist Alexander Peyer, impatient with all this talk about uterine disease in women, called attention to the role of the male genitals in producing, for example, stomach upset. In his view, masturbation and coitus interruptus irritated the mucous membrane of the urethra, which in turn acted reflexly upon the stomach. Peyer cited a young academic who would digest his midday meal poorly if, during a nap following the meal, he were to have a wet dream, or a watchmaker, thirty-four, whose gastric pain was attributed to longtime masturbation.[36]

What to do about an infant with manifest neurological disease? "You had better make a Jew of him," advised Dr. C. H. Ohr of Cumberland, Maryland, as he responded to the request of a fellow practitioner for a consultation on a fifteen-month-old boy whose joints were swollen and who had hand- and foot-drop. Doctor Ohr's diagnosis: reflex irritation of the limbs from stenosis of the penis, curable by circumcision.[37] Thus did physicians apply reflex theory to everyday medical encounters. How did these new ways of viewing the body affect patients' own representations of their internal sensations?

The Medicalizing of Women's Internal Sensations

People have always possessed some kind of implicit model for analyzing their internal sensations, and the quantity and nature of sensation have probably been historically changeless. Yet how we account for these sensations—and under what circumstances we define them as pathological, requiring medical aid—is historically quite variable. This is where the idea of the symptom pool comes in. Medically articulated, preorganized "symptoms" help individuals to make sense of their vague physical sensations. Both sexes experience internal sensations and perhaps in equal measure. Yet the bulk of evidence concerns women, although it might well be possible to write a similar analysis of men's internal sensations.

51

The following lines have a rather tentative tone, given the enormous practical difficulties of attempting a history of sensation. Yet we are not entirely without resources.

How did women in the premedical era—for the popular classes, before 1800—represent their internal sensations? A familiar notion in Central Europe was that the uterus was not a regular bodily organ like all the others but rather a live animal. Internal sensation was therefore attributed to the moving of this live animal around the body. In East Prussia the uterus was thought to be a kind of frog, or *Kolke*, so meager was popular knowledge of anatomy. Men were thought to have one too. Pain sensations in the abdomen were attributed to the frog moving about, perhaps because it was hungry or thirsty: "The frog wants to have something [*De Kolke will wat hebbe*]." Some villagers said, "If the frog climbs into the throat and gets stuck, it will choke the sick person." Others explained the pain of peritonitis by saying, "The frog is strangling him." Popular views of therapy were also influenced by this active frog. "If the frog dislikes certain dishes or odors," wrote one folklorist, "you have to avoid them. If the frog is sensitive to a chill, you have to keep the abdomen warm. Or if the frog is upset about the temperature, you have to expose the belly to warm air currents so that it will go back to its place. If the frog climbs up because it is hungry, you have to 'feed' it. Even coffee is good 'frog chow' [*Kolkefutter*]."[38]

These popular views about the normal uterus as a live animal lingered for a long time in rural areas. Even in the 1880s there were still a few villagers in the countryside about Innsbruck who thought the uterus to be a toad, and when they recovered from abdominal illness would fashion little wax toads for wayside shrines as votive offerings. These toads were called *Muttern*, from the popular word for uterus.[39]

In the course of the nineteenth century, as the popular classes acquired a grasp of anatomical facts, illness started to be attributed to an animal that had inserted itself in the abdomen. Belief in a wild animal inside one's belly would customarily count as delusional and therefore psychotic, but a number of reports concern people who bear no other obvious signs of mental illness, and one is inclined to ascribe this popular belief to the remains of a traditional belief system rather than to some psychic abnormality.

These patients would seek medical help for the creatures inside them, and represented a first stage in the process of medicalizing internal sensation. "[Hysteria patients] perceive the most peculiar and amazing sensations inside their bodies," said Dietrich Busch, professor of obstetrics in Berlin in 1840. "Sometimes it is an animal moving around inside them, sometimes a foreign body that has forcibly pushed its way inside. These bodies create all the sensations of a physical illness."[40] At some point in the 1830s Thomas Laycock saw a married woman of twenty-eight whose abdomen was swollen, her cervix uteri shortened, and her breasts engorged with milk. "She asserted she felt something alive in her, the motions of which she described; not omitting the fact that it bit her occasionally and brought on a fit of hysterics. She was firmly of the opinion that it was a snake which she had swallowed somehow or other." Doctor Laycock at first thought she was pregnant, "but I soon found, upon inquiry of her neighbours, that my opinion was not thought of much value, for she was a well-known character, was very lascivious, to a degree indeed amounting to nymphomania, and had suffered from the same symptoms for nearly a year. I never saw her again."[41]

Some of these stories recall the traditional frog-uterus tales, except that the animal is different. Hector Landouzy, a physician at the medical school in Reims and an authority on hysteria, described from his practice "a widow of fifty-six, of a nervous temperament and very irascible. She presented all the symptoms of non-convulsive hysteria, complaining constantly since the onset of her menopause three years ago of a horrible constriction in her throat caused, she says, by a worm [*ver solitaire*] which continually, except at night, climbs up from her stomach to gnaw at her and choke her."[42] On the subject of hypochondria about worms, Pierre Janet told medical students at the Salpêtrière at the turn of the century, "You rarely hear educated people talking about diseases caused by worms, but the common people of Paris continue to be interested in it a lot."[43]

With time these traditionally migrating worms diminish as a theme in reported sensation, replaced by animal stories of greater medical sophistication.[44] In other words, the unconscious mind moves with the times too. Thus in July 1906, Madame R., a married schoolteacher in Clermont-Ferrand with two daughters, appeared in Doctor Bousquet's office "with an animal in her stomach." He had seen her before for constipation, and she had spent numerous seasons at such spas as Vichy and Châtel-Guyon. In the past she had been somewhat depressed because of personal problems. But today she seated herself before him with a cheerful air, indeed triumphant.

"Finally I know what I've got," she said, "and it's up to you to cure me."

Doctor Bousquet gestured for her to continue. Standing up, she placed her hand on the right side of her abdomen, just above the liver, and said, "I've got an animal in my belly and this is where it is."

She requested an operation to get rid of it. On August 12 she was admitted to the surgical service of the Clermont-Ferrand city hospital. At admission, she stated that last March she had started to become aware of its existence, but in retrospect thought the animal probably had been present for six years. "It's definitely why I've been having this whole problem with pain, cramps and vomiting that has bothered me in recent years." She knew the animal was there because of the cries it emitted, and she proceeded to imitate for her clinicians the sounds it made when it sang. In response to a series of questions she revealed her beliefs about the animal's movements. Thus far this could be yet another traditional story of live-animal attribution.

The doctors, however, were wondering how to proceed. They hesitated for ethical reasons to do even a sham laparotomy, or abdominal incision, "but still, it was necessary to rid her of this creature." Her daughters had been begging them to do something because she was making life intolerable for the family. So the doctors told Madame R. they would be able to see the animal in an X-ray. She offered scientific objections: You will only be able to see the skeleton, and it is probably quite small anyway. But finally she was convinced. After much effort they fabricated a radiograph, which showed frog bones outlined against human viscera, and presented it to her as her own X-ray picture. "Just as I thought, the beast is right there," said Madame R. triumphantly after seeing the radiograph.

Now the doctors told her they would give her medication to rid her of the animal. Its remains would turn up green in her urine. Lo and behold, after several days of placebo medication and a bit of fluorescine and sodium eosinate, her urine turned green: *"La bête était morte."* On a new X-ray there was no trace of it. Madame R. imagined its terrible end.

But still she thought she felt some movement. The doctors were now at their wits' end. They gave the daughters some tiny frog bones, with instructions to deposit them in Madame R.'s stool. (The text is vague on exactly how the daughters did this.) Madame R. found the frog bones and was finally convinced. "Look here, doctor, I have the remains of my enemy."

That was the end of her case. Except that a male patient in hospital at the same time tried the same story, and they sent him packing, saying if they heard from him again they would call the commissar of police.[45] The story is interesting because it illustrates a basic theme of this book: The unconscious, not wishing to make itself ridiculous, brings itself medically up to date. Madame R. knew what would and would not be visible on X-rays.

In the final chapter on patients who assign internal sensations to animals, we find surgical intervention. One of Felix Preissner's patients in the early 1920s in Breslau believed she had swallowed a tadpole while drinking from a brook on a hot summer day, and that it had turned into a frog that was causing her great abdominal pain. The Breslau surgeons actually went along with the delusion, made an incision, and showed her a "wriggling beetle" they claimed to have extracted from her throat. "The result was that on the next day she declared she had even more pain than before and that an even larger creature must still be present in her stomach where it was boring and pinching." The surgeon then did a second laparotomy, and produced an even bigger specimen! She was now apparently willing to believe the "evidence" of surgery.[46]

Later in the twentieth century, the attribution of internal sensations to live animals died out or became vastly reduced because increasingly sophisticated patients found the story implausible and knew they would encounter ridicule were they to present it clinically. But even though these nineteenth- and early-twentieth-century patients attempted modern updates of their stories, the whole animal scenario remained profoundly traditional in nature.

Female patients who drifted early and firmly into the net of medical care would select more plausible attributions, believing their internal sensations came from diseased organs. Such medicalizing of internal sensation was greatly encouraged by reflex theory, which offered a more palatable, seemingly scientific explanation of bewildering sensations than toads and frogs. Reflex theory insisted that symptoms resulted from such far-distant organs as the "permanently irritated" uterus, the colon irritated through constipation, or the irritated nose. Doctors' willingness to encourage such attributions probably strengthened them in the patient's mind as well, whereas doctors were usually not willing to encourage live-animal attributions. Reflex theory accordingly offered several inducements to interpret sensation in medical rather than nonmedical terms.

Using medical evidence to construct a history of internal sensation, particularly that of women, is difficult. First of all, many of these physicians achieved little empathy with their female patients and thought of them as silly and capricious, especially when hysteria was at issue. Second, it is difficult for even the most sensitive of clinicians to grasp the subjective quality of patients' internal sensation. We might, therefore, sort the evidence into two classes: (1) how the doctors saw the patients, meaning medical generalizations about the whole phenomenon of illness attribution; (2) how the patients presented themselves to the doctors, which approaches the patients' experience more closely because the doctors are describing what they see rather than their interpretation. A third class of evidence would be how the patients saw themselves, on the basis of patients' testimony of their own sensations.[47] It is regrettable that I have encountered so little of this latter sort of evidence, and that my own account is doctor centered.

Even among nongynecologists the opinion was widespread that many female patients were fixated on their pelvic organs. In 1839, for example, Benjamin Brodie urged his colleagues to abstain from treating the pelvis on the grounds that "local" treatments demanded by reflex theory gave women pelvic preoccupations:

> I must observe to you again on the danger of treating hysterical diseases as you would other diseases. Another object which you must have in view is to withdraw the patient's attention as much as possible from the disease. This alone will do more good than anything else. In some cases it is better to treat them by doing nothing at all, because by employing local applications you draw the patient's attention to the seat of the affection.[48]

Robert Brudenell Carter, a fashionable London surgeon and later an ophthalmologist, said of women who complained of a sensation of pelvic heaviness and dragging down:

> [The complaints] are usually associated with a very peculiar moral state, arising from the habit of contemplating and discussing the sexual organs. . . . The patients have a tendency to relate their sensations in filthy and wearisome detail; often volunteering the information that they have undergone manipulation and the speculum at the hands of various doctors; and evidently loving to be questioned on matters that would make modest women blush.

Carter attributed all this pelvic preoccupation to "the recent increase of uterine disease."[49] But in fact it was probably attributable to the rise of gynecology itself—the introduction of the internal pelvic examination and local treatments of cervix and vagina.

Of course the gynecologists, who trafficked intimately with their female patients' pelvic organs, found patients to be obsessed with these organs. One must take this evidence for what it is worth—the often-misogynistic musings of men who, like many of their social class, considered women to be a separate species. And yet these observations rested on much empirical experience, so they cannot be dismissed as products of pure fantasy as the evidence of witchcraft trials might be dismissed.

In 1868 the young Munich gynecologist Joseph Amann described how attuned hysteria patients were to their internal workings:

> With what anxious attentiveness they follow the functions of their organs, thus procuring for themselves much in the way of perverse sensation. Sometimes they register a sense of constriction in the thorax, becoming short of breath and panting, sometimes there is a sense of the blood circulating poorly in the limbs. Most hysterics are further unnerved by frequent palpitations, others through the anxiety-provoking pulsation of the arteries.

Such women, said Amann, also followed anxiously their stomach and bowels, and even believed their organs were wandering. "Six years ago I treated a woman in her thirties, a mother of four, who could not be dissuaded from the idea that several times each day her liver wandered from the right to the left and back again."[50]

Why were so many nervous patients convinced they had pelvic disease? Philip C. Knapp, a Boston psychiatrist, imputed the success of his colleagues' local treatments to the patients' suggestibility:

> We know only too well how the "indiscreet youth" are led by the quacks to develop a long series of "imaginary" but none the less real and distressing sexual symptoms, which may be most difficult to cure. The sexual element plays a most important part in the psychical life of woman . . . so that the idea of "womb trouble" is fraught with every form of evil and disaster, and a woman finds plenty of evidence . . . from eminent medical authority that all her vapors and megrims [headaches, fancies] can be explained by this dreaded disorder. The suggestion of pelvic treatment may for a time relieve all these ills, and in certain hysterical conditions a tent [cervical dilator], a tampon, an application or a pessary may work wonders.

Gynecological operations, mused Doctor Knapp, might produce even more brilliant results.[51]

The belief in patients' pelvic fixation was widespread among turn-of-the-century American gynecologists. In 1908 Edward A. Weiss, a Pittsburgh physician, described the classic somatizing patient:

> Probably the most difficult class of cases the gynecologist, or in fact any practitioner of medicine, has to deal with is the neurasthenic [neurotic] without real pelvic lesion. She complains of every known symptom from the top of her head to the soles of her feet, but more prominent are dysmenorrhea [painful periods], backache, pain over the ovaries and heavy dragging pain in the abdomen.

Doctor Weiss called these patients "hysteroneurasthenics" and thought them "exceedingly impressionable." Said he: "In such cases much harm can be done by injudicious advice. Such a patient will accept almost any suggestion in regard to her condition and is always ready to attribute her suffering to some local pelvic disorder."[52]

In reality, a century of meddlesome interference in the pelvis on the basis of reflex theory had made such patients hypervigilant about their internal organs. "Let a female be told her womb is out of place, she never forgets it," said Chauncey Palmer, a Cincinnati gynecologist. "It makes a mental impression, strong, lasting. It is like telling her she has a moveable kidney."[53] These are doctors' accounts of their patients, full of the subjectivity of middle-class males operating within the framework of a completely fallacious theory of neurophysiology.

In our journey from doctors' subjectivity to patients' (which is where we really want to end up), a halfway station is the doctors' accounts of case histories. We gain some sense of the patient's world from what the patient tells the doctor after she sits down. Clifford Allbutt described in 1884 an upper-middle-class young woman from the industrial city of Leeds. In her family, "no household had been free from nervous disease. She possessed the gifts and the attractions of the neurotic diathesis [constitution], and laboured under its defects. It is possible also that she was in some degree under the stress of . . . the unconscious sexual impulse. She was restless, excitable and suffering."

So when she came to Doctor Allbutt, this was the picture: "Her pains were mostly pelvic and abdominal. She never put her feet to the ground, partly because it intensified her pain, partly because she had been forbidden to do so. She had lain on her back for months. Pessaries had often been introduced, but being intolerable to her were withdrawn." Thus she had been in the hands of the reflex theorists. Allbutt points out that she had stopped eating and was badly emaciated. Then he returned to the theme of her own internal perceptions. "Her womb had been incessantly under specular [with a speculum] and other examination for a year or two, and like nearly all such patients she had uterus on the brain." Allbutt found her pelvic region tender, the patient constipated.

How did Allbutt treat this patient? First, he got her mind off her pelvis and onto some of her other issues: "I declined to initiate any treatment whatever until she would get her feet to the ground, and thenceforth cautiously regain the use of her legs. Meanwhile, I declined to 'cure the ulceration of the womb' [her self-diagnosis] for the twentieth time." He gave her strengthening remedies, got her on horseback, and soon, in the absence of further vaginal interference, "she was mixing in general society, could ride gently to hounds [and] had regained appetite and looks."[54]

Being fixated on the uterus in this manner does not actually mean this young woman could feel her uterus, since abdominal sensation is very difficult to localize. One cannot in fact feel one's stomach, gallbladder, uterus, or ovaries. One merely has sensation from the viscera, and any imputed localization is merely guesswork on the patient's part, unless the patient learns from the diagnosis what organ is involved (hence it is often difficult to differentiate the pain of esophageal reflux, in which food surges from the stomach back into the esophagus, from that of a heart attack). Accordingly, when individuals attribute their pain systematically to their uterus, ovaries, or whatever, it is because their attention has been directed to these organs by suggestion, medical or otherwise.

Here is a fifty-year-old patient of Louisville gynecologist Vance, the spanking doctor introduced in chapter 2. "At the age of twenty-five she was seen by Dr. Crow of Louisville, on account of some menstrual disorder. He put her to bed and she had been there practically ever since. During the first six years she left the room occasionally, but for nineteen consecutive years she had never been out of bed!" Finally she came to Doctor Vance's attention:

I found the patient was quite fleshy and very flabby, with no muscular power. I asked her what was the matter with her, and she replied that every time she got up something "dropped down inside of her"! My diagnosis was chronic hysteria. I told her I would get a "contraption" that would cure her of the symptom of "something dropping down inside." This sensation was always referred to the left side at about the splenic region.[55]

Advice from the evidently reflex-oriented Doctor Crow had directed this woman's attention to a certain region of her body, and for unknown reasons she permitted herself to become incapacitated by the sensations she perceived from that region, medicalizing them in her own mind as "something dropping down" (the template for which would probably have been neighbors' tales of uterine prolapse).

This fixation on supposedly uterine symptoms was not confined to cosseted middle-class Victorian women. Raymond Belbèze, a thirty-four-year-old physician practicing in Nevers, said of his female patients in the surrounding countryside:

The rustic neurotic is above all a somatizer [*La rurale névrosée est avant tout une hypercénesthésique*]. . . . I cannot think how many neurasthenics with pseudo-metritis [pseudo uterine inflammation] I have seen. The neurotic is particularly preoccupied with her often painful periods, and we know with what mystery primitive people in general view everything that touches on the genitals. The neurasthenic woman becomes actually organized about her uterus. . . . She thinks fixedly and continually about her "uterine disease," so much so that if by chance there really is some problem with the uterus the rural woman is, as I have often seen, plunged into all the characteristics of a clinical depression. A curious attitude of embarrassment or shame becomes commingled with fear. To use a popular phrase, the patient becomes absolutely "dithered" [*frappée*].[56]

The second internal organ to which reflex theory directed patients' attention was the ovary. Among upper-middle-class women at the turn of the century, fancying ovarian origin of one's symptoms was, in fact, quite common. The following case comes from the practice of Frederick Parkes Weber, a Harley Street internist who was forty-four years old in 1907. "Parkes Weber," as he liked to call himself (although his last name was simply Weber, pronounced VAY-ber), was the son of the distinguished physician Sir Hermann Weber. He and his father both had a special interest in spas and "balneology," which explains why they attracted so many nervous patients. In the 1900s Parkes Weber had thus inherited from his father an upper-middle-class practice of individuals who demanded a great deal of attention. In 1907 he saw Miss X, forty-seven and living with a younger unmarried sister at a distinguished SW address in London. She complained of a funny feeling on the left side of her abdomen. Sixteen years earlier, at the age of thirty-one, she had nursed her mother who was dying of cancer. "After that," wrote Parkes Weber in his detailed case notes, "she went to Kenwick with a sister and felt very weak there." The particular cause of Miss X's medical misadventure, however, seems to have been an ensuing consultation with a physician who

told her she had a tumour concerned with the womb or something of the sort. Since then she has always been ailing and thinking of herself. The same doctor suggested a course of Weir Mitchell [a rest cure involving isolation, bed rest, and a special milk diet] at the time, but the result was not good, for, though she gained weight she got a dislike of food which has steadily persisted since that time. . . . The case is certainly a complicated one of neurasthenia approaching the climacteric period in a woman of susceptible nervous manner.

Over the preceding decade, Miss X had complained of symptoms in numerous organ systems, including headache. Parkes Weber did a physical examination. "I can find nil except the nervous feeling complained of on left side of the abdomen—worse after monthly period. Owing to this 'sickly feeling' [she] has to lie up all the monthly periods and a great part of every day. Has seen various doctors."

Miss X's preoccupation with her viscera reached a new chapter in 1906 when she saw Dr. Leopold Fellner in Franzensbad, a spa in Bohemia. Fellner was an old friend of Parkes Weber and part of the international crème de la crème of society nerve doctors. He would winter at the Hotel Metropole in Vienna and spend the summers seeing patients at Franzensbad. "When I saw [the patient]," wrote Doctor Fellner to Parkes Weber, "she complained of pain in the left hypochondrium, which radiated posteriorly and inferiorly in the lower abdomen. She was very emaciated, highly anemic, very nervous, suffered from complete loss of appetite and also from diarrhoea. Her menses were profuse, and hysterical phenomena were evident, also some melancholia, especially before, during and after her period." Doctor Fellner diagnosed a "floating kidney," in this case evidently a "wastebasket" diagnosis designed to placate a patient without organic disease.

Late in 1907, in spite of Doctor Fellner's prescriptions of Veronal (a barbiturate) and baths, Miss X suffered again from the feeling "as if she could lift something awry from the left side."

On December 4, 1907, Parkes Weber was called to see her at her home in ____ Gardens:

At about 2:30 P.M, in connection with the extraordinary left "ovarian" tender area, she suddenly developed an attack of vertigo and retching or vomiting—everything seemed to be going round. . . . I could feel nothing in abdomen. But she told me that any pressure on the sensitive area (always to the left of the middle line) makes her feel sick. The sensation there was never one of actual pain—it was a peculiar feeling as if there was a body there and as if she would be all right if it could be lifted away.

Parkes Weber wrote in the margin of his notes, "analogous with globus hystericus." He wondered if this sensitive area was "one of Charcot's 'hysterogenic zones.' She gets her peculiar attacks just as Charcot's patients in the Salpêtrière would get their attacks of hystero-epilepsy."

By the end of January 1908 something had to be done for Miss X, who was now depressed, anorexic, and fearing insanity. Parkes Weber arranged for the surgeon John Percy Lockhart-Mummery to examine her colon with a sigmoidoscope. From one point of view, Lockhart-

Mummery was a good choice because he was an action-oriented surgeon, known for doing colectomies for constipation and the like.[57] Nothing abnormal was found on examination, however.

In the meantime, Miss X's symptoms were worsening. Parkes Weber contemplated a consultation with Dr. George Savage (Virginia Woolf's psychiatrist). Miss X went to the seaside resort of Torquay to seek relief. On May 8, 1908, Parkes Weber noted, "I hear from her brother that Miss X is still at Torquay with a lady-companion, but she thinks that her left ovary is driving her out of her mind that it will have to be removed. I am against hasty operation of that kind, and advise dietetic and other treatment for neurasthenia at a health resort abroad, i.e. Kissingen, Baden-Baden, or near Montreux."

Resisting Miss X's demands for an operation, Parkes Weber now had her wear a special ovarian compressor belt, a product of Charcot's regime at the Salpêtrière in Paris. Putting pressure on the "ovary," it was thought to reduce reflex irritation elsewhere. Yet even the special belt was unable to prevent Miss X from "doctor-shopping" for surgeons, and she finally encountered the famous William Arbuthnot Lane, who in January 1909 operated on her and found various adhesions, which he separated.[58]

On June 9, 1909, Parkes Weber wrote, "I heard from Miss X's brother-in-law that she was at Yarmouth away from her relatives, apparently doing fairly well, though still complaining of pain etc. She herself apparently thinks that Mr. Lane's operation did her no good." Parkes Weber's notes stop here.[59]

Parkes Weber had not suggested Miss X into her obsessional concern with sensations from her "ovary"—indeed Parkes Weber tried to save her from the claws of the surgeons—her entire encounter with the health-care system had done so: the particular doctor who had first raised the unlikely possibility of womb disease in a previously healthy, unmarried thirty-one-year-old mourning the loss of her mother. It was Leopold Fellner in Franzensbad who called forth the specter of nonexistent disease from "moveable" organs. It was the entire valetudinarian universe she inhabited, with its sedan chairs, invalid companions, and special bottles of Levico water from the Levico springs in Italy (good for "nerves").

Lucky would be the individual who escaped this culture without a sense of something wrong inside. Yet this represented normal life for upper-middle-class women in Europe at the turn of the century. With little to occupy their minds save their health, women from this stratum were notorious as doctor shoppers and spa goers. Taking a "cure" became built in to one's annual rhythm, not out of medical necessity but as a source of diversion. Having relatively little authority with which to oppose the opinions of their famous clinicians, many of these women, preoccupied with internal sensations rather than external relations, ended up subject to the most astonishing procedures.

Any attempt to gain some perspective on the shift from live animals to womb disease in women's interpretation of their internal sensations must somehow take into account the rise of gynecology. The gynecologists considered in this chapter were reflex theorists and imparted to their patients some kind of implicit reflex model, which focused the patients' expectancy of symptoms upon the abdomen. Other gynecologists were more oriented toward functional nervous disease as an explanation of subjective symptoms. Both sorts of gynecologists did, however, rivet their patients' attention on the pelvis, either as a cause of disorder in the nervous system (reflex theory) or a consequence of it (central nervous theory). Thus Daniel Webster Cathell, a pathologist in Baltimore who in 1882 wrote an advice manual for physicians, advised his colleagues never to tell female patients anything that might fix their attention on their pelvic organs: "God only knows how many young women in our land are now tormented with apparitions of 'womb complaint,' which have no existence except in this or that doctor's imagination—young women that, had their minds never been fixed on womb complaints, would have lived a lifetime without even thinking of having a womb."[60]

Gynecologist August Rheinstädter of Cologne saw his specialty as helping to create these complaints. In 1884 he said:

The cause of the ever-rising level of nervousness among women is generally assigned to an increase in the so-called abdominal [gynecological] diseases. I can only give limited assent to this notion, given that such supposed risk factors as the lack of time to rest and overexposure to sexual intercourse really only apply to the poor. Moreover, the increase in diseases of the female organs of generation is only an artifact, a result of the extraordinarily swift development of better diagnosis and therapy in gynecology. Because the "abdominal diseases" [Unterleibs-krankheiten] are better diagnosed, their volume only seems to increase, and because the prognosis of treatment has improved, women decide upon a gynecological consultation more easily.

But now, a true hysteromania, a Furor uterinus, has unfortunately arisen from the previous reluctance of women to undergo a gynecological examination and from the indifference which doctors once displayed towards gynecological disease. So that every woman who suffers from migraine, stomach cramps or palpitations believes herself to have a uterine illness and indeed will find some physician willing to indulge her in the treatment of this presumed cause.[61]

In tracing the impact of medical shaping on psychosomatic symptoms, the rise of gynecology and of the reflex model turn out to have been of capital importance. Gynecological surgery, a logical extension of reflex theory, exercised a great influence on women's lives.

The Last Gasp of Reflex Theory: The Nose

As reflex theory lay dying in the 1890s, one last idea rose from its corpus to preoccupy psychiatrists, gynecologists, and rhinologists (specialists of the nose, usually part of the ear, nose, and throat specialty): the view that reflex irritation from the mucosa of the nose could cause neurosis. The doctrine claimed that the mucous lining of the nose was specifically connected to the genitals, an anatomical connection permitting many women's "uterohysterical" symptoms to be treated nasally. I do not know if this curious vogue elicited a corresponding nasal fixation among patients. Nonetheless, as the last medical chapter in reflex theory—before the whole concept of distant-body reflexes passed into the quackery of "reflexology"—the nasal reflexes merit a brief mention here.

Since virtually every other organ in the body had been implicated in reflex action, it was inevitable that the nose's turn would come.[62] The rage for treating diseases via the nose began in 1871, when Friedrich Voltolini, a rhinologist in Breslau, claimed to have cured bronchial asthma by removing nasal polyps. He invoked the mechanism of "reflex irritation."[63] Various other physicians then began to seek out what else one might cure by correcting obvious nasal pathology. Arthur Hartmann in Berlin, for example, believed he had cured epilepsy in a twelve-year-old girl who was having fits two or three times a week by correcting her deviated nasal septum.[64] In 1883 Moritz Rosenthal, a professor of electrotherapy in Vienna and owner of a private clinic for nervous diseases, described a young male patient in whom nervous irritation of the stomach was reflexly linked to a stuffy nose and to deafness.[65]

In the 1880s two "nasal-reflex" theories began to establish themselves: (1) that a thickening of the nasal mucosa over the turbinate bones, or conchi (the bones of the lateral wall of the nasal cavity that guard the tiny entrances to the sinuses and increase the surface for warming and filtering air), reflexly caused remote disease; and (2) that one could treat such disease by reducing the engorgement of the rich beds of veins in this area.[66] It is true that when those veins are filled with blood, the engorged mucosa block the passage of air through the nose and one feels stuffy, a fact that lent the theory a sort of scientific feeling. (With respect to suddenly swelling with blood, the erectile tissue of the nose is a bit like that of the penis.)

In 1883 John Noland Mackenzie, a surgeon at a Baltimore ear, nose, and throat hospital, suggested that certain areas of the nasal mucosa controlled specific distant organs. He believed, for example, that he had identified a cough-control center on the two lower turbinate bones (there are three of them) and on part of the nasal septum. He reported success in treating lung affections by removing the mucosa atop the bones so that vascular engorgement in that area would be a thing of the past.[67] The following year Mackenzie went on to enunciate his momentous theory that the nose and the genitals influenced each other. He noted that a correspondence between size of nose and size of penis had been observed in earlier medical literature. He commented on the histological similarity between the erectile tissue of the nose and the penis. Under conditions of arousal, he said, "erection of this tissue takes place." "It is the temporary orgasm of these bodies that constitutes the anatomical explanation of the stoppage of the nostrils in acute coryza [a runny nose]." Mackenzie commented on a supposed swelling of the mucosa during the menses and postulated the existence of "vicarious nasal menstruation," meaning that a nosebleed might replace or supplant menstruation. (Given that nosebleeds are statistically more common during the menses, it seemed that science had once again come to the relief of therapeutics.) Finally, Mackenzie believed that irritation of the nose could reflexly cause irritation of the genital organs, so that chronic masturbation might produce chronic nasal problems.[68]

In the same year, 1884, Wilhelm Hack, a lecturer at the University of Freiburg, published a book (which he claimed owed nothing to Mackenzie's work) announcing that many different reflex sites in the nose were connected to different internal organs. Hack argued that distant disease could produce swollen nasal mucosa and a runny nose. In sum, he said, the mucosa were both starting and stopping points of reflex arcs that encompassed the entire body.[69] His book legitimated nasal-reflex neurosis for European physicians.

After the mid-1880s a vast literature on nasogenital relations flourished among European neurologists, gynecologists, and rhinologists. A kind of pseudoneurophysiology was worked out in which the trigeminal nerve (sensory to the nose and face) carried messages from the nose to the nerve's large nucleus in the brain stem, whence subtle interconnections to other brain-stem nuclei radiated the pathological or therapeutic messages throughout the body.[70] All this was devised in the absence of any theory of the endocrine system.

Here is a typical example of nasal-reflex theory in action: In 1888 Joseph Joal, a spa doctor in Mont-Dore in France, described a young woman of twenty-three who developed a violent frontal headache each time she menstruated. She also had a runny nose. By cauterizing her inferior turbinate bone, Joal was able to relieve her symptoms, "which proves that we were dealing with nasal reflexes, themselves the result of an ovarian reflex." Another of his patients, a young merchant who had come to Mont-Dore for a cure, developed attacks of asthma every time his wife came to visit. Joal's explanation? "Conjugal excesses" resulted in nasal irritation, which in turn caused the asthma.[71]

Among the neurologists and psychiatrists early to hop on board the nasal-reflex bandwagon was Leopold Löwenfeld of Munich, who observed that a bad cold produced "cerebral neurasthenia" in one patient. In another the sudden cessation of a cold resulted in "chronic feelings of pressure in the head and dizziness," via some kind of reflex-balancing mechanism. One such patient told him, "Only when I've got a cold do I really feel in form, then my head feels so light and clear and I've got my self-confidence back and can do anything. But when the cold is over I'm weak again and tired in the head and I can't get over my timidity and anxiety."[72]

In London, Frederick Parkes Weber referred a number of patients to other London physicians for nasal treatment: Miss Z, a young servant with headaches, low spirits, and asthma, was sent to Dr. Henry A. Francis of chic Cavendish Square for his noted "nose treatment." The Reverend X, a chronic somatizer, was referred to Dr. Francis de Havilland Hall of Wimpole Street for nasal cautery (before he was sent to Grasse in the south of France). Miss Y was dispatched to Dr. Thomas Hovell at a nearby Harley Street address for nasal cautery. Miss Y then went to Ems to try a "nasal douche."[73]

A whole series of Central European gynecologists lined up to explain how removal of the ovaries might also abolish the sense of smell, or how one might stimulate the uterus in labor by tickling the nose.[74] Alexander Peyer, a Swiss urologist, reported how he had stopped the nosebleeds of a twenty-one-year-old chronic masturbator by treating his urethra with a therapy-cum-punishment device called a "psychrophor," invented by the Viennese hydrotherapist Wilhelm Winternitz.[75] Nasal-reflex therapy was thus widely embraced in the practice of medicine at the turn of the century.

Its best-known advocate in history was a Berlin general practitioner named Wilhelm Fliess. Known at the time for his nasal theories and for a crackpot set of numerological theories explaining the timing of big events in life, he became familiar to later generations because of his close friendship with Sigmund Freud. Fliess's work probably had the greatest resonance beyond rhinological circles.[76] In a series of publications dating from 1893, he pinned down "genital" and "stomach" sites on the nasal mucosa and initiated the dabbing of cocaine on genital sites as a treatment of dysmenorrhea.[77]

Fliess had close relations to some of the Berlin psychoanalysts. Alix Strachey, a marginal member of the Bloomsbury set in London, met Fliess while she was doing a psychoanalytical training analysis in Berlin in the 1920s. Her husband James wrote to her: "Is it really the great Fliess? Will you ask him to prod your Magenstelle [the 'stomach point' on the nasal mucosa]?"

Alix wrote back: "Yes, he is the great Fliess. He's very charming and old-fashioned; almost a dwarf with a huge stomach, but otherwise not fat. Much more like a Viennese, with a beard."[78]

Fliess's ideas about nasal-reflex neurosis even caught on with Sigmund Freud and his Viennese circle, physicians who prided themselves on their psychological insight into medical problems. Perhaps Freud merely wished to flatter Fliess, with whom he maintained a close friendship in the 1890s, by seeming himself to embrace reflex theory. But Freud nonetheless applied the diagnosis to his patients and to himself.

On May 30, 1893, Freud wrote Fliess, "The fact that you are inundated with patients demonstrates that on the whole people do know what they are doing. I am curious to know whether you will confirm the diagnosis in the cases I sent to you. I am making this diagnosis very often and agree with you that the nasal reflex is one of the most frequent disturbances."

Later that year it became evident that Freud had been getting his own nasal mucosa treated. November 27: "[There] came a period in which I did not feel like writing, my nose was stopped up, and I could not get myself to do it. I again let myself be cauterized, again enjoy working, but otherwise am little satisfied with the success of the local therapy."

Two years later Freud began to fall away from the camp of true nasal believers: "I discharged exceedingly ample amounts of pus [mucus] and all the while felt splendid; now the secretion has nearly dried up and I am still feeling well." Perhaps, said Freud, the flow of mucus was not responsible for distant symptoms after all, unless the nerve endings are in "a special state of excitation." Yet this was by no means apostasy, for in December 1897 Freud wrote Fliess about plans for their forthcoming get-together in Breslau, "I myself shall not bring anything along. I have gone through a desolate and foggy period and am now suffering painfully from [nasal] discharge and occlusion; I hardly ever feel fresh. If this does not improve, I shall ask you to cauterize me in Breslau."[79]

Much of Freud's circle accepted nasal-reflex theories as well, and in this regard they were like most of the physicians of their time. Adler wrote in his book on "organ inferiority," published in 1907: "Further inferiorities, which are associated with sexual inferiority, have to do with the nose (Fliess), the heart, etc."[80] In 1921 Ernest Jones wrote to Freud of the psychoanalytic conference at The Hague the previous year, "The day I joined you all [at the Congress] I was thoroughly well and active, but that evening my cold in the head began. Partly for toxic reasons and partly from my intolerance of naso-pharyngeal irritation (erogene zone, I suppose), this trouble always affects me physically, in the direction of a slightly hypochondriacal withdrawal."[81] Wilhelm Stekel, an early confidant of Freud's, cocainized the noses of his own patients on the basis of Fliess's theories.[82] And even Josef Breuer, who though certainly not part of Freud's inner circle counted as a friend and distinguished internist, sent patients to Fliess in Berlin for treatment, including his own daughter Dora. In 1895 and 1896, for example, Fliess cauterized the nasal mucosa of one patient of Breuer's, Selma B., and removed part of her middle turbinate bone for neurasthenia.[83] Freud's circle was permeated in the early years by this kind of somato-babble, with its assumption of reflex links from the nose to pelvis and brain.

Even after nasal-reflex theories had been toppled from mainline medicine in the 1920s, echoes lingered. German physicians after World War II were still following Fliess in treating the nose to arrest uterine bleeding and onanism.[84] A group of American researchers in 1950, citing favorably the work of Mackenzie and Fliess in addition to others, concluded (on the basis of three cases of people reporting how their noses felt during sex) that: "The magnitude of the changes in nasal function depended directly on the intensity of the erotic feelings—the greater the sexual excitement the more pronounced the decrease in nasal obstruction and secretion."[85] What the authors cited as physiological law was no more than the momentum of a century's worth of pseudophysiology and cultural prejudice about women as uterine-driven automata.

CHAPTER

4

Gynecological Surgery
and the Desire
for an Operation

I f reflex irritation ran all over the body, it could affect the brain as well. Between 1850 and 1900 a whole school of psychiatrists and gynecologists argued that women's internal organs could make them mad, and that the best cure for pelvic madness lay in a gynecological operation. This aberrant chapter in the history of medicine is relevant to a history of psychosomatic symptoms because so many women ended up internalizing the logic of reflex irritation and demanding operations to remove the source of the irritation.

The Pelvic Organs as a Supposed Cause of Insanity

The reflex theorists who singled out various peripheral organs could not conceivably have left the brain alone. As early as 1821 François Broussais, the Paris physiologist who thought the stomach to be the seat of emotion, had argued that irritation in the stomach produced irritation in the brain, and therewith a gamut of brain pathology from paralysis to mania.[1] A long tradition of reflex theory insisted on the bowels and their contents as sources of mental furor, a tradition scorned as "copropsychiatry" (*die Kopro-Psychiatrie*) by the great German organic psychiatrist Wilhelm Griesinger. Despite Griesinger, several distinguished late-nineteenth-century psychiatrists described "intestinal melancholy" as a disease entity, and psychotic patients would often be given enemas immediately upon admission to an asylum.[2]

69

But the uterus, ovaries, and clitoris were most often singled out for intervention, not the bowels. It was between gynecologist and psychiatrist that reflex theory brought about the firmest therapeutic alliance. Seeing the brain as a target organ of reflex irritation dated back to the earliest theorists. In 1833, the same year as Marshall Hall's first publications on the reflex, the noted Berlin physiologist and pathologist Johannes Müller argued that reflexes extended into the brain. And in 1838 Alfred Wilhelm Volkmann, another important figure in physiology, said that the brain reflected incoming stimuli outward into motor actions just as the spinal cord did, citing, for example, the act of sneezing after seeing a bright light.[3]

Reflex theorists lost no time giving these concepts clinical application. In 1833 English psychiatrist John Conolly, visiting physician to a county asylum in Warwick, considered the uterus (and the bowels) a cause of hysteria: "Of the primary irritation [in hysteria] we should say that by far the most common seat is the uterus and the intestinal canal."[4] When in 1840 the reflex theorist Thomas Laycock announced that "the brain is subject to the laws of reflex action,"[5] he handed his colleagues carte blanche for treating neurosis and psychosis by doing local procedures and major surgery on the female pelvis.

But first there had to be data. Physicians would think twice about performing radical, life-threatening surgery on hysterical and psychotic female patients on the mere say-so of some theorist. After midcentury, statistics purporting to show that pelvic lesions caused insanity began to come to light. (Of course, these data were gathered without statistical "controls"—mentally normal patients with pelvic lesions—and in retrospect it is likely that the various "irritations" were as common in the nonhysterical as the hysterical.) It would be hard to imagine more impeccable scientific credentials than those of Louis Mayer, whose father Karl Wilhelm Mayer was the virtual founder of gynecology in Germany. By 1869 the forty-year-old Louis, an assistant physician in charge of the gynecological outpatient service of his father's clinic in Berlin, had gathered information on 1,025 recent patients who had consulted for gynecological lesions in the clinic: Ninety of them, or 9 percent, had "more or less severe mental illness."[6]

A typical case of Mayer's was an unmarried patient of forty who had a history of paralysis and other hysterical symptoms. She had been melancholic and anxious until about age twenty, when her periods finally became regular. At that point her mental symptoms temporarily went away. Then around thirty-three she had started having heavy periods, at the same time showing new signs of mental disturbance. When Mayer saw her she was very anemic and also became psychically disturbed whenever menstrual bleeding occurred: "She was extremely mistrustful, rejected all social contact because people [were] bad, and considered herself to be as corrupt as possible, possessed by the devil, from whose power she could not free herself." But as soon as the bleeding ceased, she became normal again. Mayer found a uterine fibroid tumor, which he held responsible for her symptoms.[7]

In 1874 an assistant physician at the private Schweizerhof clinic for nervous diseases in Berlin-Zehlendorf found, among the 212 psychotic female patients he had seen over the last six years, suppressed menstruation in 89, overly brief periods in 13, overly long periods in 39, and so forth.[8] A Russian doctor studying in the early 1880s in Paris with Jean-Martin Charcot and psychiatrist Valentin Magnan did a study comparing patients back home in Saint Petersburg with those in Paris: of 45 Russian patients with mental illness or hysteria: 6 had stopped menstruating, 35 had various genital lesions, and only 4 had no pelvic abnormality of any kind. Further, of 155 of his insane female patients at the Sainte Anne asylum in Paris, 63 percent had some kind of genital lesion.[9]

Several English psychiatrists weighed in with statistics. Among 109 female patients who had died in the Rainhill asylum in England, serious pelvic lesions were found in 41 percent, including one patient with an absent uterus.[10] Henry Macnaughton-Jones maintained: "Of 500 private [gynecological] cases taken by me consecutively . . . 270 exhibited [nervous] symptoms, and of those 147 suffered more especially from disorders of the nervous system."[11] Many other such series surfaced from gynecologists and psychiatrists in the 1880s and later, an apparent demonstration of reflex action on the brain. As a result of such information, the proposition that abnormal menstruation and lesions in the female pelvis caused insanity won wide, though by no means universal, acceptance within medicine.

By the late nineteenth century, views of psychosis as a genital reflex were to be found among psychiatrists of almost every land. It was an article of faith among the British. For Henry Maudsley, dean of British psychiatry, hysteria and insanity were examples of reflex arcs from the uterus to the brain, thus pregnancy could tip a woman into mania.[12] Such notions found their way into practice. Sheila M. Ross, an assistant physician in the women's division of the Holloway Sanatorium, a private clinic for nervous diseases near London, said of her involuntarily admitted adolescent and postpartum patients: "It is of the greatest importance that the menses should be thoroughly re-established before the patients are considered as cured." Thus her patients would not be discharged until their periods were regular again.[13]

In France Auguste-Félix Voisin, a psychiatrist at the Salpêtrière Hospital (a combination of hospital, nursing home, and asylum of which Jean-Martin Charcot was medical director), was quite convinced that repeated pregnancies caused hysterical insanity, and that uterine lesions reflexly produced *la folie hystérique* in women generally.[14] As for Central Europe, the famous Richard von Krafft-Ebing, professor of psychiatry in Vienna, believed that every pelvic event conceivable—gynecological lesions, abnormal menstruation, masturbation, sexual excitement without orgasm—all reflexly produced hysteria and full-blown insanity.[15]

Reflex insanity was positively the bread-and-butter of gynecologists, just as rhinologists endorsed nasal-reflex neurosis. The doctrine expanded greatly the number of interventions they were qualified to make. Thus there was a group of gynecologists in every country—though the view was by no means universal—to argue that pelvic lesions made patients mentally ill. It is only surprising how many first-rank gynecological surgeons backed these views, people who by virtue of extensive experience or basic scientific knowledge might have known better. In Germany, for example, the professors Erwin Kehrer of Heidelberg and Bernhard Schultze of Jena adhered to reflex neurosis.[16] In England, Macnaughton-Jones, overwhelmingly sure of himself, mocked the disbelievers, those "pure physicians" who felt that "elucidating the nature of uterine disease . . . had a taint of impurity" about it. Laughable figures, he thought, who shrank

> from even a simple digital examination as a possible pollution of fingers educated only for gentle pressure on delicate wrists . . . or raised their hands in well-feigned Pecksniffian horror at the sight of a Fergusson's speculum. Even still, there are numbers of preeminently respectable physicians who do not hesitate, by silent shrug of shoulder or less demonstrative orbicular movement to signify their inherent doubts as to the necessity of local examinations and treatment, in those cases where uterine affections complicate more active symptoms arising in other organs and which in many instances have diverted the attention of the medical adviser from their real source.[17]

Urging his colleagues to conduct thorough local examinations was probably praiseworthy, but Macnaughton-Jones's true objective was to clear up far-distant symptoms of a mainly mental nature. Such testimony could be replicated manyfold: The gynecologist was gathering his forces to become a nerve doctor.

Gynecological Surgery to Cure Nervous and Mental Illness

It was a short step from seeing genital lesions as the cause of mental disease to repairing them as a cure for it. And in one of the most audacious leaps in the history of nineteenth-century medicine, that is exactly the step that was taken. Gynecologists began operating on their patients to cure hysteria and insanity in an era that knew no antibiotic drugs against infection and that took only cursory precautions with surgical cleanliness. Had they not been so widespread, these operations might have remained but a footnote in the larger sweep of surgical history, quite marginal to a history of psychosomatic illness.

It should be remembered that the majority of all gynecological surgery was performed for legitimate organic indications.[18] But the frequency of local treatments of vulva, vagina, and cervix uteri (carbolic acid irrigations and the like) accelerated throughout the nineteenth century, and that of major gynecological surgery rose rapidly after 1870. Thus, even though procedures for reflex neurosis may have only been a small percentage of all gynecological work, in absolute numbers they added up to quite a few.[19]

The story begins with local treatments in the 1840s and after, done to reduce spinal irritation and reflex neurosis. A precondition for applying caustics, leeches, and cautery irons was persuading women to abandon their traditional fear of having their private parts manually examined by a male doctor, and especially their fear of the speculum.[20] Overcoming this resistance was part of the general medicalizing of women's internal sensations considered in the last chapter, and by the 1860s local vaginal procedures had become quite common. In 1853 London surgeon Robert B. Carter recalled a chance conversation in a railway carriage. "A stranger . . . said without knowing the profession of his fellow-passengers that he had applied caustic to the wombs of twelve women on that morning, making the statement with an air of great exultation, and proceeding to describe himself as a country general practitioner."[21] In the second half of the century, the literature on advice to physicians is filled with references to the doctor as the woman's special friend because of his "intimate" association with her, an association established by legitimating his right to examine and treat the pelvis.[22]

Much of this local treatment was done in the name of curing reflex neurosis and insanity. In 1872 New York gynecologist Fordyce Barker described a thirty-year-old married patient with a retroverted (backward-tilted) uterus who had taken to spitting at family members:

> One evening, after an absence of four days from the city, I found an urgent call to visit her. . . . From the mother, who lived with her, I learned that she had been suffering for three or four days with pain in the back and head, and what was never before seen in her, she had been excessively irritable and ill tempered.
>
> That morning she, whose sweet affectionate nature had always been remarkable, had beaten her little girl most cruelly. After doing this she had spoken to no one.

Later that day, however, she began spitting at her mother, and "when her husband returned and attempted to greet her with a kiss, as was his wont, she not only spit in his face but violently seized his hair, and it was with a great deal of difficulty that her hands were detached." When Dr. Barker entered the room she began spitting at him as well.

Barker examined her vaginally and found the uterus firmly retroverted, "so that it required some force to replace it. As soon as this was done, she loudly ejaculated, with a kind of satisfied grunt, 'there now!' and at once ceased spitting, and became perfectly quiet and before I left the room she fell asleep." A Hodge pessary, an instrument placed in the vagina to support a backward-tilting uterus, prevented recurrence of this behavior.[23] Clearly she expected to be cured by the pessary and believed that her own behavior was caused by her uterus.

Heinrich Laehr, chief physician of the Schweizerhof private asylum for women and a disbeliever in uterine-reflex theories, noted how many of his patients had had gynecological treatment before their admission. Of 436 patients, "the majority had been physically examined by gynecologists and treated for a considerable time; nonetheless their psychoses had worsened and they were brought into the asylum."[24]

The advance of surgery in the nineteenth century entirely changed the nature of these interventions. Now gynecologists would not stop at topical applications but advanced to major operations, especially the removal of the ovaries. (Many different procedures were done in the name of curing mental illness, such as stitching retroverted uteri to the anterior abdominal wall or performing hysterectomies.)

Although the first successful ovariotomy, or removal of the ovaries, was done in 1809 by an American frontier surgeon named Ephraim McDowell, only in the 1840s in England did the operation acquire real currency.[25] It was the pioneering operation in the history of abdominal surgery, the early ones performed mainly for ovarian tumors and massive serum-filled cysts. Then, in the summer of 1872, two surgeons on opposite sides of the Atlantic, unknown to each other, removed the healthy ovaries of young female patients in order to cure problems of an essentially psychological nature or, as with perimenstrual pain, problems having an admixture of the physiologic and psychological. On July 27 Alfred Hegar, professor of gynecology at the University of Freiburg, removed both ovaries of a twenty-seven-year-old woman from Kenzingen who had been suffering "unendurable" abdominal and thigh pain at the time of the menses. "After having tried all possible systemic therapies for more than two years [including two spa visits], the patient herself demanded the operation." She died several days later of peritonitis.[26] Then on August 17, 1872, Robert Battey, a forty-four-year-old surgeon in Rome, Georgia, who had done postgraduate work in Paris, removed the ovaries of a patient who had been a chronic invalid. A single woman of thirty, she had been in bed for sixteen years. Although she had apparently menstruated only twice in her life, her menstrual molimen (an old-fashioned word for premenstrual tension) was said to be "excessive, accompanied by headache, suffused countenance and usually convulsions which were epileptiform in character and left the patient in a semi-comatose state." She became septic after the operation but later recovered, all nervous phenomena having vanished.[27]

What to call this operation—the removal of healthy ovaries in young female patients—provoked some head scratching. Battey initially christened it, quite accurately, "normal ovariotomy" but later abandoned the term because he did not like its sound. "Oophorectomy" was often used, to indicate ovariotomy for reasons other than ovarian disease. But it was Battey's colleague James Marion Sims, the founder of gynecology in the United States, who in 1877 proposed that the operation be called "Battey's operation."[28] The name stuck, giving rise to the phrase "to Batteyize a woman," meaning to remove her ovaries. Although both Battey and Hegar were at pains to point out that the ovaries were often "diseased" (meaning they had small cysts, a virtually normal accompaniment of ovulation), the indications for castrating the patients were clearly psychological, including, said Battey, "long protracted physical and mental suffering, dependent upon monthly nervous and vascular perturbations."[29] "Gynecology," as Hegar put it, "represents the bridge between general medicine and neuropathology."[30]*

*It became standard usage to call "ovariotomy" the removal of ovaries having tumors or cysts, "oophorectomy" the removal of ovaries with some kind of pathology though not necessarily large tumors (or ovaries which had been promoting disease elsewhere such

Battey's operation spread rapidly in the late 1870s and 1880s in the Anglo-Saxon world and in Central Europe. The great English ovarioto-mist Lawson Tait, who had been doing ovariotomies since 1857, reaching by June 1880 his thousandth case, let slip that some had been for nervous problems: among Tait's 28 ovariotomies from July 1879 to June 1880, two had concerned "menstrual epilepsy and mania," and twelve had been for painful periods.[31] In June 1878, the Edinburgh gynecologist Alex-ander Russell Simpson did the first Battey's operation in Scotland. His patient, a woman of thirty-six from Dundee who had long consulted him for menstrual complaints, had asked him, "Can't you do here what the doctors in America can do?"

Simpson told her the operation "was by no means free from danger." He put her off.

She returned two months later and looked him in the face, "If I funked it before," she said, "I think you're funking it now."

He repeated that the operation could be fatal.

"One in three of the patients die, don't they?" she asked.

"Yes, and you might be the one," he said. "But how do you know?"

"Oh, I've been reading all about it," she responded.[32]

The exchange is interesting because it suggests that even in 1878 the patients' world was full of information about the wonders of being Battey-ized.

In April 1879 surgeon Heywood Smith of the Hospital for Women in London did the first Battey's operation in England.[33] By 1879 in Ger-many enough surgeons had performed it that the subject could be dis-cussed at a September meeting of gynecologists in Baden-Baden. Karl Schröder, an otherwise quite progressive professor of gynecology in Ber-lin, had removed the normal ovaries of a "mentally-ill girl with nympho-mania," whereupon she recovered from her mental illness. Hermann Freund, that Strasbourg fan of reflex theory, had removed three sets of ovaries that were producing hysteria (by causing uterine myomas to grow), and one set of ovaries causing "hystero-epilepsy." One of the four patients died. Four further professors reported their varying experiences with Battey's operation, which they called Hegar's operation.[34]

It was among American gynecologists that Battey's operation had its longest run. Even early on, it was performed not just by obscure surgeons in places like Rome, Georgia, but by members of the nation's gynecologi-

as breast cancer or uterine cancer), and "castration" the removal of both ovaries to bring on early menopause. Battey's operation was thus a form of castration, but was often classed under oophorectomy as well on the grounds that the ovaries did have some kind of lesion.

cal elite, such as George Engelmann of Saint Louis and William Goodell, founder of the Philadelphia Obstetrical Society.[35] Throughout the 1880s in the United States the indications for Battey-izing expanded steadily. By 1884 small-town surgeons, such as a Doctor Barss of Malden, Massachusetts, were removing young women's ovaries for hysteria, in this case a twenty-nine-year-old who was bedridden with a backache, a right-sided hysterical paresis, loss of sensation, and fits.[36] In 1888 J. Taber Johnson of Washington, D.C., removed the ovaries of a twenty-eight-year-old for nymphomania. She had been confined to an asylum for four years, and her family was quite unable to control her behavior.[37] This surgical onslaught would continue for another decade at least.

How many Battey's operations were ever done in the United States? In the absence of an official registry, one can only speculate. Yet there seem to have been many. For example, in1895 Robert Edes, staff physician at the Adams Nervine Asylum, a fifty-bed private clinic founded in 1880 in the Jamaica Plain suburb of Boston, said that among recent female patients, twenty-seven at some point before admission had "had both ovaries removed for the relief of nervous symptoms."[38] "Many ovaries have been removed," said Frank Billings, a distinguished Chicago physician in 1904, "when there was no good reason for their removal. I could cite many examples." He remembered a young "neurasthenic" woman from Wisconsin he saw about 1892 who had long-standing complaints in multiple organ systems. Billings could find nothing wrong, so the woman went to New York, where both of her ovaries were extirpated. "Her engagement was broken off because of the operation, and she is as much a neurotic today as before her ovaries were removed. The woman's life is ruined. There was no more reason in my opinion for removing her ovaries than for removing her ears."[39]

Another American physician, the Georgia internist William R. Houston, remembered in 1936 how casually his colleagues had once removed patients' ovaries:

> I recall having been able to rescue more than one girl from a double ovariectomy proposed as a cure for her hysterical seizures. . . . These were merely instances of the bias that money-mindedness can give. It must be hard for an expert tonsillectomist to weigh with perfect nicety the etiological and pathological problems of the pharynx in the child from a wealthy home.[40]

Statistically, on the basis of article titles in the *Index-Catalogue of the Library of the Surgeon-General's Office, United States Army,* 51 percent of all articles about oophorectomies in the 1889 edition concerned mental and nervous disorders, 42 percent in the 1907 edition.[41] These figures indicate that Battey's operation was not a marginal procedure conducted by a handful of crackpots, but central in the arsenal of late-nineteenth-century gynecology.

Battey's operation enjoyed a somewhat less extended run in Central Europe. In 1884 several German gynecologists sounded the alarm at a medical congress in Copenhagen, which included an audience of enthusiastic Americans; in Berlin also that year warning bells went off.[42] But even so, Battey-izing enjoyed fair currency in Central Europe in the 1880s and early 1890s. Typical of these years were a series of peasant women on whom Hermann Klotz, a member of the gynecology department of the University of Innsbruck, operated in the early 1880s. Here is a sample case:

Frau A. O., thirty-eight and single, a farm worker in the Sellrain Valley, sought out Doctor Klotz in August 1881 for deep pelvic pain. She also had a history of chronic vomiting and "general convulsions" resembling catalepsy every three to six weeks, which were accompanied by a feeling of tightening up in her insides. Her periods and gynecological examinations triggered the convulsions. In addition she had a history of hysterical aphonia, dysphagia (difficulty swallowing), a burning feeling over her entire body, and migraine. "From internal medications there was little further to expect, as she had already swallowed half of the pharmacy." Because life had become "torture" for her, Klotz operated on February 2, 1882. She recovered smoothly. When he saw her three months later she enjoyed glowing health, had experienced no more vomiting or fits, was eating copiously, and was again capable of work.[43]

That such gynecological tinkering with nervous and mental patients in Central Europe was common in the mid-1880s emerges from the remark in 1883 of Josef Peretti, a young assistant physician in a Prussian asylum, "It is rare to find female patients, above all middle-class patients, admitted to asylum who have not already been either the object of gynecological treatment or regarded as presumably suffering from pelvic-organ disease."[44] As late as 1887 Max Schede, a member of the department of surgery of the Hamburg General Hospital, was removing the ovaries of nineteen-year-olds for "epilepsy."[45] In 1891, Sigmund Gottschalk, chief physician of a private gynecological clinic in Berlin, called the reputation of the Battey-Hegar operation "over the last fifteen years ever more brilliant."[46]

Only in France did Battey's operation fail to make much headway. Although it was called to the attention of French surgeons in 1878, the first one was not performed until 1880.[47] By the mid-1880s several surgeons were doing the "opération d'Hégar et de Battey," among them François Villar at the Salpêtrière. Villar's opinion: "If hysterical fits have a clear point of departure at the ovary, one might attempt it. Unfortunately, most commonly neuralgia originates in the central nervous system and castration produces no result." Among the nine Villar had so far conducted, two had been for ovarian pain and *accidents nerveux*.[48]

If operations for nervous disease did not sweep the field in France, it is probably because Charcot opposed them, just as Charcot was unenthusiastic about reflex theory and spinal irritation. He believed hysteria to be a disorder of the central nervous system and advocated treatments such as spa going to reduce "central" irritation. The greatest concession the Charcot school made to ovarian-reflex theory was the introduction of the ovarian compressor belt mentioned in the previous chapter, a belt to hold in place ovaries that were responsible for "ovarie," meaning fits originating from the ovary. Charcot's student Georges Gilles de la Tourette labeled ovarian operations "absolutely wrong" as a treatment of hysteria.[49]

Gynecology in the Hands of Psychiatrists

It was only logical that psychiatrists not leave pelvic operations to chance encounters with outside gynecologists but commission surgery right there in the asylum. The possibility now existed that a woman, admitted to an asylum for a mental disorder, might leave minus her ovaries.

Some asylums in North America actually had staff gynecologists. Among the first to Battey-ize insane inpatients was George Rohé at the asylum in Catonsville, Maryland.[50] In 1895 the London Asylum in London, Ontario, appointed A. T. Hobbs to conduct pelvic surgery.[51] By the early 1890s the State Hospital for the Insane at Norristown, Pennsylvania, was removing the ovaries of female inpatients.[52] Riding high in the saddle, these psychogynecologists ridiculed the timid neurologists who rejected reflex theories of insanity. Rohé, by this time superintendent of an asylum in Sykesville, Maryland, crowed in 1897, "To the neurologist the suggestion that a mental state may be a reflex of a morbid bodily condition has somewhat the traditional effect of shaking a red rag before the eyes of a bull or sprinkling his Satanic Majesty with the consecrated water of the Church." He mocked the neurologists for their therapeutic nihilism. "Those of us who believe . . . that pelvic disease in women has an etiological relation to mental disease urge the importance of gynecology in hospitals for the insane, primarily upon the ground that the insane woman has the same right to be treated for bodily disease of any kind as her sane sister has."[53] Asked in 1900 whether they agreed that "malformations and traumatisms of the female genital apparatus [are] causes of insanity," all but one of the American asylum superintendents who were polled answered yes. The response of Walter P. Manton in Detroit was typical: "If disease of the reproductive organs is included, I have seen and operated on quite a number of cases of hysteromania and nymphomania, which were cured or greatly relieved by the removal of diseased ovaries."[54]

An interesting feature of the American landscape not found in Europe was the large number of American female physicians who performed, commissioned, or approved of Battey operations. In 1879 Margaret Cleaves, a staff physician at an asylum in Mount Pleasant, Iowa, urged her fellow female physicians to undertake "psychical gynecology" in their asylum work. Much insanity in women, she said, was located not in the brain but represented a reflex disturbance, "capable of cure by removal of the primary cause."[55] Alice Bennett at the Norristown asylum advocated therapeutic castration, which staff doctors Joseph Price and Marie B. Werner carried out.[56] An unnamed female physician at the Adams Nervine Asylum in Boston also recommended the Battey operation.[57] Mary Jacobi, a New York physician with a psychologically oriented practice, who was a "staunch feminist" and advocate of women in medicine, recommended, in the presence of reflex irritation, the "removal of the ovaries for intractable hysteria." Jacobi said: "I have known of two cases where Battey's operation was performed with entire relief to an immense train of morbid symptoms, which in one case included eight years' paraplegia. In neither did the ovaries appear abnormal to the naked eye."[58] The point is not to indict these female doctors with the advantage of a hundred years of hindsight, but rather to indicate that if women physicians themselves advocated the operation, how little female patients must have been able to object.

The sustained nature of the enthusiasm for Battey-izing in the New World was perhaps a result of life on the periphery. Yet in the very center, among German professors of psychiatry, a brief but passionate vogue for Battey's operation may also be noted. Paul Flechsig, professor of psychiatry in Leipzig, director of the university psychiatric clinic in that city, and one of the epoch's pioneers in the study of cerebral localization, reported in 1884 the case of a patient with "hysteria magna" whose ovaries one of his assistants had removed in July of that year.[59] In 1878 the great Berlin neurologist Karl Friedrich Westphal, codiscoverer of the knee-jerk reflex, urged his colleague Karl Schröder, a gynecological surgeon at the Charité Hospital, to remove the ovaries of at least one hysterical patient.[60] Moritz Benedikt, the idiosyncratic but world-famous Viennese neurologist and psychiatrist, became angry in 1903 at Bernhard Krönig, codirector of a private gynecological clinic in Leipzig. Krönig had suggested that nervous problems might cause, rather than result from, such phenomena as ovarie and various pelvic sensations. Krönig was among the first gynecologists to venture such a heretical view. Benedikt insisted that gynecological operations could indeed cure hysteria and maintained that it was "completely childish"—indeed, *"Denkdilletantismus* [intellectual dilettantism]"—on Krönig's part to see pelvic lesions as incidental in nervous complaints.[61]

The general medical rush to repudiate these pelvic-reflex theories and their surgical corollaries that occurred later tends to eclipse the support they once enjoyed. Only that support makes comprehensible some of the patterns of illness behavior that developed.

Clitoridectomy

One last surgical correlate of reflex theory was clitoridectomy, or the surgical removal of the superficial portion of the clitoris. A procedure not as widespread as Battey's operation, in its very occurrence it was profoundly indicative of a willingness—or, indeed, desire—on the part of women to let themselves be operated on. Clitoridectomy, one of the oldest operations in the history of medicine, was performed by the ancient Egyptians and is frequently mentioned in Roman texts for clitoral hypertrophy and for nymphomania.[62] Late in the eighteenth century, clitoridectomy was being performed occasionally for "nymphomania," which usually meant chronic masturbation. Here is a typical case from Paris around 1800:

A young woman was so given to masturbation that she was close to dying from exhaustion [*marasme*]. Although she understood the danger of her situation she was too weak-willed or too swept up by its pleasures, truly enslaved by them, to be able to resist. In vain her hands were tied. She was able to gratify herself by rubbing against some protruberant part of the bed. Her legs were tied. She had only to move her thighs, rubbing one against the other, or wiggle her pelvis and hips in order to achieve numerous orgasms [*pollutions*]. Her parents took her to Professor [Antoine] Dubois. Following the example of [André]

Levret, he felt justified in proposing the amputation of the clitoris. The patient and her parents readily agreed. He resected the organ with a single knife stroke. The stump was cauterized with a hot iron, thus stopping hemorrhage. The operation was completely successful. The patient, cured of her pernicious habit, quickly recovered her health and her energy.[63]

Until well into the nineteenth century nymphomania continued to be the main indication. Robert Thomas, a physician in Salisbury, noted in 1816 in a widely read textbook, "As the clitoris is the seat of pleasure during the act of coitus, nymphomania might possibly be cured by extirpating this organ."[64] In 1822, for example, the distinguished Prussian military surgeon Carl Ferdinand von Graefe clitoridectomized a disruptive fifteen-year-old girl whose chronic masturbation could not otherwise be halted.[65] In the early 1840s Dietrich Busch rather grudgingly accepted clitoridectomy in the treatment of nymphomania in his big textbook on the sex life of women.[66] And in 1851 Claude-Marie-Stanislas Sandras, specialist in nervous diseases at the Beaujon Hospital in Paris, suggested clipping back the labia minor in nymphomania and cutting down an overgrown clitoris.[67]

These traditional clitoridectomies occurred in the context of a general busybody approach to the vulva, perhaps tickling the clitoris or stitching the labia together to achieve various therapeutic objectives. In 1802 Jean-Baptiste Louyer-Villermay, who had just received his medical degree in Paris and was presumably up on the latest procedures, wrote that one could stop hysterical fits by tickling the clitoris, "a shameful practice" he described only in Latin.[68] In 1856 Raoul LeRoy d'Étiolles, another Paris physician, described tickling a patient's clitoris as a test of whether she had total body anesthesia, a supposed inability to feel skin sensations: She did not realize they were doing it until she removed her blindfold, at which point she reddened.[69] Thus, it can be seen that medicine had always practiced an intermittent kind of clitoral meddlesomeness of both surgical and nonsurgical varieties.

The modern history of clitoridectomy begins with the rise of reflex theory, which provided justification for increasing the number of interventions from this traditional episodic level. This increase is not well documented, perhaps because the operation itself—the surgical mutilation of young women—went so much against the grain of the profession. But there are occasional references, such as the veiled allusion of Jacques Lisfranc, a surgeon at the Pitié Hospital in Paris, to certain "shameful procedures" his colleagues were doing to arrest hysterical fits, procedures Lisfranc himself rejected completely.[70] The indication for the operations to which he referred was not nymphomania, the traditional justification for clitoridectomy, but hysterical convulsions, an implicit application of reflex theory.

In the mid-1860s in England a medical scandal exploded that made it apparent that quite a number of clitoridectomies were being conducted, largely in the name of stopping reflex hysteria originating from "irritated" clitorises. This scandal was associated with Isaac Baker Brown, a noted London ovariotomist, member of the Obstetrical Society, and founder in 1858 of a private gynecological clinic. Brown was forty-nine in 1861, when he published a new edition of his book *On Surgical Diseases of Women,* in which he recommended excision of "enlarged" clitorises in "high abnormal irritability." He wrote: "Experience has taught me that . . . the irritation of the clitoris and its horrible results may frequently be cured."[71] Five years later in another book, *On the Curability of Certain Forms of Insanity . . . in Females,* Brown recommended clitoridectomy for the therapy of mental illness.[72]

What apparently provoked a crisis was Brown's unlawful detention in his London Surgical Home of a mentally ill woman whom he was about to clitoridectomize or had already clitoridectomized. The Commissioners of Lunacy complained about this infringement of the law under which the insane might be detained in nonasylums. Brown's developing dementia, apparently from neurosyphilis, might perhaps be blamed for this particular lapse in judgment and for his generally reckless approach toward clitoridectomy in those years.[73] In March 1867 the London Obstetrical Society met to consider whether he should be expelled, not for doing the operation, which numerous members, who had been performing it themselves, defended, but for not being frank with the patient, the family, and the family doctor in advance about what exactly he was going to do. On April 3 he was expelled by a vote of 194 to 38.[74]

Not just Brown, but many English doctors in these years were routinely doing clitoridectomies. Tyler Smith said at the trial:

It appears to me the great vocation of the meeting tonight is to defend women who have been and are liable to be injured by the practices in question. There are a great number of females in London, and scattered throughout the country, who are in this case, and I may say that for the last two or three years I have never gone into the country to see a patient without having complaints of cases made to me upon this matter of clitoridectomy. There are numbers of families where the husband is annoyed, and the wife made wretched for life, by this operation having been performed with or without the consent of the patient and her husband. Then there are a number of young women upon whom this operation has been performed . . . and these young women are in as deplorable a condition as can be imagined. If they are honourable, should any proposal of marriage come to them, the parents are obliged to tell the parties proposing that they have been mutilated, and thus they are obliged to expose themselves to the possibility of being treated as imperfect persons.[75]

In October 1866 an anonymous physician had, as "William Smithers Taliacotius" (after a sixteenth-century Bologna surgeon named Tagliacozzi who described an operation to restore noses that had been cut off), written ironically to the medical press:

It is well known that during the last few years many London Surgeons have been in the habit of amputating the clitoris for the cure of most of the imaginary ailments to which women are liable. To such an extent has this operation been performed that it will soon be somewhat rare to meet with a woman whose sexual organs are entire. Just as we commonly inquire of our female patients if the bowels act daily . . . so it will soon become necessary to ask, "Has your clitoris been removed?"[76]

There were many references to clitoridectomy in the medical press. After describing in 1866 how "ovarian irritation" could poison the mind, William Murray, a Newcastle gynecologist, said, "In the female the practice of masturbation is not uncommon . . . a disease which is dependent on a morbid irritation of the clitoris and adjacent parts, and which is curable by removing that organ or subduing its irritability."[77] That year a doctor in Maida Hill wrote in, complaining that against his advice the operation had been performed on a fifteen-year-old patient of his who had had epilepsy since the age of seven.[78] Thomas Tanner, a physician at several London hospitals and founding member of the Obstetrical Society, described several cases he himself had clitoridectomized—for example, Miss X, age thirty, who had been "in bad health for years" but without any specific disease. Feeling unable to do anything, she had suffered from back and abdominal pains and was "very nervous and hysterical." By 1865, when she first saw Doctor Tanner, "she was always suffering either from headache, neuralgia, piles, prolapsus of the rectum, or spinal pains, et cetera. In fact she was, in her own opinion, a martyr to disease, spending most of her time in bed, living alone in lodgings, and never going out into the air unless positively obliged." Tanner was convinced that her problems were attributable to masturbation and operated on her around March 1865, the results being a complete failure.[79] Robert Harling, a consultant in London's Portman Square, treated a seventy-three-year-old woman who had "a sense of irritation in the external organs of generation." "She often expressed apprehensions of approaching madness, longed for relief by death, and yet betrayed great consternation at the intrusion of any new symptom upon the dismal routine of her miseries." He treated her with clitoridectomy.[80]

Enough has been said to suggest that by the time the Brown affair broke, clitoridectomy had become a not-unfamiliar operation to doctors and their patients, certainly in England and possibly elsewhere as well.[81] Its history before this time is a bit unclear, but three points might be made about its vicissitudes after 1867.

One is that it did not disappear in England, as perhaps might be thought, but continued to be performed—at a low level of frequency—until the turn of the century. (Brown himself, who died in 1873, operated as late as 1869.[82]) At a meeting of the British Gynecological Society in October 1890 it emerged that a number of members were still doing clitoridectomy.[83] I have seen no more references to it in England after that date.

Second, the discredit into which removal of the clitoris fell after 1867 catalyzed a boom for cauterizing and putting caustics on the clitoris. As one London practitioner explained, caustics were superior, "because the effect of the caustic can be kept up for as long a period as the medical attendant pleases, and may, if necessary, be reapplied; whereas with regard to extirpation, directly the part is healed peripheral irritation [masturbation] may be had recourse to again over the remaining branches of the pudic nerve."[84] In 1883 the distinguished Viennese electrotherapist Moritz Rosenthal advocated "energetic cauterization" of the clitoris in cases of hysterical vomiting.[85] And in 1901 London society gynecologist Henry Macnaughton-Jones related the following case: An unmarried woman "who had done good public work" began masturbating and then became alarmed about it after reading a gynecology textbook. She was unable to stop, and Macnaughton-Jones assured her he could cure the condition. He "freely cauterized the clitoris and the surrounding area with glavanocautery. The effect was, that she abandoned the habit, and her will-control over it was permanently established." The author concluded, "It was not the effect of the cauterisation that effected a cure, so much as the influence on the patient's mind of the assurance that it would do so, and the time afforded for her will-power to assert itself."[86]

Finally, the vogue for clitoridectomy lasted far longer in the United States than in Europe, once again the effect of location on the periphery.

Some surgeons in the 1870s and 1880s were clitoridectomizing prepu-bescent girls for "reflex paralyses" of an obviously organic nature.[87] Turn-of-the-century homeopathic publications praised manipulation of the clitoris, an organ that served, they said, as a kind of telephone station on the reflex pathway.[88] The mainline publication of American gynecolo-gists and obstetricians, *The American Journal of Obstetrics,* from its founding in 1869 right up to World War I, contained numerous articles praising and reporting clitoridectomy.[89]

No other country in Western society has a record even approaching America's. The preoccupation of American physicians and surgeons could not fail to affect how the patients of these men saw their bodies, caus-ing women to incriminate their pelvic organs as a cause of physical symp-toms and to seek out surgery for relief. In 1943 Walter Alvarez of the Mayo Clinic in Rochester, Minnesota, recalled "a stout, unattractive, middle-aged farmer's widow" who had come twice to him with a vague account of indigestion. "Because it did not occur to me that an uninteresting woman of her type and age could have sexual problems, I did not ask about such matters," and so she had not been able to tell him what was really on her mind. But she later wrote him a letter. "What had hap-pened," Alvarez said, "was that the death of her husband had left her with a sexual hunger that tortured her day and night. A friend suggested that the removal of the clitoris might help, but each time she came to have the operation done she was too bashful to come out with what was on her mind."[90] In other words, she had learned—sometime in the late 1920s or 1930s in small-town America—that clitoridectomies might help persons such as herself. She thought Alvarez would do one for her. Pa-tients were now seeking out surgery for their symptoms.

The Desire for Surgery as a Psychosomatic Symptom

The fixed belief that one requires an operation represents a psychoso-matic symptom. The patient has coalesced the various ill-defined sensa-tions that plague him or her into a fixed diagnosis and is seeking help on the basis of that self-diagnosis. This new desire to seek out surgical help seems to have been a direct result of reflex theory, and of the orgy of pelvic operations on women done in the name of that theory.

In writing the history of women's subjective awareness of their internal sensations, a major practical problem for the historian is gaining insight into the intensely private domain of what patients actually experienced. First, there is common medical opinion. Of course the physicians—in the main, those who wrote articles were jaded older men—scorned their patients' complaints and behavior. Yet the rather cynical advice the doctors gave one another does represent the distillation of one kind of experience, to be taken for what it is worth. Second, there are actual tales of the patients coming in to request operations. At least such accounts tell us that this behavior is not a medical figment, and that the patients, whose reasons were entirely opaque to the physicians, truly did seek out operations as part of a larger pattern of somatization.

On the first kind of evidence: In the late nineteenth century doctors in every country cautioned their colleagues about operation-seeking women. As Carl Backhaus, a Leipzig gynecologist, warned in 1901 at a professional meeting about local treatments to the genitals for hysteria: "We have learned that women—and this applies absolutely to hysterical ones— are psychically heavily influenced by the news that something is not quite right with the genitals. Such women tend to drift from one gynecologist to the next, are ready for every operation and are usually made sicker than they were before by this kind of gynecological busy-work." In Backhaus's view, gynecologists should learn the symptoms of hysteria so as to recognize such patients.[91]

William Priestly, said to have the largest maternity and gynecological practice in London, urged his colleagues in 1895 at a meeting of the British Medical Association to ignore the pleas of women for gynecological operations. "Caution in this respect is the more necessary because there are always discontented women who magnify their sufferings, and some neurotic patients will submit to any martyrdom for the sake of evoking sympathy. They much prefer an active and energetic doctor."[92]

Similar advice was given in France about neurotic or neurasthenic women who demanded gynecological operations.[93] And in the United States many physicians with a conservative approach to surgery felt they had had their fingers burned by their patients' pelvic mania. Thus Carlton C. Frederick, chief surgeon at the Woman's Hospital in Buffalo, said in 1895 it was patients' neuroses that caused pelvic symptoms, rather than the other way around: back pain, thigh pain, painful urination, loss of sexual appetite, and so forth being neurotic symptoms. "These women come to us expecting us to pronounce the verdict that the uterus, tubes, or ovaries in some way are the direct cause of their ills." Do not operate on them, he urged his colleagues.[94] These quotes must be taken as the dour assessments by powerful males of powerless women, males who also had the power to withhold operations.

Many patients did seem to be fixated on operations. Not all these women were uninfluential or easily subject to medical intimidation. Mrs. X of Washington, D.C., forty and a mother of three, had by 1885 "suffered a constant burning pain in the left ovary for twenty years, and for the past few years in the right ovary also. . . . She had been under treatment for many years and had spent," she told Washington's Doctor Johnson, "over $10,000 to obtain relief from this constant gnawing, burning pain, without success. She was practically bedridden three weeks out of every month, and had little if any enjoyment in life. Her pains all culminated about the time of her period. Constant nausea and neuralgia, both reflex, made her life a burden which she refused longer to bear."

At this point, the very image of a lifelong somatizer, she sought relief from Doctor Johnson:

> A lady friend, in about her condition, had been operated on and cured, and she calmly and deliberately made up her mind to have her offending organs removed. I demurred, and begged her to stand it five years longer, until nature would come to her rescue in change of life. She replied that she had stood it just as long as she could, and that, unless she obtained relief, she would be in her grave or an insane asylum in less than a year.

Johnson relented and removed her ovaries.[95] Perhaps it was because the patient died six days postoperatively that he emphasized to his readers that she had been the one to demand the operation. In essence, however, she had self-diagnosed her problem as in her ovaries and, a woman of wealth, had hired a surgeon to do her bidding.

Paul Mundé was born in Germany, trained in medicine at Harvard, and returned to Vienna for postgraduate study. In 1881, at the age of thirty-five and already very much a society women's doctor in New York City, he became consulting gynecologist at Mount Sinai Hospital. He seems to have been a magnet for self-diagnosing female patients who demanded surgery. Here is a typical case: a twenty-two-year-old patient, "while returning home one evening from a party, during the menstrual period, was seized with what was called a fainting fit and was unable to walk." Thereafter she remained paralyzed in the lower limbs, with some strength restored in the affected limbs but unable to rise from bed. Three years later when she saw Doctor Mundé she was an emaciated, bedridden invalid. She was anxious for Battey-izing but Mundé and her other physicians opposed it, believing her to have myelitis, an inflammation of the spinal cord. Three more years passed in which the patient was plagued by "ovarian" pain.

Now, at twenty-eight, she noted in a copy of the *Zentralblatt für Gynäkologie*, the German journal in gynecology, the case of a woman with symptoms like hers. The German woman, who had been unable to walk for seven years and was able to eat only through a tube, had had her ovaries removed and made a perfect recovery. After the operation this German woman could walk six miles.

Mundé acceded to his New York patient's request and removed her ovaries on January 6, 1884. "The patient, who was an unusually intelligent lady, called his attention, four days after the operation, to the fact that she was able to move the toes of the left foot, which she had not been able to do during the preceding seven years. About a week later, she was able to bend the left knee." Then she actually got out of bed, and two months after the operation "walked the full length of the double room without assistance, and apparently as well as anybody could."[96] Thus Mundé had unwittingly cured a woman with hysterical paralysis by removing her ovaries.

Though the persistence of reflex views in American gynecology probably made these cases commoner in the United States than elsewhere, they were not a peculiarly American phenomenon. Baroness S., a Berliner of thirty-two, had been sick since her first menses, having fits around her monthly periods and otherwise vomiting everything she ate except "Champagne frappés." She also suffered from urinary retention and catheterized herself once daily. When on July 26, 1881, Karl Schröder examined her gynecologically, she had a major fit, going into *opisthotonos*, or rigid hyperextension of her neck, back, and leg muscles. "She is very emaciated, quite miserable, and deeply unhappy." She showed some improvement after he excised her ovaries a week later, but over the next year demonstrated repeated "nervous phenomena," including inability to swallow. She also became a morphine addict in this period. Other physicians removed her coccyx, and to relieve her of the need to catheterize herself daily, performed some procedures on her urethra as well. Finally, believing herself cured by the operations, Baroness S. returned to normalcy.[97]

Many similar cases establish that patients' operatic craving is indeed an important theme in the surgeon-patient relationship. Two variants of it, however, are of particular interest. In one, the patients expressed a continuous desire for abdominal surgery of any type. They tended to end up, years later, with the "battlefield abdomen" characteristic of polysurgical patients who have had many organs removed; they may have had a host of other procedures as well, such as laminectomies (on the spinal vertebrae) and operations on the temporomandibular joint (the hinge of the jaw). "There are men and women," wrote George Bernard Shaw in 1911, "whom the operating table seems to fascinate: half-alive people who through vanity, or hypochondria, or a craving to be the constant objects of anxious attention or what not, lose such feeble sense as they ever had of the value of their own organs and limbs." Shaw might have had some of Paul Mundé's patients in mind when he added, "There is in the classes who can afford to pay for fashionable operations a sprinkling of persons so incapable of appreciating the relative importance of preserving their bodily integrity (including the capacity for parentage) . . . that they tempt surgeons to operate on them not only with huge fees, but with personal solicitation."[98]

German doctors called this need to be operated on the "mania operatoria passiva." "If the problem earlier was patients' reluctance to undergo an operation," said Albert Krecke, chief surgeon at a private clinic in Munich, in1925, "today we fight against the inclination for operations." "One can even talk of a mania for operations [Operationswut]. I often hear patients say, 'Don't I have to be operated on?' or 'Isn't there some operation that will get rid of my problem?'"[99] According to Rudolf Schindler, a colleague of Krecke's, an internist in Munich who also was struck by this "mania operatoria," such patients constituted virtually the only category of somatizer inaccessible to psychotherapy. "These are the unhappiest individuals," he said in 1925, "trapped in a horrifying milieu, their lives filled with burdens, torment and lack of appreciation—and therefore mainly women. They see, unconsciously of course, in an operation the only possibility of finally finding rest, maybe even sympathy and respect."[100]

In 1922 a woman of twenty-three was admitted to the Pitié Hospital in Paris with evident symptoms of multiple sclerosis. She told of a turbulent neurological history, half her body paralyzed at one point, spasmodic contractures of the muscles on one side of her face, also on occasion pneumonia and the tympanitic, or gas-filled, abdomen of peritonitis.

The residents were horrified to see her abdomen when she undressed. It was plowed by scars (she had already had nine laparotomies). "The uterus and oviducts, the gallbladder, the appendix, the cecum and a meter of colon had vanished. Fluoroscopy showed a perfectly functioning gastroenterostomy [surgical creation of an artificial passage between the stomach and intestines] from some previous operation. Of course all the removed organs had turned out subsequently to be healthy."

In the belief that she had multiple sclerosis, they did a spinal tap, gave her a careful neurological examination, and the symptoms vanished. She was discharged from hospital. "Once again, the symptoms had been played out right up to the end," wrote Pitié consultant Paul Chevallier. "Right up to the definitive procedure or to the overwhelming public demonstration, even for the patient herself, of the normal working of her organs. . . . Some reader of this journal will probably find her hospitalized somewhere in France at this very moment," he said.[101]

In 1934 Karl Menninger, a psychoanalyst and psychiatrist in Topeka, Kansas, recalled a patient who had thirteen operations in thirteen years. Engaged to a physician, just after the engagement she let him operate on her for "chronic appendicitis" (which often meant abdominal pain of a non-organic nature). "Less than a year later she had her tonsils removed. A few months later she developed an ectopic pregnancy." She then gave birth with ensuing perineal repair. Three months after delivery she had a breast abscess opened, then an infected toenail removed. There followed more repair of her perineum. "Four years later three impacted wisdom teeth which had caused her no trouble whatsoever were removed at the suggestion of the dentist. This was the first operation performed by anyone other than her husband. . . . The following year her tonsils were again removed." Then she had several ectopic pregnancies and abortions. "Finally, just before beginning her analysis, although she is a handsome, well-formed woman she insisted that her abdomen was too protruberant and had her husband remove the adipose panniculus [fat roll]." Menninger concluded she was suffering from penis envy.[102]

Whatever the actual cause of her distress, this patient represented a characteristic American phenomenon: addiction to surgery as a sequel of half a century of medically suggesting the population into the belief that vague, nonspecific physical symptoms were the consequence of reflex phenomena from peripheral organs. In 1953 Mandel Cohen and coworkers described a group of fifty Boston women who had undergone an average of 3.8 operations each by the time they reached an average age of thirty-seven (in contrast to a control group of healthy working women who by age thirty-seven had had 1.2 operations each). This article situated the addiction to surgery, which began in the 1880s, in the context of larger patterns of neurosis.[103]

A second variant of the demand for operations is different from the first only in that the psychological mechanism is more conscious in the patient's mind. It involves deliberately simulating medical or surgical illness in order to be admitted to hospital for an operation and is called "Munchausen's syndrome," after an anonymous pamphlet that appeared in 1785 in London, *The Adventures of Baron Munchausen*. In fact, the German Rudolf Erich Raspe, a former professor, then penniless in London, wrote the story, partly based on the adventures of the very real Hieronymus, count von Münchhausen, who in the service of the Russian army before 1760 achieved some fantastic feats as a soldier and sportsman.[104] "Munchausen's syndrome" became the term for patients who had fantastical stories and who faked illness in order to be operated on. New York surgeon Joseph Bryant (who once had operated on President Grover Cleveland's jaw) encountered a typical case of Munchausen's syndrome in 1892, although he did not call her that but rather a "laparotomy fiend of the highest order." Miss N. N., twenty-two, was admitted to Bellevue Hospital in February of that year, describing a history of "inflammation of the bowels," as she called it. Each of three previous attacks had resulted in an exploratory operation (laparotomy).

Now she again had lower-abdominal pain, chills, fever, vomiting of blood, and bloody stools. In the hospital they gave her an enema containing the tracer methyl violet, and twenty seconds or so after its administration she vomited up some methyl violet, suggesting a large fistula, or hole, somewhere in the gastrointestinal tract, in which the lower part of the bowel was somehow in contact with the stomach (X-rays had not yet been discovered). Yet they could find nothing. Puzzled, they closed her up to await developments. The abdominal incision then began to leak feces; shortly thereafter she started vomiting fecal matter as well, indicating various obstructions and ruptures in the gut. All the while, she developed symptoms of "great nervous excitement," was unable to open one eye, and cried violently. By now highly suspicious, her medical attendants stripped her, tied her in bed, and placed "a continuous watch over her." At this point she confessed to having sneaked some of the methyl violet "while it was in a dish placed on the stand by her bedside" so that she could be ready to spit it out and thus fake a fistula, just as she had procured her own feces in order to simulate a perforated colon. "There can be little doubt," wrote Doctor Bryant, "that those who were previously in charge of this patient were led to perform laparotomy upon her because of the presence of simulated obstruction or other phenomena which she then exhibited."[105]

The chickens had now come home to roost in the form of Munchausen's syndrome. Taught to see surgery as the answer to problematical physical sensations, patients had begun simulating symptoms that would be recognized as medically legitimate in order to receive access to the life-giving knife. Of course there was nothing intrinsically life-giving about the surgeon's knife, but half a century of emphasis on reflex disorders had made it seem so.

Sexual Surgery on Males

Were no operations done on men? Were only women singled out? Reflex theory called for the existence of "genital irritation" in both sexes, and while the pelvic organs of women were thought to be permanently irritated, masturbation and other conditions could nonetheless cause reflex neurosis in men too.

Castration of men was exactly comparable to oophorectomy, and while it was not done often, it was indeed carried out. For example, in January 1859 an American of forty-four, Eli B., was admitted to Westminster Hospital in London to be castrated for epilepsy. His fits had begun at the age of ten, soon after he started masturbating, and he had acquired gonorrhea in New York City at sixteen. Thus the preconditions for reflex epilepsy were present, thought staff surgeon Carsten Holthouse. Married at twenty-four, Eli B. plunged with his wife into sexual excess. His fits, during which he broke a number of limbs, became worse than ever. Applications of silver nitrate to the urethra did some good, but sexual intercourse seemed the true villain. Mr. B. finally came to Europe seeking relief. After asking, unsuccessfully, several surgeons to castrate him, he finally happened on Mr. Holthouse (in England surgeons were called "Mister"), who performed a double orchidectomy on January 4, removing his testes. Eli B.'s fits continued thereafter, although they were milder.[106] Richard Krömer, director of the Prussian asylum in Neustadt, was a well-known advocate of removing women's ovaries for mental illness. But he also came out in favor of castrating males, and in fact conducted several such operations in his asylum, although for medicolegal reasons he did not publicize them.[107] Richard Dewey, owner of a private clinic for nervous diseases in Wauwatosa, Wisconsin, said in 1907 that he had seen grave operations undertaken for hysterical pains—ovariotomy, appendicitis, and the like: "In men I have seen circumcision and castration under like circumstances."[108]

Why were as many castrations not done on men as ovariectomies on women? Male surgeons, though driven by reflex theory, probably shrank back psychically from mutilating patients of their own gender in a way they were perfectly willing to do to women. One must consider also the resistance of male patients, much more forceful than that of the females. As Archibald Church, a neurologist at Northwestern University in Evanston, Illinois, said in a discussion at a joint meeting of obstetricians and other specialists in 1904: "Men do not accept mutilating operations upon the genital tract with the equanimity which is presented by the gentler sex, who peaceably accept unsexing operations without much question as to their effect, provided they can be relieved of some trivial or temporary ailment."[109]

A second, less destructive class of sexual surgery in males involved freeing the prepuce, or foreskin, of the penis when it was adherent to the glans penis (head of the penis) below. This was done in children, for example, to cure reflex paralysis.[110] In 1870 the distinguished New York surgeon Lewis Albert Sayre, said to be the founder of orthopedic surgery in the United States, touched off a vogue of circumcising boys—removing the prepuce—for "reflex neurosis." He said, "I am quite satisfied ... that many cases of irritable children, with restless sleep, and bad digestion, which is often attributed to worms, is solely due to the irritation of the nervous system caused by an adherent or constricted prepuce."[111] There was, therefore, no shortage of surgical meddlesomeness with the male genitals.

It is an ironical footnote that one physician who assailed the male scrotum for hysteria and the like was later convicted in court for assaulting his female patients for the same conditions. Moritz Wiederhold, owner and chief physician of a private nervous clinic in Kassel-Wilhelmshöhe, in Germany, administered electric jolts in 1891 to the scrotums of male patients whose nervous problems were attributable to varicocele, a swelling of the venous plexus in the scrotum. He was convicted the following year for beating up his female patients.[112] Thus reflex theory had led Doctor Wiederhold to equitable treatments for both sexes.

Even though men did find themselves entangled in the net of the urologist as women were, in Allbutt's phrase, in the "net of the gynecologist," on balance the overwhelming number of surgical victims of reflex theory were female. It is a striking phenomenon that women in this period manifested these hysterical symptoms and sought out surgery for them. It cannot be unimportant that this behavior occurred at a time when women were constrained in their sexuality, their mobility, and their expression. The stress of their pent-up lives manifested itself in a physical paralysis or passivity, which doctors saw as irritation of their sexual organs. What else but their own sex could have caused it?

CHAPTER

5

Motor Hysteria

Of the various forms of somatization, symptoms attributable to the motor side of the nervous system underwent major changes during the nineteenth century. Hysteria is the old-fashioned term for somatization, and these classic forms of hysteria—paralysis of limbs, eyelids, vocal cords, and the like—made the nineteenth century the century of motor hysteria.[1] Some of these types, such as paralysis, probably increased in frequency. Others, which had been around for centuries, such as pseudo-epileptic fits, persisted throughout the nineteenth century without necessarily becoming still more frequent. Thus there are two questions: Why do these new forms of paralysis occur? And how may we understand the survival of traditional fits in a new era?

The rise of reflex theories may be a key, for the concept of the reflex arc encouraged the formation of motor symptoms. In the reflex arc, a sensory signal automatically gave rise to a motor response, without the intervention of mind or will. Attributing the paralyses of motor hysteria to an automatic consequence of the reflex arc—no question of shamming or it being "all in one's head"—proved irresistible to both patients and doctors. The reflex paradigm thus offered a perfectly legitimate "medical" explanation of symptoms that otherwise might have been hard to take seriously.

Yet these changes in symptoms ran through the lives of many individuals across Western society. It would be stretching the power of a medical paradigm to believe that transformations of such magnitude are caused merely by medical ideas alone. Given that hysterical paralysis affected mainly young women, larger cultural and social changes bearing on women's lives generally also played a role. If nineteenth-century culture prescribed what it meant to be an "ideal woman," perhaps it dictated as

95

well the physical symptoms that rebellion from this ideal might entail. Here "culture" enters patients' lives. The ultimate template on which symptoms are forged is what the culture prescribes as "legitimate" and "illegitimate" symptoms. The doctor is merely an agent of that larger culture.

Hysterical Fits

Fits remained the commonest form of motor hysteria throughout the nineteenth century. Of one hundred cases of hysteria seen around 1890 at the St.-André Hospital in Bordeaux, for example, forty-three were *attaques,* meaning episodes of sudden onset. Of these forty-three, thirty-four were proper fits (*attaques convulsives*), eight were attacks of "sleep," and there was one attack of *délire.*[2] These statistics highlight the predominance of the fit.

There were two main variations of hysterical fit: falling into a fainting trance called "catalepsy," and uncontrolled motor activity such as thrashing about, jerking, and trembling. Frederick Simpson, a doctor in Hartford, Connecticut, who had started practicing in the 1880s, remembered the first fit he had ever seen in his practice.

On a Sunday-school picnic a young lady was noticed by her friends to act queerly. She stopped talking, became absent-minded, stared about her in a dazed way, began to walk off in an automatic fashion, turning now this way and now that. . . . We led her on board the steamboat and got her to lie down in a berth in a stateroom. She was only half conscious of her environment. She soon began to get rigid and her face flushed. Then she commenced to go through various irregular movements of the body. She thrashed with her arms and kicked with her legs, threw her head from side to side, arched up her back and rolled about with such force that several of us had to hold her to keep her in the berth.

She had these paroxysms for two or three hours before recovering consciousness, and the next day said she could remember nothing.[3] Was she having an epileptic fit? Probably not, although one cannot be sure in the absence of an electroencephalogram performed during the attack. This kind of purposive, highly coordinated straining against restraint is unusual in epilepsy, which results from the spontaneous, uncoordinated discharge of electrical activity in the brain. She was probably having a hysterical fit.[4]

The purposive quality in a convulsion qualifies it as hysterical as opposed to epileptic. Pierre-Adolphe Piorry, professor of medicine at the Pitié Hospital in Paris, described in 1850 pelvic movements in hysteric fits almost as a kind of orgasm: "There is a close analogy between these pathological movements and those which a woman makes during a venereal orgasm or while giving birth." Further:

Very commonly during fits a woman will grasp her throat with her hands as if to tear it open in order to remove a foreign body strangling her. . . . The hysteric woman strikes out at the things around her and even at the back of her bed, in which she seems to be bouncing up and down. . . . You might see a slender young woman, her limbs rigid, holding her own against a number of strong men trying to pin her down. She sobs, cries out, screams, cuts off her words, rages angrily about things that have vexed her or about the man she loves.[5]

This quality of volition and deliberateness accordingly characterizes the hysterical convulsion. As Joseph Amann wrote in 1868 about such fits, "If the patient's hands are left free, they beat mightily upon the breast, the face or grasp at the throat, as if they wanted to free up a constriction there. The patients try to tear out their hair, to tear their clothing to shreds, and try to bite and strike out at bystanders." They may pause, exhausted, then resume. Sometimes laughing and crying are combined with these fits.[6]

These fits corresponded to some kind of model in the patient's unconscious mind of "genuine" physical symptoms caused by demonic possession or by ungovernable reflexes.[7] The inventive unconscious mind can therefore devise an enormous range of behavior to match the presumed causes. Yet there are certain consistent central features. Psychiatrist Pierre Briquet accumulated data on around 450 patients with a diagnosis of hysteria at the Pitié Hospital in Paris over the period 1849–59. His findings on these patients represent the single largest pool of information on hysterical conversion disorders in the nineteenth century. Of these 400-odd female patients, roughly two-thirds suffered from fits of gradual onset. Briquet described the typical course as follows: onset marked by paleness, leading to loss of appetite and loss of weight; a host of pain symptoms ensue, headaches and epigastric pain in particular. At this point two routes may be taken. The epigastric pain may lead to pain in the left side, the spine, and the abdomen, causing a sense of strangulation, spasms, and fits. Or the various pains may lead to mood changes, which then give rise to strangulation and so forth. Briquet gave an example: A girl of eleven sees a dog, which she believes to be rabid rushing at her. Her limbs begin to tremble and she feels a sense of oppression and stomach pain, which last for about three months:

> At the end of this time a violent, constant headache commences, epigastric pain, pain in the back and the left side, shortness of breath, palpitations, a feeling of continual strangulation. She vomits violently all that she eats, then experiences attacks of lethargy which last twenty-four hours, leaving in their wake an extreme feeling of debilitation and a loss of muscular force to the point that she must remain in bed. These symptoms persist unabated for three years.[8]

As for the precipitating symptoms: Of 142 patients whose attacks began with a fit, 25 percent had had a sudden fright, 16 percent some kind of emotional shock, 12 percent had been the victims of physical abuse on the part of husband or parents, 12 percent had been subjected to "des passions tristes, fort vives et du peu de durée" (sudden feelings of sadness), and 5 percent began convulsing after seeing other persons struck with hysteria or epilepsy.[9]

Because these fits virtually vanish in the twentieth century, it is important to try to gain some kind of psychological fix on them in the nineteenth. Were the patients able to control their behavior at all? Had the unconscious mind seized the reins entirely? At what point does the presumably unconscious mechanism spill over into simulation?

Many of these fits did have a manipulative element, or feature of secondary gain, which does not necessarily mean they were factitious, merely that they served some purpose in the patient's life. Jean-Baptiste Louyer-Villermay related the following case from the Napoleonic years: A young and highly impressionable girl of middle-class origin fell in love at fifteen, without wanting to admit it to herself. She kept her passion secret, "with truly heroic courage, for she had the firm resolution of avowing it neither to the object of her love nor to her parents, for fear of injuring those most dear to her." She then received a blow on the head, which led to a violent headache and a general malaise:

> Thereupon, at the sight of her loved one, she fainted, uttering plaintive cries and sobbing involuntarily as she drifted in and out of somnolence. As she slipped into total unconsciousness, uncoordinated contractions of her upper limbs began, a convulsive twitching of her chest, violent palpitations and spasmodic contractions at the throat, with a feeling of strangulation and "globe hystérique [lump in the throat]," also a tetanic contraction of her lower jaw and occasional convulsions of its muscles.

Dr. Louyer-Villermay feared at first she might bite her tongue off but then recognizing the hysterical component, asked her parents if she were in love. No, came the answer.

Upon awakening, she decided to avow her love to her parents and to the young man himself. "Political events delayed the declaration and prolonged the convalescence but finally the consent of her parents and the natural course of events [*le voeu de la nature rempli*] returned her to perfect health, providing her with the occasion of furnishing society with a model of all the social virtues."[10] What could more soften the hearts of hard parents than fits in a fifteen-year-old daughter (fits that "lent her countenance a soft melancholy")?

But even when secondary gain is not evident, certain kinds of behavior are so "overlearned,"or deeply ingrained, that they might surface in the most profound hysteric fit to govern the patient's actions. Thus Thomas Emmett, a New York gynecologist, attempted to revive patients from their hysterical trances by giving them enemas, hoping that efforts to cope with not soiling the bed would suffice to waken them:

> I was present on an occasion in my private hospital where a young lady had been lying in apparently an unconscious state, after a hysterical convulsion, and had taken no notice of my presence, although I felt satisfied that she was aware of it. The nurse had just introduced the rectal tube as I entered the room, and the patient began an attack shortly afterwards for my benefit. She suddenly threw herself into a position of opisthotonos, but before head and feet could be brought under her, a loud escape of flatus took place from the tube, and continued with a steady but lowering note for several seconds, as she gradually straightened herself out, and the colon became empty. I was in a position to see her as she opened her eyes, and the appearance of astonishment and mortification depicted on her face, as the flatus continued to escape, was intense. I quietly asked if she had lost all the delicacy of her sex, in making such an exhibition before me, when she burst into tears and covered her face.

She never again repeated an attack of hysteria.[11]

Moritz Benedikt in Vienna, in his enormous private neurological practice, was quite adept at playing on patients' fears as they lay apparently unconscious. (One remembers that the unconscious wants to be taken seriously and not be made a fool of.) A young woman, the daughter of a professor at a provincial Austrian university, was brought to Vienna in the company of her mother, suffering from terrible "exhalational screaming" *(Ausatmungsschreikrämpfe)*, in which she had to be implored to

99

inhale or she would suffocate to death. There were terrible scenes, in which Benedikt and a colleague kept a twenty-four-hour watch over her. Finally one evening as Benedikt was about to depart at the end of his watch, the mother broke down in despair.

Benedikt said scornfully, "'The ladies should calm themselves, the comedy [die Komödie] will soon be over'. . . . The word 'comedy' struck the ladies like a bite of a viper. I pretended not to observe its effect. The next morning I was coolly received."

He then explained to the irked mother why he had used the expression "comedy": "It's not a tragedy because she's going to get better."

After Benedikt had left the next night, the daughter asked the mother if perhaps the moment the professor indicated had finally arrived. Indeed it had. The following morning the two ladies went to the art gallery in the Belvedere Palace and then returned home.

Benedikt, who had rather a low opinion of his female patients, was full of such stories. But so was Mrs. Benedikt. As Mrs. Benedikt and her daughter were visiting the church of Saint Anthony in Padua, the custodian was clearing the parishioners out. "Suspecting that something unusual was happening, the two ladies remained behind. A peasant woman having terrible fits of convulsive screaming appeared." The screaming lasted for an hour and a half. As the exhausted priest unsuccessfully summoned a second priest to come and relieve him, Mrs. Benedikt said to the custodian that, since nobody was available, "Why don't you suggest to the priest he tell her that St. Anthony will punish her if she doesn't shut up at once." The priest did so and the woman fell silent.

The priest asked the custodian who had offered the good advice. "A stranger," said the custodian.

"It was not for nothing that my wife was married to a neurologist," said Benedikt. "She was hard as nails on hysterics, often unfairly. She once said to me, 'You'll never learn. These hysterics will always lead you around by the nose.' She also gritted her teeth against the most intense pain, in order not to be considered 'hysterical.'"[12] Mrs. Benedikt represented a quite unsympathetic assessment of patients with hysterical fits, considering them simulators.

Yet patients had a range of degrees of insight into their symptoms, just as we noted a range in patients' motives for seeking operations, from a genuine conviction of illness to Munchausen's syndrome. Psychiatrist Robert Wollenberg remembered seeing during World War I a letter that a rifleman in Upper Silesia had sent to a patient in Wollenberg's field hospital in Strasbourg about how to simulate hysteria. "I already wrote you in Hirschberg about what you have to do to get into a military hospital," the letter said, "so you know the routine. You have to throw yourself to the ground, clench your teeth together and roll your eyeballs far back in your head. At the same time you have to roll around on the ground holding your arms and legs stiff. At most they'll try to look into your eyes, but keep the eyes steadily upwards and don't move them. If you do that every day once or twice, you'll get into the hospital. . . . Another thing, you do your duties and then while on duty work it out so that your hands and feet shake. Understood?"[13]

Two supplementary points might be made about hysterical fits.

Although I am aware of no important class difference in their occurrence at the beginning of our period, by the time they went away in the 1920s and 1930s, fits had become very much a working-class phenomenon. The late eighteenth century saw reports of hysteric convulsions from all social classes. Said Henry Manning of the "hysteric passion" among London society people in 1771, "This disease chiefly seizes women who are delicate and endowed with great sensibility. The unmarried and widows are more subject to it than those who have husbands, in so much that many have been relieved from it by entering into conjugal life."[14]

Thus an example of upper-class fits. But around the same time Adrian Wegelin, a physician in Saint Gallen in Switzerland, described the following case: In February 1785 a peasant woman, twenty-three, consulted him for perimenstrual complaints. She was pale and thin with "extremely irritable nerves," and was also constipated because she ate so little. She had a history of having fits in church and other public places. Wegelin suspected masturbation to be the cause, but she would confess nothing. Several days later in a repeat visit she fell into a fit in his office, "her body making curious movements; uncontrollable laughter interchanged with loud crying and shaking of hands and feet. . . . During the fits I noted the patient looking rapturous [*ein besonders verliebtes Wesen*] and pressing her hands together with great emotion." Now she confessed to masturbating in a group with the other village girls. After a long illness, she went on to recovery.[15] The worlds of Saint Gallen and Saint James's could not have been more dissimilar, yet the fits resembled each other. Reports from both kinds of settings are common.

By the years between the two world wars hysterical fits had become basically a working-class phenomenon. In 1925 the neurological department of a public insurance hospital in Breslau was still seeing quite a bit of convulsive hysteria. "It is unsurprising," wrote medical supervisor Felix Preissner, "that almost daily the entire gamut from innocuous feelings of dizziness to extreme agitation or epileptiform convulsions and twilight states comes in. . . . Almost the daily bread of the division are 'hysterical attacks' that usually unfold in the following manner: during rounds, at lunch or at evening prayers a patient will sink, with or without previous commotion, to the floor and begin to moan and groan, the limbs trembling. . . . The eyes are closed tightly or the eyeballs screwed up wards."[16] These were mainly working-class patients. As late as 1936 classic fits were still the commonest single symptom in the neurology division of Vienna's large General Hospital. Between the years 1925–35, of the 2,400 male patients with hysteria of various kinds, 13 percent had epileptiform symptoms; of the 1,500 female patients, 36 percent.[17] These patients, again, came largely from the working class.

As for fits among the middle and upper classes, few were reported in these years. Israel Wechsler, who graduated in medicine in 1907 and by the 1920s had a middle-class neurological practice in Manhattan, had seen only two in his whole professional life.[18] Among the hundreds of nervous patients who passed through Frederick Parkes Weber's Harley Street practice between the 1890s and World War I, not a single patient's chief complaint was hysterical convulsions.[19] Hysterical fits had passed in the course of a hundred years from being a generalized expression of psychic unease to a highly class-specific one.

The Rise of Hysterical Paralysis

Previous chapters contained many references to young women who were "paralyzed" and cured of their paralysis by various procedures such as Battey's operation. In contrast to fits, which are an age-old kind of psychosomatic symptom, paralysis was uncommon before 1800, increasing greatly thereafter. In 1883, at age 35, Margaret Cleaves, an American psychiatrist who had been a staff physician at an asylum in Mount Pleasant, Iowa, came to New York. There she established an electrotherapy clinic and served as president of the Women's Medical Society. Sometime after her arrival in New York, she took a trip to Europe, where she herself developed hysterical paralysis:

My physician had warned me, that if I did not stop work, he could not answer for the integrity of my intellectual centers. . . . Before the steamer was out of New York harbor, the inevitable had occurred. It seems to me that every neuron was for the time *hors de combat*. As for courage, willpower, motor ability, all that makes us capable sentient beings, I was temporarily at least without them. I literally grovelled in my mind. I could not eat, never could very much for that matter, could barely dress and undress myself, and had no right to do that even. My head hurt, and my mental anguish was great. No one about me understood what I was suffering, in fact the suffering of the true neurasthene is but little appreciated at any time, not always by the attending physician even. The exhaustion implicated my left cerebral center, as is usually the case. My right leg and arm had no reserve of strength, and a few moments' effort was enough to bring about a condition of motor inability. The sensation in my right leg from above the knee was as though my stocking were constantly slipping down and a few moments' effort aggravated the condition to such an extent that I was confident I should never walk again.

She did, however, land in Europe and commence her itinerary. At Fontainebleau, near Paris, trouble struck again. "I undertook the visit without a thought of disaster, the only thing concerning me was the good-for-nothingness of my right leg." Inside the château she felt a sensation of horror as though the walls were closing in on her:

The impending helplessness of my right leg was so great that I turned to the door and fled incontinently to the grounds of the château. Never shall I forget how wearily I crept down the massive and beautiful Escalier du Fer à-Cheval and how heartbroken I felt. It seemed to me that there was nothing to be gained by trying any longer to keep up the weary struggle for existence.

On the voyage back things became still worse. "So profound was the exhaustion of my left motor centers that the loss of strength and the feeling of being paralyzed, extended throughout the entire right side of my body, invading the left after a day of tempestuous seas." Further on she noted, "I had lost my toes again."[20]

Margaret Cleaves's account of her own illness illustrates several aspects of somatization: the patient's heartfelt conviction of organic disease, the involvement of other kinds of psychological distress such as depression, panic attacks, and chronic fatigue, and a background of personal dislocation against which the symptoms are projected. Doctor Cleaves was not typical of her time in attributing her symptoms to a specific cause—the exhaustion of her "motor centers"—but in the symptoms themselves, she was a daughter of the nineteenth century.

Doctors' accounts permit us to map the rise of a virtual pandemic of these hysterical paralyses.[21] The pandemic began at some point late in the eighteenth or early in the nineteenth century and came to an end in the years between the two world wars. When exactly paralysis shifted from being an isolated item in the symptom pool to a pandemic is difficult to say, given the dispersed nature of the sources. But the impression is that the last quarter of the eighteenth century was the turning point, and that the upturn took place first of all in France. In 1770 Jean-Baptiste Chevalier, the local surgeon at the Bourbonne-les-Bains spa in the Champagne region, reported an almost epidemic outbreak of paralyses and fits, which prompted young women to come and take the waters. In 1764, for example, Madamoiselle de Serrière, seventeen, of Sarre-Louis, had become paralyzed and anesthetic in her lower limbs after fainting from a bloodletting. "Her paralysis was so extreme that she felt nothing from a needle plunged deeply into her legs and thighs." Two days after her arrival she developed screaming fits so powerful that it took four men to hold her down. The paralysis thereupon reappeared. She was cured by taking the waters. Chevalier reported numerous other young women, paralyzed in half their bodies (hemiplegia) or in their lower limbs (paraplegia), all cured by the waters.[22]

From the spas of Europe came a steady stream of cured paralyses in the years ahead. "How often," wrote Louis Verhaeghe in 1850, "do we see patients with paralyzed arms, legs, the side of the face or even a more limited area such as one or two fingers, problems attributable to an unequal distribution of nervous fluid." Organic paralyses, perhaps? "It is individuals of a pronounced nervous temperament, subject to hysterical fits, *somnambules* [people who believe themselves to be in a psychological "second state"], persons subject to shameful habits [masturbation] or who abuse the pleasures of love, who are most likely to experience these paralyses." He cited a young countess who suffered first a hysterical aphonia, then a paraplegia "of such a nature that she was unable to walk without crutches and even then had much difficulty. Sent to Ostende, she was able to take sea baths for two months and had, soon after returning home, the good fortune of recovering her voice and then the use of her limbs. Now married, she has experienced no recurrence "[23]

Similar to hydrotherapy as one of the placebo forms of physical therapy was electrotherapy (except that it "recharged" rather than "soothed"). From electrotherapy as well came a flutter of reports in the last quarter of the eighteenth century of cured "paralyses." Between 1749 and 1799, there were twenty-three publications in France and elsewhere on the use of electricity in what were evidently hysterical paralyses (electrotherapy would not have cured organic paralyses). Seventy percent of them were published after 1780.[24]

By 1838 hysterical paralysis had become frequent enough in the daily practice of medicine that Charles Despine, a spa doctor in Aix-les-Bains, described a young female patient who was "scarcely able to get a foot on the ground or take a step without feeling sick or falling into a faint." He continued, "The tendency to collapse *[défaillance]* in rising from the horizontal position, also a weakness of the lower limbs, and a kind of demiparalysis of the limbs affecting both sensory and motor functions, are phenomena we frequently encounter in young women disposed to hysteria and who are sanguine [of temperament] and nervous."[25]

In the mid-1830s hysterical paralysis began to drift from the hypnotists, hydrotherapists, and electrotherapists who had previously treated it to the attention of the professors of medicine. Pierre-Adolphe Piorry, professor of medicine in Paris, started collecting observations "around 1835 or 1836," as he later recalled, on these cases, and in 1844 Maurice Macario published an article based on Piorry's cases. Macario, who rejected Piorry's own rather organic views, saw hysterical paralysis as a reflex phenomenon, coming perhaps from a loss of "nervous fluid" in the uterus. A typical case was Virginie Joannot, fifteen, who one evening in her home village thought she had seen a young man dressed in a shroud appear before her. Terrified, she began convulsing and for forty-eight hours cried out, "He's coming for me, he wants to get me." She continued to have intermittent fits, even after moving to Paris a year later and getting a job in the garment industry. Now seventeen, her left side had recently become paralyzed so that she could walk only with crutches; she also experienced episodes of aphonia, which were cured by bleeding at the neck and by steam baths. Piorry's service admitted a number of similar cases, all young women with paralyzed limbs, most of whom were cured by the placebo therapies of the day. Macario himself, following the logic of the symptoms, later became director of a water-cure clinic at Serin near Lyon.[26] His article in 1844 is generally acknowledged as having introduced hysterical paralysis into medical discussion in France. Thereafter reports multiplied.

In England as well, reports of paralyzed young women began to accelerate toward the end of the eighteenth century. John Abernethy, a renowned London surgeon who attributed nervous symptoms to the stomach, said in 1809 that over the years "a paralytic affection of the lower extremities," resembling spinal TB but without lesions, had caught his attention. Sometime before the 1790s he had seen "a young lady with weakness of the lower extremities and pain in the loins." "This lady could scarcely walk." Abernethy thought she must have vertebral disease (which she apparently did not). He blistered her back on each side of the spine "and kept up a discharge from the surface." She recovered, relapsed again, recovered after the same treatment, and stayed well for the next seventeen years.[27] The case sounds like a psychogenic paralysis.

In Edinburgh, John Abercrombie found the cases about which his late friend Doctor Monteith used to tell him something of a medical marvel. Dr. Abercrombie had never encountered such stories before: young women without apparent lesions who developed the most remarkable symptoms, for example, a young lady of seventeen, whose complaints began as a violent headache that confined her to bed in exhaustion. "Soon after, she first complained of pain in the spine, and this was speedily followed by a sudden attack of most excruciating pain in both lower extremities, extending over every part of them, and accompanied by such increased sensibility that she could not bear the weight of the bedclothes upon them, and the slightest touch with the finger made her scream." Nor could she bear to extend her arm long enough to have her pulse felt. Then her lower limbs began to "draw up" under her, so that her knees were folded tight to her body. "She now became much emaciated, pale and debilitated." Abercrombie continued: "Dr. Monteith said, she was not moved in bed six inches [because of all the pain]. At the end of four years, this lady began to improve and to get out of bed a little daily; but at this time her legs were so much bent upon the thighs, and the knees so rigid, that no force could bring them to a right angle." (She had, at last, acquired an organic condition: flexion contractures from disuse.) Doctor Abercrombie visited her once. "I certainly never saw a case which gave me more the impression of deep-seated and hopeless disease."

There was much more from Doctor Monteith's practice: ". . . particularly [patients with] long-continued and uncontrollable vomiting, fits resembling epilepsy and catalepsy." "There was in general a remarkable aversion to light, and one of his patients lay in a state of almost total darkness for more than a year." One patient with uncontrollable vomiting also went blind off and on several times."[28] Doctor Monteith was clearly a magnet for somatizing patients.

Of course, any of these patients might have had an organic illness as the cause of her symptoms. The doctors of the day were unable reliably to disentangle the somatogenic from the psychogenic, to say nothing of historians with their retrospective diagnoses being able to do so in individual cases.[29] Yet it is the pattern that counts. The massive occurrence of paralyses in a population of otherwise healthy young women suggests that most of these paralyses were psychogenic, or hysterical, in nature. Two criteria are applicable in trying to determine if given cases were psychogenic or neurogenic: (1) response to placebo therapy (though of course there may be spontaneous recoveries from diseases such as multiple sclerosis); (2) the presence of a combination of symptoms unlikely to be explained by an anatomical lesion, such as sudden blindness in a patient with paraplegia.[30] These two characteristics formed a pattern that became increasingly common during the nineteenth century.

In England and France early in the century, many cases of spinal inflammation and spinal irritation, whose supposed causes we saw physicians devising, turned out to have paralysis. Here is a case from some time before 1824, which Edward Sutleffe, a London surgeon, diagnosed as spinal inflammation: "Miss Sarah P. of Brixton was brought by her anxious parents for my inspection. The only complaint made by the parties was an incapacity for walking. The knees were accordingly examined, it being supposed that the seat of weakness was there; but instantly recognizing the law of sympathy, I replied that the disease was in the spine." He leeched and bled her spine "till she could jump and hop about the room." Three years later, "the young lady bids fair to rival in elegance of form and activity the most admired of her sex."[31]

Many of these early paralyses seemed to represent a bridge from fits, for the patients began with convulsions, presumably the conventional item in the symptom pool, and then progressed to paralysis, a relative novelty. In 1860 Arnold von Franque, a spa doctor in Bad Kochel, described a thirty-four-year-old woman who had had a long nervous history ever since an attack of chlorosis (a term for iron-deficiency anemia) at fourteen. She started having fits with the onset of menarche at fifteen. The fits had since recurred regularly at every period. In the summer of 1856, when she was thirty, constipation began. By November, it had worsened to the point that she had not moved her bowels in three weeks. When a bowel movement finally eventuated, it occurred with terrible pains, more fits, and fainting. As she awakened she noted that she was paralyzed and anesthetic on her left side. Hydrotherapy at Dr. von Franque's spa abolished all her symptoms by August of the following year.[32]

Contemporary writers noted that fits often segued smoothly into paralysis. After an account in 1842 of fits seen in patients at the Pitié Hospital, surgeon Jacques Lisfranc said: "Violent and extended fits [crises] may be followed by attacks of mania for several months; one also sees paraplegias ensue which may last for several years, persistent spasmodic retractions [of joints], chorea, and paralyses of one or more of the special senses [vision, hearing, and so on]."[33] For Hector Landouzy, fits and paralyses might alternate. Almost invariably as a prodrome of a fit there would be, "shaking limbs, a feeling of coldness or heaviness, an unusual weakness, the persistence of acute pain." Anticipating Charcot's doctrine of hysteria in which fit-like attacks could temporarily suspend the permanent "stigmata," Landouzy said fits could even abolish paralyses.[34] So much did fits represent the essence of hysteria that some authorities felt compelled to point out that paralyses counted as hysteria even in the absence of fits.[35]

When paralyses finally replaced fits among middle-class people, the question arose of what had happened to these once-spectacular outbursts. In 1895, Robert Edes blamed "the more modern habit or manner of repression, of keeping the feelings concealed, a habit which increases with civilization and fashion, with higher social position, and is especially strongly marked in our Anglo-Saxon race." This habit of repression, said Edes, "has . . . a good deal to do with the diminished prevalence of the more outspoken and striking forms [of hysteria], and the substitution therefore of the quiet, insidious, obstinate paralyses which are so closely counterfeit organic disease, and are in reality so much more serious than a good old-fashioned hysteric 'fit' which comes on slight provocation and is soon over."[36] Some of these psychological issues will be examined again later. What is of interest here is seeing one symptom piggyback on another and then replace it entirely.

A Picture of Paralysis

Characteristic of the pandemic were several kinds of deficits involving the voluntary muscles, especially those of the lower limbs. There are really four kinds, two of them involving paralysis or paresis in which the muscles worked too well, resulting in a spastic contracture, or worked not at all, causing a flaccid paralysis. Third comes joint pain, which is not really in the category of paralysis yet is equally disabling. Finally there is astasia-abasia, meaning the inability to maintain oneself upright (astasia) and walk (abasia).

Not only were paralyses of the lower limbs symbolically powerful—the young woman who cannot walk and is trapped passively in bed—they were also quite frequent. "Of all the manifestations of hysteria," said two Parisian staff physicians in 1876, "paralysis is one of the commonest."[37]

What exactly was paralyzed? In the absence of a central register, a few broad traits emerge from the chance observations about commonality. Among the limbs, hemiplegias were commoner than paraplegias.[38] And among the hemiplegias, the leg was more commonly affected than the arm.[39] As for the issue of two limbs or one, monoplegia versus hemi- or paraplegia, authorities were quite divided.[40] But perhaps the disagreement had to do with the nature of their samples, the country in which they lived and the years in which they made their observations. What matters is that all these phenomena were common and increased in frequency in the course of the nineteenth century. There were also endless clinical subtypes, involving such issues as the presence of cutaneous anesthesia or "ovarian" pain. None of these conditions could be said to represent an independent disease entity, and all corresponded to varying concepts of the unconscious mind as to what represents "legitimate" organic paralysis.

The issue, however, of spastic contracture versus flaccid paralysis is an interesting one, for it represents two alternative concepts of paralysis present in the symptom pool. In the spastic version of paralysis—doubtless based on centuries of folklore about demonic possession—muscles were supposed to move uncontrollably in devilish displays of supernatural power. Small-town patients in Kentucky at the beginning of the twentieth century had a definite conception of a limb "drawing up" all on its own. Margaret M. of Louisville was thirteen when her left leg first "drew up," the thigh flexing itself on the abdomen, the knee bent. Doctor Vance extended the limb under an anesthetic and put a plaster cast on it to hold it straight. "This was done simply as a matter of suggestion." Three days later when he went to remove the cast, the girl cried out: "It is going to draw up; it is going to draw up."[41] In small-town Georgia, people referred to such contractures as a "drawing spell," often preceded by globus hystericus.[42] Thus these patients had some notion of limbs that contracted on their own, a perfectly natural event as far as they were concerned.

Flaccid paralysis, the opposite of spastic, seems to have had as a folkloric template reaching far back in time the phenomenon of catalepsy. Catalepsy involves a trancelike, indeed deathlike, state, with or without changes in mental functioning. Many patients had their paralysis just "come over them," in the same manner in which catalepsy once struck. Representative of these victims of flaccid paralysis for whom everything suddenly went blank was Matilda B., a patient of London physician William Gull's (he was among the first to describe anorexia nervosa). She was seventeen when admitted to Guy's Hospital in January 1862:

Twelve months before admission the patient suddenly became insensible while lying awake in bed, about nine o'clock at night, and was found in this condition by her mother. The absolute unconsciousness lasted about two hours, and during that time the mother supposed her dead. On returning to consciousness, she found she could not move her arms or legs, and had lost sensation over her whole body up to the neck.[43]

Here the pattern for the attack seems to have been the patient's notion of a trance: In a trance one is as though dead and even later can move nothing. Both concepts, then, of demonic "drawing up" and trancelike conditions, had long been available to Western culture and helped model the new epidemic of paralysis.

Two other forms of paralysis, not related to muscle activity, deserve mention. One is inability to walk because of joint pain: The muscles and joints are not paralyzed but it simply hurts too much to walk. Arthritis would be a perfectly legitimate reason for such a complaint, but these pains occurred in young women, not greatly at risk for arthritis (the incidence of rheumatoid arthritis is low in women under thirty-five[44]), and they seem to have spread as part of the larger epidemic of paralysis. In a discussion of hysteria, English psychiatrist John Conolly said in 1833: "Pains of the limbs are not unusual, and they are now and then united with an impairment of the motions of the hip or the knee. . . . In very young but precocious females we have seen the curious complaints combined with strange affections of the sight and of the voice." He recalled a case some years previously from the Edinburgh infirmary: "The subject of it was a girl of thirteen, and the lameness and partial blindness, and an appearance of fatuity, all disappeared under a steady application of Dr. [James] Hamilton's purgative treatment."[45] But it was usually the surgeons rather than the psychiatrists who saw such patients, and weighed whether to amputate the limb. Thus the influential London surgeon Benjamin Travers commented in 1835 on the difficulty of treating "pain which affects the joints in those slow and obscure changes to which young females are especially liable. . . . Such cases go on for years, and the patients are cured by perseverance in bandaging or a residence at the sea coast, or in some cases of humble life, it is to be feared, by a sacrifice of the limb at their own earnest request, to enable them to procure the means of subsistence."[46]

Benjamin Brodie, at St. George's, had had extensive experience with "hysterical" joint affections of young ladies, which he saw almost daily in his large consulting practice. "I do not hesitate to declare," he wrote in 1837, "that among the higher classes of society at least four fifths of the female patients, who are commonly supposed to labour under diseases of the joints, labour under hysteria and nothing else." Brodie described the physical exam. "The patient winces and sometimes screams when you make pressure on the hip; but she does the same if you make pressure on the ilium [the crest of the hipbone] or on the side as high as the false ribs, or on the thigh, or even on the leg as low as the ankle."

Brodie believed the pains were not organic because the patients could be distracted from them by conversation (some physicians used conversation in French to distract), while the physical examination went on unremarked. Nor was there any muscle wasting.

These pains nonetheless confined Brodie's young patients to the couch. The symptoms of a young woman he had seen in 1834 continued "nearly unaltered for almost two years, when one night, on turning herself in bed, she said that she had a feeling as if something had given way in her hip, and from that moment she was quite well."[47] Such early cases initiated a torrent of description that continued in Britain and on the Continent for the rest of the century.

Another disabling affliction was the inability to stand up and walk, astasia-abasia. Here there was no paralysis, and the legs functioned perfectly when the patients were examined in bed. But as soon as the patients were up they fell over or collapsed after a few steps. Early descriptions originated from physicians at the Paris teaching hospitals, who saw many other forms of gait disorders as well. Ernest Mesnet, a student of Pierre Briquet's in 1852 at the Charité, said: "Sometimes they are obliged to remain in bed because their legs collapse as soon as they are upright."[48] In 1864 Sigismond Jaccoud, a staff physician at the Pitié Hospital, baptized the condition "ataxia from a lack of automatic coordination," but the term did not catch on (although one later writer suggested calling it "Jaccoud's syndrome").[49] Numerous cases of astasia-abasia appeared at the Salpêtrière hospice under Charcot's regime during the 1880s. A student of Charcot's, Paul Blocq, proposed calling it astasia-abasia in 1888.[50] Thus in that year it stood freshly hewn as an independent disease entity.

But old hands at nervous disease, far away from the hothouse environment of Paris teaching hospitals, realized that the inability to stand upright and walk was just another form of hysteria. Silas Weir Mitchell in Philadelphia, who knew it as "hysterical motor ataxia," said: "The disorder . . . adds many recruits to that large class which some one has called 'bed cases,' and which are above all things distinguished by their desire to remain at rest."[51]

Astasia-abasia is the boundary line between gait disorders as such and chronic invalidism, which might keep individuals bedridden for decades. In 1919 a Stockholm telephone operator of twenty-five fell ill in the great influenza pandemic. She also became engaged that year:

Her fiancé wished to marry, but she opposed this as she was compelled support her mother. Engagement [was] broken off, after which the patient made an attempt to commit suicide in 1928. During the ensuing period in hospital astasia-abasia developed, and the symptoms have persisted ever since. Was treated in 1932 in Serafimer Hospital [in Stockholm] under the diagnosis of hysteria. The patient has lived alone for the last twenty-five years, and for periods of many years she has not been away from her home. Visited, but only very occasionally by a distant relative. During the follow-up investigation on April 14, 1953, she tottered about the room supporting herself with sticks. Noisy, dramatic, theatrical and given to self-pity. Extremely thin and has convulsions in arms and legs, especially when observed. . . . Somatically normal, neurological state normal, but with lively reflexes.[52]

It is evident that hysterical paralysis could take on several different forms. Yet all had a "final common pathway"—the inability to walk normally. How might such a symptom arise?

Triggering Paralysis

Of the many different life situations that could set off a hysterical paralysis, three in particular stand out: a personal shock, a traumatic injury, and adoption of the symptom as a kind of mannerism.

"Paralysis from horror," or *Schrecklähmung,* was familiar enough to establish itself in German as a separate diagnostic term. Semi Meyer, who directed a private clinic near Danzig, said in 1911: "The typical picture of monosymptomatic hysteria is, in my opinion, *Schrecklähmung.* . . . Anyone can become speechless from fright, and also become crippled. . . . It is for me the purest form of hysteria."[53]

The shocks ranged from the bothersome to the perfectly horrible. Four days after Christmas in 1904, Helene T., a sixteen-year-old servant in a Berlin household, was startled by the noise of an attempted break-in. She tripped on the stairs, slid forward, then walked trembling to her room. For the next several days she was fine. Then, on New Year's Eve, she drank a glass of punch and suffered a colossal frontal headache. On New Year's morning her limbs were so weak that she could not even get dressed. Two days later she was admitted to the Charité Hospital with flaccid paralysis of all four limbs.[54]

Paralysis might also supervene on receipt of bad news. In April 1850, Maria Fischer, a servant aged twenty-two, was admitted to the Holy Ghost Hospital in Frankfurt am Main for a limping gait and agonizing leg pains. Her story? Four months previously she had received news that her brother, her only living relative, had died in a railway accident. At

112

the time her knees became weak, but she found it impossible to cry. Then she had a small fit and missed a period. In the coming days, insomnia, anorexia, a shaky gait, and various pains appeared. After the funeral all symptoms vanished except the weakness in her legs, especially the right one. Her period had still not returned, however. As the weeks passed, pain began in her right ankle, spreading to her left leg. The right leg became stiffer; chorea seized her arms. By the time of her admission to hospital the patient was unable to rise from bed, even though she could move her legs in bed. By September 1850 her period was still lacking, but her symptoms had nonetheless improved to the point where she could be discharged. "No great debate is required," said Theodor Clemens, a staff physician at the hospital, "to designate the case as a reflex neurosis caused by genital irritation."[55]

Disturbing encounters could trigger paralysis. In March 1892 a seventeen-year-old woman named Jeanne L. was admitted to the Lariboisière Hospital in Paris with a diagnosis of astasia-abasia. Almost the entire family was said to be "nervous," and indeed the patient herself, in boarding school from age ten, was thought to be a troublemaker. At fifteen and a half, a failed apprenticeship in the garment trades behind her, she went to live with her grandmother in Lyon. There, while riding on a bus, she sat in front of a drunk who made threatening gestures with a knife. "She became frightened, tried to get off the bus, and fell into a faint," remaining unconscious for two hours. In the coming days she had a series of fainting fits ("crises"), and after one such fit awoke incapable of walking. Sent to Vichy, where she went into a kind of cataleptic sleep, she was awakened for only a few hours every four days or so to be fed through a tube. From Vichy she was transported to the Lariboisière Hospital, where again she could not walk, by now having a hysterical contracture of both lower limbs and being "incapable of movement of any kind."[56] A major episode of psychopathology had been triggered by a drunk with a knife.

There were awful family tragedies, too. Evelyn L.'s knee pains began at the age of fifteen in Huddersfield after her father attempted suicide.[57] The problems of a patient of Albert Charpentier's at the Pitié began in 1892 at age forty-five when she saw her husband shoot himself "a number of times with a revolver." Thereafter she was unable to go out alone. "Her gait became hesitating and difficult. She consulted a doctor who said, on the basis of what she had told him, that she would not recover from her paralysis. Months passed; she walked less and less, her anguish growing at each new effort."[58]

A young patient of the Paris hydrotherapist Alfred Beni-Barde had witnessed her mother trampled to death in a panic at the Opéra-Comique. Several days later the daughter felt that a tight belt was encircling her entire body; "an enormous lassitude made walking almost impossible."[59] The Salpêtrière psychiatrist Auguste-Félix Voisin remembered a young woman of seventeen who, during the 1871 siege of Paris by loyalist troops from Versailles, was crossing the rue de Grenelle with her mother when a shell exploded, decapitating the mother without injuring the daughter. The daughter became amnesic for the event, started having convulsions, and passed from the convulsions into paraplegia.[60] All these seem quite understandable reactions to grief and shock and would later be classified under the category grief reaction or posttraumatic stress disorder. Except that these young women dealt with their grief and shock by becoming paralyzed. The point is that paralysis as a response to loss, mourning, and trauma was not often seen in the eighteenth or the twentieth centuries. It was a culturally specific nineteenth-century mode of processing extreme emotion.

The above examples involved severe psychic shocks, but physical trauma as well could unleash a hysterical paralysis. There is a large literature on such phenomena as "railway spine," the development of apparently psychogenic paralysis by patients who had been in derailments and other such accidents. Debates between psychogenic and neurogenic schools of thought over "traumatic neurosis," a synonym for railway spine, dominated the pages of medical journals in the 1880s and beyond. These debates spilled over into an argument during World War I about whether shell shock represented a genuine but invisible injury of the nervous system or whether it was a form of hysteria.[61]

Here is a typical "traumatic neurosis." Sometime in the 1860s a young lady in London, age twenty, fell down in her drawing room, injuring a knee. Dennis de Berdt Hovell, a London surgeon, found some swelling and inflammation. Four years later she was still incapacitated:

She finds going up stairs especially productive of pain; can walk a short distance without disability, but beyond a certain distance the pain becomes intolerable. . . .

She is neither fanciful nor hysterical, but simply weak and nervous; and I see no reason to question the validity of her complaint. One peculiar feature in this case is, that before her accident this patient was fond of music; now it distresses her so much that she cannot bear it. A street organ is intolerable. On one occasion she had lodgings in the same house with a gentleman who played the harmonium: her friends were obliged to tell him that either he or she must leave the house.[62]

Possibly her paralysis involved a mix of somatic and psychological factors, yet clearly she had permitted it to change her entire life.

Especially interesting are hysterical paralyses resulting from medical encounters. Th——, an unmarried seamstress of twenty-two, gave birth for the first time early in 1857 in Paris. She developed a postpartum infection, for which she was cauterized "eight or ten times" at the Necker Hospital. She also suffered an anal fistula, for which she was operated on. Admitted in great abdominal pain in July 1857 to the Charité Hospital, she was diagnosed as having a uterine inflammation and a periuterine abscess. On July 17 her uterus was catheterized internally with silver nitrate. "Some moments later, the patient lost consciousness, and upon recovering two hours later, found that her right leg was paralyzed. In bed she was not able to move it, either to flex it or lift it. The left leg was fine."[63] After a long series of emotional and physical shocks, in other words, the right leg had finally cried, Enough!

In the case of Doctor Douglas, an Australian physician who had hemorrhoids, it was not the leg that cried out. After an attack of dysentery in January 1864, he began to experience "great inconvenience from piles [hemorrhoids]," and on February 28 "had a ligature placed on a pile."

Doctor Douglas said that thereupon, "I experienced intolerable pain, with indescribable sensation in the nates [buttocks] and rectum while sitting."

On March 5 the pile sloughed away. Doctor Douglas then "experienced a sensation of numbness on the left side of the body, and in the perineum."

By June the symptoms had increased. "There was oppressed breathing, restlessness, complete loss of sensation and motion in lower extremities.

"July 10, quite helpless, cannot move either hands or feet." By February of the following year he was able to move about slowly, and eight months later had recovered.[64] Th—— and Doctor Douglas had both experienced the same ailment—a hysterical paralysis following painful surgical procedures whose very nature terrified the imagination: tubes with caustic passed into the cavity of the uterus, pieces of string bound tightly about one's secret parts.

A final precipitating cause of paralysis seems far more banal than these tragic separations and traumatic procedures. It was paralysis as a kind of mannerism, a symptom that one chooses almost because it is in style and seems the thing to do. Louis Stromeyer, a German surgeon of great experience, remembered two sisters, both governesses aged about twenty-four to twenty-six, who came down simultaneously with back pain, "which acted so disadvantageously upon the lower extremities that both had to remain constantly recumbent, able to take only a few steps in the room." They became sofa cases, spending years in bed. Called in as a consultant, Doctor Stromeyer sent both of them to Bad Driburg to take the waters:

> The older sister returned somewhat improved, yet the younger one remained in a wheelchair, as poorly-off as ever. But the girls were intelligent and listened to my advice. I convinced them they were not destined to permanent paralysis and encouraged them to walk. Then an accident came to my aid, in the form of an invitation to a wedding [in another town], which of course both wanted to attend and the more so because the family doctor did not want to hear of it. The younger sister did not quite have the nerve to appear at a wedding after spending years on the sofa, but the older sister went and returned from the trip fully restored and very agile. The younger sister then said to the older one, I'm going to the next wedding.[65]

At the Charité in Paris, Pierre Briquet had numerous young "hysterical" patients—by which Briquet understood an invisible but real organic disease of the nervous system—who seemed to flip in and out of their paralyses as it suited them:

> One young girl on my wards was struck with hysterical paraplegia. After much therapy, we finally got her to the point of balancing upright. Then one day she found out that someone very special to her had come to Paris. She requested a pass-out, which was granted to her without delay in the belief that she would not be able to make use of it. Not at all. She went out, and this girl who could not walk four steps on the wards went by foot from the Charité to the Austerlitz bridge where the person was awaiting her. She walked around in this way for a week, and then upon hearing a piece of bad news again lost the use of her legs, recovering it later. After doing this several times, she finally recovered completely.

A doctor in a provincial town wrote Briquet about a young female patient who had recently become paraplegic as a result of worry. Briquet advised him that it was probably hysteria. The girl's father, who himself had studied medicine, later wrote back to Briquet, "You would like to know the outcome of this case which you considered very interesting. My daughter has been cured, and radically cured. After she had been in bed around two months, our family doctor became convinced that she was suffering from progressive paralysis [a synonym for neurosyphilis] and initiated the appropriate treatment." Then apparently Briquet's letter arrived stating the opinion that it was hysteria. "In two days she was out of bed and started running and dancing, and even taking long walks in the cold air from which she returned feeling great. It was hard to believe she had ever been ill, the more so because after this miraculous cure she feels better than she ever did before."[66]

All this is not to say that hysterical patients were silly or simulating, merely that the symptom of paralysis in this second half of the nineteenth century was easily available to all those who wished to become symptomatic. And for young women, subject to the many constraints on behavior and movement that society imposed, paralysis seemed the appropriate physical response.

Male Hysteria

If hysteria was a result of reflex irritation, males could get it too, for men could have irritated colons, gall bladders, and so forth. It was only that in women the pelvic organs were permanently irritated, while in men a urethritis or gastritis would be transitory. Thus the view that men were susceptible to hysteria goes right back to the end of the eighteenth century, when the precursor of reflex theory we saw in chapter 1 insisted that nervous diseases were dependent on the nerves rather than on the uterus. Jacob Isenflamm in Erlangen, for example, said in 1774 that hysteria (the women's nervous disease) and hypochondria (the men's nervous disease) were almost identical, and that each sex could get the other.[67] At Bourbonne-les-Bains, Jean-Baptiste Chevalier believed that even if men could not be called *"hystériques,"* they sometimes got the symptoms of hysteria.[68]

With the advent of full-fledged reflex theory in the nineteenth century, doctors ceased to be surprised when encountering hysteria in men. For Benjamin Travers, writing in 1835, the playing field was level for both men and women: "The condition of system termed in females 'hysteria' exists under certain modifications in the male sex. It is a morbid condition of the nervous system." Further: "The breast of the female and the testis of the male are particularly liable to be affected with preternatural irritability in young persons. . . . It has been properly called the irritable breast, and the irritable testicle." He continued: "The successful employment of remedies of the diffusible stimulant and tonic character, and their perfect though often slow recovery, show clearly that the disease is of the neuralgic class modified by the sexual organization."[69] The implication was that irritation could produce hysteria as easily in the one gender as the other.

At Reims, Hector Landouzy, one of the main French reflex theorists of hysteria, had no problem making the diagnosis in males. "And if we do find hysteria in men, is that a reason for denying that in women its seat is in the genitals? May not the genital ganglia of the male be affected in a manner analogous to the woman?. . . . In almost all cases of hysteria in men I have seen, the point of departure for the symptoms may be found in the genitals."[70] Moritz Romberg, the great German authority on nervous diseases, allowed that men could have hysteria too, but only briefly, masturbation and other transitory irritations of the male genitals being but a passing cloud compared to the massive, permanent irritation of the female genitals.[71] Thus, from the late eighteenth century onward, theoretical license for male hysteria came from many authorities.

To what extent did motor hysteria actually occur in males? That is to say, how often is it found before 1885, when Charcot began to make male hysteria a fashionable diagnosis? In 1859 Pierre Briquet at the Charité reported seven cases of male hysteria (including one case of lead poisoning and one fatal case that sounds like neurosyphilis). One of his more psychogenic cases was Ernest Langlois, a butcher of twenty-five, said to be of highly romantic temperament and often on the verge of tears. Three years previously—this must have been in 1851—he had received a visit from a former girlfriend. An argument ensued in which he lost consciousness and began convulsing, so that "a number of people were needed to hold him down." The next day he found himself paralyzed and anesthetic on the left side of his body, a paralysis that vanished in five or six days.

Then early in November 1854, Langlois entered the Pitié Hospital to have a benign cyst removed from above his left eye. There were a few complications, from which he recovered. As he was set to leave the hospital on November 28, he had a bath that was too hot. "In climbing from the bathtub he felt dizzy, began sweating, and fainted. There were more fits in which he tried to strike his attendants and grab hold of nearby objects." He also had a sense of strangulation. He ended up after this attack, as after the first, sobbing. This touched off a series of nervous accidents, including contractions and more convulsions, lasting for more than two weeks, after which he was discharged well.[72] Thus a typical case of male motor hysteria.

There were many cases of male hysteria from midcentury. To give the reader a sense of them: when Louis Stromeyer was a surgeon in Munich in the early 1840s he saw a lawyer, thirty-eight, who had already been bedridden for three months with a slight inversion of his left ankle. The foot seemed all right to Stromeyer, who examined it carefully:

> But the patient believed himself unable to move his toes, and was finally able to do so after I had manipulated the joint a bit. Then he tried to walk, supported by someone on either side. That seemed to go well and I reassured him about the condition of his foot. Then, because it was evening, I stayed a half hour to smoke a cigar with him. As I took my leave he had forgotten his sick foot and accompanied me, lantern in hand, right to the stairs. I told him that after this accomplishment he probably would require my help no longer.[73]

Maurice Krishaber, a physician born in Hungary and educated in Vienna, Prague, and finally Paris, settled in Paris after getting his M.D. in 1864. Krishaber acquired a practice filled with wealthy psychoneurotic patients. At some point in the late 1860s he treated a twenty-four-year-old intellectual who had been asked by a friend to join a club. The evening of the invitation the young man and his friend went to dine with a dozen other members. They ate well, but then after dinner the "club" turned out to be a secret society opposed to the government of Napoleon III. The young man became outraged at the duplicity, stalking away after a stormy discussion. "Accompanied by his friend, he went home, but was able to walk only with difficulty. Things spun about, he saw double." There were violent palpitations and a feeling of strangulation.

Once at home and in bed, he continued to experience all the symptoms of what was evidently an anxiety attack. But in addition he felt pain in his shoulders and arms. "He could scarcely move them, and soon his lower limbs were in turn affected. They were not painful, but seemed to him paralyzed." The young man remained symptomatic for several weeks, and ended by losing all his hair.[74]

Were such incidents in men truly frequent or extraordinary anecdotes? John Ogle, physician at St. George's Hospital in London, ventured in 1870: "There can be no doubt that any physician who has seen much of hospital practice will agree that cases of true hysteria are to be met with in men."[75] Montrose Pallen, a gynecological surgeon in New York, thought hysterical symptoms in men very similar to those he saw in women, merely requiring a different name, for male hysteria arose from disorders in the circulation of the brain rather than reflexly from the pelvis. He proposed the term *neurospasia* for hysteria in men. Clearly he would not have deliberated on the point had he not believed hysteria in men to be common.[76]

In sum, these scattered reports show that male hysteria definitely existed before the 1880s. It is quite misleading to believe, as some writers have proposed, there was no male hysteria before the shell shock of World War I, or that Charcot was the "inventor" of male hysteria. Men too were inclined to express psychic unease in the form of motor hysteria. Yet to go by the frequency of reports of male hysteria, men selected this particular symptom from the pool somewhat less than women did. This relative infrequency of reporting male hysteria may just be an artifact of medical prejudice about "hysterical" women: Perhaps doctors more often interpreted a given constellation of symptoms as hysterical when encountered in women. It is also possible that some factor other than a distortion of the medical gaze is at work here. Historically, men may have expressed stress in other ways. But at some level male hysteria existed for both doctor and patient.

The Family Psychodrama

What larger cultural factors, aside from changing medical diagnosis, might account for an increase during the nineteenth century of symptoms that affected the ability to walk? Details of the psychosocial circumstances of patients are sparse indeed in the case reports. But vast social changes swept through family and personal life throughout the century. To what extent might these be invoked?

The tableau of symptoms in the foreground is set against a deep background of increasingly sentimentalized family life. Family relations before 1800 might generally be characterized as cool, oriented more toward the preservation of family name and dynastic possessions than toward the nurturing of togetherness. Then, late in the eighteenth or early in the nineteenth century, depending on the country and social class, new ties of intimacy started to form between the spouses, uniting parents and children more closely. Such phrases as *une famille bien unie* (family togetherness) or *chacun chez soi* (our home is our castle) became common. Personal sentiment and attraction started to replace the calculus of familial advantage in choosing a partner, and the success of marriage itself would be judged by the extent to which it had enhanced the happiness of the spouses rather than their property and fortune. These were enormous changes in intimate life, and they had the effect of converting the family into something of an emotional pressure cooker. This "modern" style of family life charged with affect ties that previously had been emotionally more neutral (of necessity, because whether husband and wife loved or

120

hated each other, they had to get on with the common tasks of farm or craft shop).[77]

The passage of the family from a relatively porous institution, open to community inspection from all sides, to a site of deep privacy is illumined by one of Freud's failed cases. He had been treating with hypnosis a young woman who had a hysterical paralysis, and as the hypnotic suggestions had been unavailing, Freud tried a "psychical analysis." Her father, himself a physician, had been attending the sessions with her.

"So I desired to know," wrote Freud in 1895, "if any emotional upset had preceded the onset of the disorder. Now she explained (under hypnosis and without any sign of agitation), that just previously a young relative had died whose fiancée she had regarded herself for many years. This revelation changed nothing in her condition. So in the next hypnotic session I told her I was quite convinced that the death of the nephew had nothing to do with her condition, that something else had happened that she had not mentioned. Now she permitted herself to make a single allusion, but scarcely had she said a word before she fell silent, and the elderly father who was sitting behind her began to sob bitterly. Of course I did not press the patient further, but I never saw her again."[78] This was the new, nineteenth-century family, inward-looking, intimate, and freighted with secrets.

Given that the patient's unconscious mind deliberately selected the symptom of paralysis over a host of others, paralysis evidently served a symbolic purpose. If symptom formation is seen as a way of solving problems, the following kinds of problems in the psychodrama of family life might require a solution: extracting oneself from acute problems, from chronic misery, and the need for revenge.

Few problems in family life are more acute than being discovered in some marital trespass. The Berlin internist Ernst von Leyden recalled a young musician who suddenly became quadriplegic:

As I tried to interrogate his relatives, especially his temperamental wife, about the circumstances of the illness, it turned out that the couple did not live in a very harmonious marriage and quarreled often. The young husband had bumped into his wife quite unexpectedly and suddenly either very late at night or very early in the morning as he tried to steal unnoticed into the house. Perhaps it was the pangs of conscience, or merely fear of new eruptions of his wife's anger, in any event it is clear that as soon as he saw her, he sank in a faint to the floor, crippled in all four limbs.[79]

In Riga, Latvia, the neurologist Valentin von Holst had as a patient a young woman who at seventeen had married for love and was living happily with her husband and two small children. When she was about twenty-one, "she met a young man who impressed her deeply. And to her horror, it slowly became clear to her that her relationship with this young man was boring like a poisoned thorn into the happiness of her own marriage, and that she had not the moral strength to free herself from the man." There arose within her an agonizing conflict

> which made her all the more desperate because she was forced continually to deceive her husband, who adored her. In this struggle she deteriorated not only mentally but physically, though no one in her entourage, not even the family doctor, was able to guess the reason. Finally she forced herself to confess all to her husband. That was a terrible psychic shock for her. The result was that before she even got to the end of her confession she fell into a deep faint, from which she awoke paraplegic, anesthetic in one leg up to mid thigh, in the other to the knee.[80]

Also, obligations to one's parents sometimes called for the solution of paralysis. In the late 1920s or early 1930s in the United States, a student at Bucknell University who was an ex-nun married secretly, then developed a paralysis of her right arm so that she could not write the news home to her parents. She next acquired a hysterical aphonia, so that she could not confess the problem to a priest.[81]

Apropos male hysteria, on July 27, 1926, a young man of nineteen was brought to the Mayo Clinic in Rochester, Minnesota, with both legs paralyzed. About three weeks earlier he had complained of fatigue; then one day he could not get up from the dinner table. "He was helped to his bed with his limbs dragging helplessly behind him." Once in bed, he was found to have a complete paralysis of the lower limbs. The family doctor pronounced it incurable spinal inflammation.

As he hobbled about the clinic on crutches, "it was obvious . . . that firm contractions of the muscles of the lower limbs and pelvis were necessary and actually these could be seen contracting and relaxing normally." Nor did he have any neurological findings or bladder problems. He also displayed "indifference" to his symptoms: "His limbs seemed no longer part of him." On the fourth day of his stay in hospital, "he was commanded to get up and walk. He suddenly left his bed and walked unaided, at first hesitatingly and like a child, but later, confidence being restored, within an hour he was almost running to the telegraph office to send messages to his father, his sweetheart, and his friends that his paralysis had gone." The conflict? He had wanted to become a medical missionary but instead had to teach the next year "in a very disagreeable locality" in order to help out the family financially.[82] None of these conflicts would have arisen in the absence of family life valuing attachment to spouses and parents above all else. Unable to renounce the attachment, the participants found themselves paralyzed.

But not all families were so happy. Maria Rivet ran a private nervous clinic in Paris that her father, the famous psychiatrist Alexandre Brierre de Boismont, had founded in the rue Neuve-Sainte-Geneviève near the Pantheon. Here is one of her patients, Mme. N., whose husband made the mistake of taking his wife for granted:

> Mme. N., who had a remarkable intelligence, was basically a nervous type as a result of her almost pathological impressionability. . . . She was married to a dynamic man, whose business affairs did not permit him to spend time with his wife. As with many big financiers, Monsieur N. did not think it was possible to be unhappy if the market was up, and that a husband who kept his wife informed about all his deals and required her to calculate the profits had done everything possible to make her happy.
>
> This unhappy woman suffered in the kingdom of profit and loss, buried in figures whose importance necessitated all of her attention. [And when she wanted to go out socially] she found herself in the presence of a husband floored with weariness and ignorant of all the needs and the délicatesses du coeur of a woman; he was a husband who, after a review of the day's operations, fell asleep and snored.

"It was a horrible struggle," Mme. N. later told Mme. Rivet. Mme. N. imagined she was going mad. Then after a sudden disappointment, Mme. N. "acquired a nervous disease whose downhill course left her with only one thought: suicide." It sounds as though Mme. N. became depressed. She also developed violent headaches and neuralgic pains that seemed increasingly to situate themselves in her joints. "I have so often seen her rejoice at not being able to move her legs," wrote Mme. Rivet of Mme. N.'s hospitalization. "I have so often seen her pray to God to increase her pain in the hope of losing consciousness." Her illness relapsed over the years, and Mme. N. finally escaped from her marriage into the sanatorium.[83]

The chronic unhappiness of Fräulein E. S., a twenty-two-year-old unmarried mother from the countryside near Saint Gallen culminated one morning as she was to appear in court to testify against her former boyfriend in a paternity suit. From a large farm family in which the father had died early, she had had an unremarkable life until she became pregnant out of wedlock. Depressed during pregnancy, after the delivery she was, according to her mother, filled with "anger, regret and shame." Then the boyfriend refused to help support the child. On the morning of April 2, 1906, two weeks after giving birth, she was unable to arise from bed, paralyzed hand and foot. "Similarly her speech was incomprehensible and mumbled. She was able to understand us quite well," wrote her physician, "and made efforts to move her limbs, but in vain." The doctor was obliged to certify that she would be unable to appear in court and testify.[84] In these cases paralysis served not so much as a means of avoiding family confrontation as a way out of hopeless binds: a loveless husband, or a humiliating court appearance because one had "sinned."

Finally, in the family psychodrama, paralysis was a form of revenge: You have made me unhappy, so I will make your life miserable. The classic full-blown revenge seeker was the chronic invalid, pounding on the floor with her cane. But there were more acute forms of punishment. A young Liverpool woman of twenty-three unburdened herself to Albert Davis, a hypnotherapist there, sometime during World War I. "She and her mother (a widow) were practically alone in the world; she had a young man of whom she was fond, but her mother discouraged the affair and would not speak of him. He had joined the army and was about to proceed to the front."

So she acquired a hysterical paralysis of both legs and her left arm. "Her other symptoms were depression, loss of appetite, and occasional fainting." The mother was being punished for thwarting the romance. When Davis saw the patient ten weeks later, he gave her a psychological pep talk. "I pointed out the cause to the patient and her mother, I broke down the reserve that was between them." Mother and daughter became friendly again and in five days the daughter was "walking steadily and well without help. Grip of left hand strong."[85] The message to the mother had been: Cripple my relationship, cripple me.

What message was the following woman giving her mother? She was a thirty-eight-year-old patient of the distinguished physician John Thomas Banks in Dublin, bedridden since the age of twenty-two.

> Her lower extremities were perfectly powerless. She had not attempted to put her legs under her for years. She was prepared for a life such as she had been leading, and had made all the arrangements which people make when they are doomed for life, having her birds, books, and animals about her. She had a good appetite. For years it was supposed that she laboured under paralysis of the rectum. She had no power of expulsion, and three times in the week her mother removed the contents of the rectum.[86]

The crime of the mother, who disempacted her hysterical daughter three times a week, must have been awful indeed.

A new quality in nineteenth-century family life gave family members this kind of leverage over one another. That quality was, I think, the sentimentalizing of family relations, so that the threat of debility (as in paralysis) or self-destruction (as in anorexia nervosa) thrust new weapons into intrafamily struggles for emotional control.[87] These weapons were largely lacking in peasant and working-class families before 1800, and in middle-class families on the whole at some point before the middle of the eighteenth century. Perhaps in the traditional family, where all lived close to the margin of existence, the threat of self-starvation would have been received with disbelief, or the threat of staying abed "paralyzed" for months or years greeted with a beating. Such retrospective attempts to link changes in family life to changing symptom patterns are quite speculative, yet cry out for further research.

The Doctors' Dislike of Hysterical Paralysis

It is ironic that a symptom which medical theories themselves had done so much to call into existence, should have met with such loathing among physicians. But hysterical paralyses had a large "downside" for the physician in that: (a) they were hard to cure, and (b) if the doctor failed to effect a cure, he would further lose credibility when the patient was cured by a quack. William Osler, then a professor of medicine at Johns Hopkins University, said of hysterical joint ailments in 1892, "Perhaps no single affection has brought more discredit upon the profession, for the cases are very refractory, and finally fall into the hands of a charlatan or faith-healer, under whose touch the disease may disappear at once."[88] Harry Parker of the Mayo Clinic noted that, in taking on hysterical paralyses, the profession was competing against "the vast array of crutches and canes" at religious shrines, and against electrified revival meetings where "recoveries take place in those whom grave and learned physicians had prognosticated would never use their limbs again."[89]

When an apparently hysterical patient limped in, the physician was in a double bind. On the one hand, what if the paralysis was really organic? "There is a deep and troublesome fear that [the doctor's] diagnosis may be mistaken," continued Parker. "To make a frank diagnosis of hysteria always means that the burden of proof rests on [the doctor's] shoulders, and the only proof is that he has the ability to cure the disease by simple psychogenic means." On the other hand, "To pronounce the paralysis incurable and to hear later that the patient has drifted into the hands of a charlatan whose pompous power of suggestion removed the paralysis is enough to cast a slur on the reputation of the physician and the power of his healing art."[90]

If the downside risks of false diagnosis and embarrassment had no compensation, few doctors would have taken on these cases. Fortunately there was an upside as well: The doctor might acquire a reputation as a master healer, a useful foundation stone for a practice in what one might think of as neuropsychogynecology. Byrom Bramwell, a well-known senior consultant at the Royal Infirmary in Edinburgh, gave the medical students some advice on the management of hysterical paralyses in 1903.

He began by demonstrating a patient. "Gentlemen, you will remember this patient—the case of functional paraplegia and hemianaesthesia which I brought before your notice and discussed at some length last Wednesday. I told you that I expected she would be quite well today. I am glad to say that this expectation has been fulfilled. . . . The day after the clinique she ran up and down the long female ward." Her ovarian pain had disappeared too. And the next day she clipped three seconds off her record, doing the ward in seventeen seconds. "Excellent time. I timed her in order that she might have a definite object and goal before her."

There was a lesson in all this for students, said Bramwell. "Now, suppose that soon after you get into practice, a case of this kind should come under your care—it is of course a chance, but it may occur to any one of you—suppose the result should turn out to be as successful as the result has been in the present case, your reputation would be at once made. A single case like this would do you immense good. It would certainly bring you many patients."[91] Of interest in these remarks is Bramwell's almost palpable contempt for his female patients. It is as though the medical students were being invited into a sewer in hopes of finding gold.

Organically trained physicians felt deep ambivalence about these cases of paralysis, the more so because, as men who were not atypical of male culture in their day, they glimpsed the whining woman behind the female patient. Silas Weir Mitchell said as much, describing typical patients with hysterical paraplegia as, "women with a low, whining, bleating voice that is by itself a tell-tale of the kind of will-less ataxia which seems to cripple the mind no less than the body."[92]

Even more striking evidence of their savage impatience with hysterical women—even more savage than Battey's operation and clitoridectomy—was the ease with which physicians once amputated "paralyzed" limbs. In 1818 Benjamin Brodie was invited to consult a "lady in the country on account of a disease of the knee." There were no obvious local findings; he recommended a course of treatment that failed, and the symptoms became aggravated. "She suffered more than ever, so that she became anxious to undergo the amputation of the limb." Brodie advised against it. "However, her wishes remained unaltered; and two surgeons of eminence in the country, yielding to her entreaties, performed the operation." On completion of the amputation they were surprised to see that they had removed a normal joint.[93] Brodie's colleague Frederic Skey remembered in 1855 how it used to happen that, after such limbs had been amputated, the paralysis would spring up again elsewhere.[94]

Nor were such amputations done in England alone. Against Louis Stromeyer's advice, in 1830 surgeons in Hamburg amputated the "clubfoot," evidently hysterical in nature, of a "pretty young girl of twenty."[95] In the absence of solid physical findings, the notion of "hysteria" must have entered the minds of these surgeons. It is impossible not to see in these ruthless amputations a desire to punish the young female patients for their misbehavior.

Some of the therapeutic tricks used to cure hysterical paralyses, although effective in their application, do indicate a certain conception of the doctor-patient relationship that infantilizes, to say the least, the women. Using all the medical authority of an honorary Viennese "professorship," Moritz Benedikt would simply order them out of bed.[96] There is the story of Silas Weir Mitchell in Philadelphia and the patient who refused to arise from bed. "Dr. Mitchell had run the gamut of argument and persuasion and finally announced: 'If you are not out of bed in five minutes—I'll get into it with you!' He thereupon started to remove his coat, the patient still obstinately prone—he removed his vest, but when he started to take off his trousers—she was out of bed in a fury!"[97] Abraham Myerson, a Boston psychiatrist with a large society practice, was treating in his office a forty-four-year-old housewife with a hysterical paralysis of the left leg: "[I made] the rather bold statement that she would not be allowed to go home until she used the left leg as well as the right."[98] A prisoner!

Yet of all physicians treating paralysis, few could have been more abusive than Louisville's Doctor Vance, who generally behaved with his patients as though he were at a wrestling match. A sample: In dealing with Miss G., paralyzed and confined to bed for six months, Vance said:

I went to the infirmary and walked into the ward where I found a very comely young woman, rosy cheeks and otherwise looking very well, lying on her back in bed.

I remarked, "You do not look sick to me."

Her reply was, "But, yes, I am; I cannot do anything."

I then asked her to turn over on her face, and she replied that she could not do so. Without any further comment, I took her by the hips and jerked her over on her back, saying to her, "The devil you can't," and immediately told the nurse to remove her from the ward where there were too many old women sympathizers, to take her to a room in the infirmary and I would burn her back from the nape of the neck down. The next day when I called she was up and able to walk about the halls.[99]

Doctor Vance had no particular medical warrant for slapping and threatening his patients, merely that, as a powerful man used to dealing with compliant women, he knew these techniques to be effective. There is similarly something in the entire picture of hysterical paralysis that lifts it above the immediately medical and makes it a symbol of male-female relationships in the nineteenth century. The Victorian woman, stereotyped in her day as weak and passive, was able to communicate with a world dominated by powerful males often only by becoming "paralyzed."

CHAPTER

6

Dissociation

When the mind "splits," it creates a special opportunity for causing havoc in the body. This kind of splitting, which is often accompanied by psychosomatic features, is known as dissociation. Dissociation means that one part of the mind has supposedly lost track of what another part is doing, as, for example, forgetting what happened under hypnosis, or having "multiple personalities," some of which do not know of the others' existence. Far from being an exotic footnote in the history of psychiatry, such dissociation was once common. The physical symptoms associated with it represent a distinctive chapter in the history of psychosomatic illness—distinctive because this kind of splitting changes greatly from one historical period to another.

Whether dissociation really exists as a special psychological process in the brain is a moot question. It is unclear whether thought truly has the capacity to compartmentalize in such a manner that one area of conscious thought is ignorant of another.[1] But patients have always believed that dissociation exists, and many doctors have been willing to accept it as a genuine disease entity. By describing new forms of dissociation, doctors may even "create" new forms of illness and thus encourage patients to take them on.

In the nineteenth century, patients often believed themselves in some kind of "second state," or dissociative state, as the result of encounters with hypnotists and "magnetizers." Magnetizers used metal rods and dramatic gestures to influence "magnetic fluid," originally conceived of as a kind of physical fluid circulating in the body. Physical symptoms arising during these second states were then ascribed to the effects of the fluid. The symptoms accompanying dissociation, far from being distinctive to second states, were drawn from the larger symptom pool of Western society, and changed over the years in accordance with general shifts in patterns of somatization. Accordingly, the hypnotic phenomena of the nineteenth century tended to be drawn from motor hysteria. As hysterical paralyses then began to vanish from history, the kinds of motor catalepsy and coma states associated with hypnosis became discredited as well. With the shift in somatization from the motor side of the nervous system to the sensory, the belief arose toward the end of the nineteenth century that one might go through life "permanently benumbed" in a kind of sensory second state, or that one might have a "multiple personality."

Spontaneous Somnambulism and Catalepsy

Even before the ascent at the end of the eighteenth century of the magnetizers, forms of hypnotic phenomena had always been known.[2] For centuries two of these phenomena in particular, somnambulism and catalepsy, had been symptoms of a dissociative state.

Once the hypnotists incorporated somnambulism into their jargon, it would take on quite a specific meaning. But before that happened, two forms of traditional somnambulism existed. There was an innocuous version, sleepwalking, possibly while under the influence of the moon. It is, however, the pathological version of somnambulism that is of interest here, for in this state the patients were physically symptomatic. This pathological version of somnambulism entailed dissociation (a fugue state forgotten afterward) and somatization (in particular, hyperexaltation of the sensory side of the nervous system).[3]

How did spontaneous somnambulism present itself to doctors? In September 1834 a young lady of twenty appeared at the Farringdon General Dispensary in London with a roving set of physical symptoms, including pains that suddenly came and went, convulsive breathing, total blindness now and then, and a jaw clamped convulsively shut. "The most peculiar feature in this mélange," said John Jacob, "was a kind of hysterical somnambulism, under whose influence my patient has performed correctly on the pianoforte her favourite pieces, walked up stairs, undressed, and imperfectly fulfilled many accustomed domestic duties, unconscious of all around her, with no recollection after the paroxysm of what had transpired."[4] Thus one part of her mind seemed dissociated from another, in a manner Doctor Jacob considered "somnambulism."

As for catalepsy, it too entailed both altered mind and body states, or dissociation and somatization. Persons under catalepsy might go into an apparent coma, as well as demonstrating such physical symptoms as "waxy rigidity" of the limbs, meaning that the limbs stay in the position in which someone else puts them, or in which they were at the onset of the coma.[5] In catalepsy, the patient lay in a virtual stillness of death, insensible to stimulation, yet jaw clenched and often all muscles rigid. Pierre Pomme described this in 1763 as a kind of "hysterical attack": "In some women the pulse is totally extinguished, and respiration is so unapparent as not to cloud a mirror [a test of death] or disturb the flame of a candle held near the nose. The stiffness of the body has caused it to be confused with death more than once, and the ghastliest of accidents [burying someone alive] may result from failing to note it."[6]

John Maubray, a London physician, described early in the eighteenth century various ways to tell if a woman were dead or merely having an "extreme fit of this [hysteric] passion": These included objects "such as lint, feathers, or burnt paper being held to the mouth; if moved, the patient breathes; a glass of water being set upon the breast; if stirred, there is some motion and dilatation still in the breast." The only certain test, however, was "when the body begins to send forth a cadaverous smell."[7] In the early nineteenth century John Conolly told the story of Lady Russell, a century before, "whose funeral having been postponed for a longer period than usual, afforded time for her happy recovery [from a hysterical coma], which took place while the bells were ringing for prayers; the supposed dead person exclaiming that it was time to go to church."[8]

From the late eighteenth century onward, these hysterical death spells frequently became described as part of the larger phenomenon of catalepsy. In 1794, for example, Franz Xaver Mezler, court physician to the princely dynasty in Sigmaringen (southwestern Germany), was called to see a young pregnant woman having lower abdominal pains. "I discovered at once that since childhood she had been subject to nervous diseases and twitching," and now had fragile health. She had complained of a sense of something climbing into her throat. So Doctor Mezler attempted to awaken her as she lay in apparently peaceful sleep, "but she was stiff as wood as I tried to move her hand. This lasted for a few minutes, then she came to herself and complained of nothing. Everything was fine." She vaguely remembered something stuck in her throat. "Sometimes it comes over her so quickly that she spends the entire attack in exactly the same position as when it began. If one exerts slow, steady force, one is able to shift the position of an arm, for example, which then remains in the new position until she awakens." What caused these strange attacks?

131

Doctor Mezler once observed an attack come on as she was kissing her husband. "He was thus obliged to remain in her arms until she came to herself again."[9]

On Whitsun Monday, 1878, Doctor Munk in the little Hungarian town of Verebély was called to see young Albert Schwartz, an apprentice to a local merchant, who had fallen ill. After being sought everywhere, Schwartz had been found in the basement of the shop apparently asleep.

In the belief that he was asleep, he was left as a joke to slumber on. But the siesta lasted too long and moreover the staff remembered that he had complained of a headache several days previously. . . . Schwartz was given a shaking and yelled at to stand up, but he emitted no sign of life. An errand boy who still thought this a trick—Schwartz was known as a practical joker—lifted Schwartz up, led or dragged him into the office, and stood him against a desk. Schwartz now leaned motionlessly against the desk, whereupon this lunatic errand boy threw a glass of water in his face. When at this point Schwartz remained lifeless and failed to grimace, the affair was taken as deadly serious and I was sent for. I found Schwartz lying on the couch.

Doctor Munk examined the patient, ordered rubbing of the skin, and returned in half an hour. "[The patient] was insensible to the strongest stimuli, such as knife- and needlepricks. His limbs remained in the positions in which they were put. I forced open his eyelids and found the eyeballs turned up. . . . There was no response to loud shouting. Consciousness seemed quite suspended. He easily swallowed a teaspoon of water poured into his mouth. It was clear that we were dealing with an episode of catalepsy."[10] Many similar cases were reported from the European literature.

In nineteenth-century America too this "death-spell" style of catalepsy was a not-uncommon occurrence. During an interview Weir Mitchell provoked such a death spell in one of his patients, a young woman with a previous history of aphonia.

She said to me, "I am going to have an attack; feel my pulse. In a few minutes I shall be dead."

Her pulse, which just before was about 100, was now racing and quite countless, while the irregularity and violence of the heart's action seemed to me inconceivable. With the interest of an hysterical woman in her own performances, she said to me, "Now watch it; you will be amazed."

This certainly was the case. Within a few minutes the pulse began to fall in number, and . . . in some fifteen minutes was beating only 40. Then a beat would drop out here and there; the pulse meanwhile growing feebler, until at last I could neither feel it, nor yet hear the heart. In this state of seeming death, white, still, without breathing or perceptible circulation, this girl lay for from two to four days.[11]

The symptom of a death spell was still apparently familiar enough in the United States that a Wisconsin housewife, sometime after World War I, felt it could be convincingly simulated. She lay "motionless" in bed for six days, it was said "to force her husband to employ a maid." The husband, faking a departure for work, hid in the hall closet and caught her up eating and going to the bathroom.[12] If the community had not still believed in death spells that went on for six days, she would not have attempted it.

While the dissociative component of catalepsy captured the imagination, it was the motor component, the waxy rigidity of the limbs, that established the diagnosis. Even without unconsciousness, the physician's ability to sculpt the body into place would establish the case as one of catalepsy. In the late 1830s a Jewish girl* of fourteen or fifteen came into the city hospital, province of Galicia, in Brody, unable to speak and giving no history:

> She lay in bed like a statue, gaunt, white, her cheeks slightly red but cold as marble. Breathing and pulse were scarcely perceptible, the latter spasmodic and delayed. The eyes were open and rigid. . . . Hearing, smell and sensation seemed to have vanished entirely. . . . I could not discover how long the illness had already lasted, for she remained in the same condition the entire week she was in hospital. Thus *Catalepsis continua* without a doubt.

So the doctor began doing experiments: He would raise her arm, and it would stay up for a while, slowly sinking down by itself. And if he pressed it down, it stayed down. There was a second such patient who came in around the same time. Her limbs seemed contracted in a terrible paroxysm. But when the doctor stroked them a bit he was able to put them at will in any position. His friends would look on in amazement as he carved out for her various postures as she lay in bed, "sometimes a threatening field-marshal with a command baton in hand, other times an Apollo playing the lute or a supplicant at prayer."[13]

---

*Physicians of the day considered Jews to be at special risk for such illnesses. In a future volume we will see if this is so. Both the doctors and the population in general considered religion a fundamental category of social organization.

Thus spontaneous somnambulism and catalepsy qualify for inclusion in a history of psychosomatic illness. Along with other forms of motor hysteria, they seem to increase in frequency from 1800 until about the 1880s, as they become caught up in the climate of suggestion surrounding "animal magnetism" and hypnotism. When deliberately putting individuals into second states started to become fashionable, as in the rise of hypnotism, the patient's unconscious mind would seek out the symptoms of somnambulism and catalepsy to express the dissociation that both doctor and patient firmly believed was occurring.

The First Wave of Hypnosis

This part of the story began in 1766, when Franz Anton Mesmer, at age thirty-two, graduated in medicine from the University of Vienna, having written a thesis on "The Action of the Planets on the Human Body." Born in a village on Lake Constance, Mesmer had drifted, Faustlike, between philosophy and theology before settling on medicine. After finishing his thesis he settled in Vienna as a general practitioner. Eight years later he was inspired by an astronomer friend to investigate the therapeutic uses of steel magnets, which seemed to be in the same general vein as planetary action. In 1775 he published his first work on "magnetic cures." This was the birth of "animal magnetism" (as opposed to mineral magnetism)—the belief that humans have in them a physical fluid whose distribution may be adjusted with the application of magnets, and that this magnetic fluid may pass invisibly from those who have an ample supply of it (the magnetizer, or hypnotist), to those who have too little (the "medium," subject, or patient).[14]

Mesmer's writings on magnetic cures after 1775 aroused enormous interest. Not only did he acquire a large practice in Vienna, he traveled all over Europe consulting and improving his technique. He determined, for example, that the magnetizer might readjust the magnetic fluid by making "passes," stroking motions with his fingers. Insulted by the criticism of nonbelievers in Vienna, Mesmer left Vienna for Paris, arriving there in February 1778. He enjoyed enormous popularity in the French capital, and began after 1784 to extend his movement throughout France in the form of "harmonic societies," of which more than forty were founded, with hundreds of members. Unfortunately, also in 1784, trouble began in the form of a disbelieving royal commission that had been summoned to consider his doctrines. Physicians referring patients to him were now threatened with the loss of their licenses. Five years later the

Revolution broke out. Mesmer fled to Germany, and ultimately ended up settling as a family doctor in the small Swiss town of Frauenfeld, close to Lake Constance, where he ended his days a forgotten figure. He died in nearby Meersburg in Germany in 1815.[15]

Mesmer's doctrine, however, was not forgotten. His own patients seem to have been the standard kinds of somatizers, with hysterical aphonias, abdominal complaints and the like. Yet some of the Parisians, receiving fill-ups of their magnetic fluid as Mesmer stroked their abdomens or looked into their eyes, started falling into "crises," or second states. One of Mesmer's disciples, Armand, marquis de Puységur, then cultivated, or shaped, this propensity for falling into trancelike states. During the states he might ask patients to undertake all kinds of bizarre activities, and they would awaken from the states cured of whatever had ailed them, with no memory of what had transpired. This was the formal birth of what James Braid in 1843 would promote as hypnotism. Puységur and several generations of followers referred to it as "artificial somnambulism," in contrast to the spontaneous variety.[16] Mesmer's animal magnetism and Puységur's somnambulism thus boil down to the same thing: the capacity to act on the infinite suggestibility of certain kinds of patients, tricking the unconscious mind into the belief that it has achieved a second state, or dissociation. Both animal magnetism and induced somnambulism became known by the shorthand label "Mesmerism."

The spread of Mesmerism within the medical community after 1800 may be measured by the number of publications on it. The medical bibliography compiled by the U.S. government, the surgeon general's *Index-Catalogue,* charted only 16 references to animal magnetism in world medical literature for the decade 1800–1809, 71 for 1810–19, then an increase to 190 references for the decade 1840–49.[17] Thus, after an initial setback, Mesmerism recovered well, growing steadily in popularity with physicians until midcentury. Carl Kluge, a surgery instructor at the Prussian military medical college (the Pepinière) in Berlin, noted in 1811 that despite its initial discrediting, animal magnetism was now thriving in Germany, merely that German physicians were reluctant to write up their results. He preferred the term *animalischer Magnetismus* to the more properly German *thierischer* [animal] *Magnetismus,* because it sounded nobler.[18]

Although the Austrian government had officially forbidden the exercise of animal magnetism in 1795, Austrian physicians continued to perform it anyway. When in 1845 the government of Lower Austria (the province in which Vienna was situated) asked the Viennese medical faculty for an opinion on the subject, the great majority spoke out in favor of it, and by a vote of 125 to 3 in that year recommended that restrictions on its medical use be abolished.[19]

In France, despite the negative assessments of various royal commissions, several professors of medicine employed Mesmerism clinically. Jacques-Étienne Belhomme recalled that when he had interned in 1821 at Bicêtre Hospital in Paris, fellow intern Philippe-Frédéric Blandin—later a famous surgeon—was actively hypnotizing patients on one service. "One patient had insomnia despite being given opiates, and Blandin magnetized him every evening so that he slept all night. One patient with rickets who had been on the ward for a long time received a quite extraordinary magnetic effect: whenever Blandin entered the ward, he fell immediately asleep."[20] Pierre-Adolphe Piorry at the Pitié had recommended hypnotism to his residents and had used it himself since at least the 1840s.[21] Even at the academic heights, therefore, hypnotism had a certain following in the first half of the nineteenth century.

But at the medical grass roots the doctrine was extremely popular. A whole corps of true believers flourished, spreading the contagion in a manner not unlike the physician-enthusiasts of spinal irritation or ovariotomy, or of chronic fatigue syndrome today. Doctors who themselves were convinced that magnetic fluid circulated in the body would end up shaping the symptoms of their patients, who sought physiological explanations of disturbing psychic phenomena.

Hypnotic Catalepsy

Under the hands of the magnetizing physicians, the symptoms of catalepsy and somnambulism became transformed. Although a magnetized patient might be expected to produce both catalepsy and somnambulism in the course of an episode, the concepts themselves remained distinctive.[22]

Now catalepsy could be induced and abolished by means of hypnosis (as opposed to being just a natural disease state)—explicit evidence of the hand of medicine shaping the symptoms. Juliana Neumann, a fifteen-year-old Jewish girl from Schleimingen in Hungary, was sent in August 1851 on account of deafness to Vienna for a magnetic consultation with Dr. Johann Schoder. She sounded as if she might also have been depressed, asking forgiveness for sins she had never committed and the like. Schoder magnetized her and attempted to cure her by blowing into her ear and by rubbing her temple and jaw. After three weeks of this treatment she began staring fixedly, became deeply sad, refused food, would not speak or respond to questions, and had insomnia. She had probably become even more depressed. Schoder diagnosed homesickness and recommended she return home.

Once back in Schleimingen on September 3 she became even worse: mute, cried a lot, could not hold herself upright, and had to be put to bed. At this point a local doctor diagnosed catalepsy, observing that she retained for some time every position into which she was placed. By September 11 she was much better, except that she believed herself to have been "under a spell" *(verzaubert)* in Vienna and could not stand to hear Schoder's name. Thus all the conditions of medical suggestion were present: She had learned the name of a new disease—catalepsy—and discovered what symptoms qualified for it: rigid muscles and weird behavior. It is therefore unsurprising that on October 1 she relapsed, not into the symptoms of depression but into those of catalepsy: suddenly emitting as she lay in bed with her sister that night "a horrifying groan, and from that moment on remained motionless with eyes and mouth wide open. She was sleepless for forty-eight hours, and held food firmly that was placed in her hand, without looking at it." Sent back to Vienna on October 29, she was admitted to the clinic of the famed Joseph Skoda, where she lay "motionless in bed, her eyes open, directed immovably ahead. . . . From her closed mouth flowed foul-smelling saliva." All muscles were uncontracted, save those of the neck.[23]

The most striking feature of the new catalepsy was an exaltation of one or two of the senses, such as vision or touch. Authorities reasoned that the general suppression of the senses occurring in catalepsy might nonetheless result in heightening just one of them, indeed transporting that sense to another part of the body entirely. Thus in a cataleptic "crisis," vision might be shifted from the eyes to the stomach. Or the sense of touch might become hyperexalted, concentrating itself in the tips of the fingers so that one could read by simply running one's fingers along the page.

Although some of these perfervid psychic feats had already been seen among Mesmer's and Puységur's patients, the true codifier of the new doctrine of catalepsy was the Lyon physician Jacques-Henri-Désiré Petetin, forty-three in 1787, when he wrote "Notes on the Discovery of the Phenomena Produced by Catalepsy and Somnambulism, Both Being Symptoms of Basic Hysteria."[24] Opposing Mesmer's views for a long time, Petetin ultimately had come around to them, and indeed was reproached for having tried to smuggle Mesmerism through the back door with his notions of "animal electricity" and "hysterical catalepsy."[25] What was hysterical catalepsy? When individuals went into "crisis," or states of self-hypnosis, the concentration of their electrical energy in just one sense, such as vision, gave them special powers: They might see through solid objects, read minds, glimpse interior organs and even diagnose disease. Even though cataleptics were apparently dead, all their other senses and all movement having been extinguished, their vision had merely been transported to the area of the stomach and the tips of the fingers and toes, and from there was observing the external world.[26]

The presentation of hysterical catalepsy was very much a product of Petetin's own medical vision. On December 23 of an unstated year, he was called to see a married woman of nineteen who had been having fits and now seemed dead. Suddenly, before the eyes of her astonished parents, she arose and began singing. Next she began convulsing (giving rise to the diagnosis hysteria). Four men could scarcely hold her. Petetin plunged her into a cold bath, where she recovered. She was put into bed, thereupon fainting. Petetin gave her a tobacco enema. She began singing again. After much furor, he discovered he could communicate with her by speaking not to her ears but to her stomach. Petetin had established that "the sense of hearing, destroyed in its proper organ, has been transported to the region of the stomach." He realized that catalepsy did not just mean loss of movement.

The next day the young woman's husband urgently summoned Petetin again: His wife had been singing loudly for half an hour and could hear only through her stomach (a first triumph of medical suggestion). Just speaking to her stomach did not now suffice, so Petetin addressed that organ through a kind of speaking tube formed by his hands, which stopped the singing.

Why was she singing? To distract herself from the spectacle of being able to see her entire insides. He discovered he could also speak to her through the tips of her fingers and toes. In the course of the illness she produced many more symptoms, all of which could be abolished through the development of similarly new techniques. It became evident that the ferocity of her symptoms stood in direct proportion to the number of minutes that had passed since someone had attended to her, for Petetin noted at one point, "After I had ceased to occupy myself with her for five or six minutes, she would begin to hum, and as nothing was to be feared so much as her starting to sing again, I would speak with her at once." She began seeing into Petetin's body, knowing by clairvoyance when he had a headache. She even successfully predicted the course of his headaches.

In addition to these psychic symptoms, she produced a number of physical ones, such as "remarkable weakness in the lower limbs, being unable to stand upright on her legs. If she persisted in the effort, she would break into a convulsive cough up to the point of suffocation." The attacks of catalepsy occurred regularly throughout the day, three in the morning and two in the evening. Petetin, beginning to tire of the case, now ardently desired a resolution, and finally cured her by putting his hand on her head and breathing into her nostrils. After a week of this, the catalepsy disappeared.[27]

Petetin did not treat her with mesmeric "passes," but it was evident to readers of his book that similar patients might be cured with electrotherapy or with animal magnetism. The book was widely read among physicians and evidently among patients as well. One medical reader of Petetin was Charles Despine, whose father, Joseph Despine, had in 1787 become medical director of the decrepit spa at Aix-les-Bains, then called Aix-en-Savoie, accomplishing a highly successful renewal. Charles was born in 1775, got his M.D. in 1800, and after helping his father for thirty years succeeded him as director of the spa in 1830. In 1825, as part of the vogue for animal magnetism, Charles hypnotized his first patient.[28]

What kinds of patients were attracted to Aix in these years? There was Françoise Millet, of a nearby mountain village, twenty-three at the time she had "a fright," upon which she started having attacks of catalepsy. These attacks continued for four years. When Doctor Revil of Faverge came to her village, people spoke of *la morte* (the dead woman). Revil saw her and diagnosed "the disease described by Petetin." In 1820, now thirty-three, she came to Aix to take the waters. Her chief complaints: "Apparent death, insensibility, hearing at epigastrium and at her feet." When awakened from the *crise,* she had no memory of her symptoms. She also had visions of monsters, hell, sorcerers, and little figures carrying candles.[29]

Mlle. Annette de Roussillon of Grenoble was more typical of the middle-class patients of Aix. Her family had lost all its money in the tumult of the end of Napoleon's reign. When she was seen at Aix in 1822 at age twenty, she demonstrated all the symptoms of "catalepsy, ecstasy, hysteria and somnambulism." ("Ecstasy" meant a kind of trance or state of rapture.[30]) All her senses had been transported to various bodily organs. When not in crisis, she had a partial paralysis (hemiplegia), but while in somnambulism walked quite normally. She could read easily with her fingers or copy letters in the dark. She saw the walls of her room as "diaphanous as glass," and could also see far away, having "double vision of the Hebrides."[31] Among the thirteen patients on whom Doctor Charles Despine reported in detail, there were many such stories. These patients had clearly been suggested into catalepsy by friends, neighbors, or previous medical attendants.

One patient of Doctor Despine's, however, was of particular interest: Micheline Viollet, a twenty-one-year-old seamstress from Annecy, seen in 1823 and who returned in following years as well. She had developed various nervous symptoms *("lypothimies")*, for which local physicians in Annecy had treated her without success. One had almost amputated her left breast after it became painful and discolored. Because she had heard of Françoise Millet and of another cataleptic patient successfully treated at Aix, she had decided to seek help there herself. Having no money, she was hired as a servant in Doctor Despine's home.

Micheline up to this point had symptoms of ecstasy and somnambulism, but no sign of catalepsy until it was suggested to her. The symptoms appeared suddenly after a visiting physician said to Doctor Despine, apparently within earshot of Micheline, "But if there's no catalepsy, why do you call these patients cataleptics?"

"Because," said Despine, "if these phenomena that one considers as characteristic of catalepsy do not yet exist, they surely will one day appear." Micheline thereupon developed hers.

Micheline and the other patients began spinning for themselves a kind of subculture of catalepsy, a subculture that ultimately would take magnetic phenomena somewhat beyond Despine's medical control. Micheline had an assertive personality: If someone she did not like looked at her, she would instantly become immobile with catalepsy. She and another patient, Nanette Roux, began creating their own language with each other while *en crise*. Micheline also evidenced great interest in therapeutics, as she could not stand "galvanism," meaning electrotherapy from a battery or the application to the body of metal plates. Static electricity turned her rigid as a statue. But she had her own *formules magnétiques* to cure pain and to plunge herself into "lethargy."[32] At this point Micheline vanished from the published sources.

Years passed. In September 1844 a Mme. Joséfine L. of Neuchâtel and Geneva wrote to Charles Despine, asking if she might come as a patient. Twenty-nine at the time, with several children and unhappily married to a Swiss businessman who frequently was abroad, Mme. L. was a "spa-shopper," going continuously from spa to spa, or doctor to doctor, until she finally found one who would recognize how sick she really was ("No one can understand my sufferings," she wrote). In 1844 she had started at the new private clinic in Boppard am Rhein that Doctor Schmitz had opened four years before. Then after a spat with Schmitz she moved on to Albisbrunn, a small spa near Zurich. Now she needed someone who could restore her magnetic fluid. When she arrived in Aix in September 1844, she complained of a bad headache *(le clou hystérique)* and various neuralgic pains. She had tried to magnetize herself but was too exhausted and upset to succeed. "I only succeed in recycling vitiated fluid which does me no good: I have quite a lot [of fluid] but it is badly distributed. I believe that it has accumulated in my heart and, on the basis of my mental suffering, in my head too."[33]

Mme. L. had no need to come to Aix to immerse herself in a culture of magnetism: She brought it with her. She had read Petetin and discussed learnedly with Despine the thesis that cataleptics are able to view glass only through the eyes of other people about them. Shortly after she arrived in Aix, the mother of Pauline, one of Dr. Despine's servants-cum-healers, had just died. Mme. L. wanted to hypnotize Pauline to help her deal with her grief, but Pauline refused. Later on Mme. L. did experiments on the feet of her servants, making magnetic gestures with her fingers and then glimpsing "vapor" at the tips of the toes. She even wrote to an unspecified member of the Bernoulli dynasty of mathematicians and scientists, soliciting his opinion on some point. Mme. L. had clearly immersed herself in magnetic and cataleptic lore. She signed one of her letters to Despine, "votre . . . cataléptique Joséfine."

Mme. L.'s life in Aix illustrates the culture of suggestion surrounding magnetism, as well as establishing the profoundly neurotic nature of many of the patients, such as Mme. L. herself, who sought out this scene. Mme. L. settled into a comfortable life of bathing, electric sessions, and magnetization. She was constantly symptomatic and reproached everyone for ignoring her condition or making it worse. On November 16, 1844: "A thousand excuses my dear Doctor that I have been unable to come to the 11 a.m. appointment to be electrified. Pauline proposes, and my nerves dispose. In arising from bed my legs, though wanting to do so, refuse to carry me and collapse." On November 24: "This morning I have been tortured by pains and spasmodic cramps from the uterus that bend me in half. I am unable to find a position in which I am comfortable. My cupping *[vésication]* was so painful that I asked Pauline to forget the second round. The first was very productive and, given that it yielded much water and stuff *[matière]*, I thought it would suffice for two." But perhaps Pauline might magnetize her instead, she asked. It emerged by mid-December, in fact, that Pauline was really in charge of the case.

In March 1845, after Mme. L. returned to Aix for further treatment, her letters took on an increasingly irritable note:

"If I had known that you were coming immediately after my bath," she wrote Despine, "I wouldn't have been so alarmed. I become worse after the slightest noise; the slightest upset is hurtful to me, and you, without thinking of my poor nerves which are in these circumstances so irritated, you turn on all your electric machines! You rush about me while the slightest vibration of the air exhausts me, and what is worse you permeate me with your fluid! [She had refused to let Doctor Despine magnetize her because his fluid was "too old."] Then you rustle a newspaper after the noise of the machine! All that just for much too long and how could I not have suffered. Martyr!!!"

Mme. L., for all her exasperating personality, demonstrated some sensitivity to psychological motivation. She lectured Despine: "To cure a disease like mine, you have to remove the memory of the causes that produced it." She cheerfully admitted to Despine that her husband bored her and that she would like to find a wealthy replacement at Aix. "You understand," she wrote Despine on May 6, 1845, "how urgent it is for me to get well before decrepitude sets in." She also had little time for her children, and would have liked to find a wealthy spinster to take on one of them.

By September 1845, Mme. L. was quite depressed, or perhaps merely awash in self-pity. "My poor nerves are so excited and irritated that my limbs are constantly stiff." She complained of the noise in her inn. "I have repeatedly asked the Duvernays [the innkeepers] to put sand in the laneways of the garden because the noise of the gravel underfoot is insupportable. They have promised to do it but haven't done it. . . . Are you going to come see me soon? Please put on a suit as little impregnated with the emanations of others as possible."

Mme. L.'s stay at Aix also reflects the theme of women's empowerment through magnetism to the status of "healers." Not only did Mme. L. consider herself simultaneously a patient and a healer, but the servants became healers as well. In September 1845 and possibly sooner, Micheline Viollet was succoring Mme. L., who had momentarily rejected Pauline's fluid as too weak. Thus it emerged that Micheline, who came to Aix as a patient in 1823 at the age of twenty-one, now twenty-two years later and still a servant of Despine's, had become an important magnetizer. Until Mme. L.'s final departure Micheline and Pauline often magnetized her.

On September 9, 1846, Doctor Despine bade Mme. L. farewell. After a few pleasantries he expressed the hope that she would find a doctor

such as you desire. . . . The doctor that you need is one who remains waiting at the door and portico, who will accept all your whims and little tasks attentively [she had constantly asked Despine to intervene with the innkeeper etc.], who will be able to bow to your will, if I might say so. You need a doctor who will occupy himself with you alone and whose nervous and magnetic effluents are in sympathy with yours. This may not be easy to find.

We all understand you more or less, although you may have a different opinion. But everybody is simply not able to bow to the demands you feel appropriate for your nervous state . . . and which actually are quite characteristic of another kind of disorder. In this regard you will never be in agreement with your physicians, given that your needs, which you believe to be wholly immutable, are actually quite fleeting and subject to change. . . . As for those *monsters of perfidy* [*scélérates*] as you call them, Pauline and Micheline, and the perfidious father Despine . . . oh well!

Doctor Despine wished Mme. L. a safe trip home.

There is no reason to think Mme. L. atypical of many middle-class spa-goers in the first half of the nineteenth century or Doctor Despine, in his belief in animal magnetism, atypical of physicians. Their encounter is distinctive merely because his own published case records are more complete than most, and because this remarkable correspondence has survived. Several features in the encounter call for comment. Far from being a passive patient, Mme. L. took her own treatment immediately in hand; she knew what kind of magnetic fluid she wanted, and bent to Despine's medical authority only on the subjects of baths and electrotherapy. Thus there was little of the passive woman about her. Second, she possessed an unshakable illness attribution: maldistribution of magnetic fluid, fluid that, moreover, required renewal by sturdy servant magnetizers. Third, even though she was only twenty-nine, she displayed all the characteristics of a confirmed valetudinarian, and although we do not know what happened to her (save that she died at sixty-two), she may well have progressed to further years of spa shopping and complaining about others' lack of comprehension of her condition. Fourth, the case demonstrates the extent to which the culture of animal magnetism offered self-confident young women such as Micheline and Pauline the ability to advance their status by virtue of their superior "magnetic fluid": It was Micheline and Pauline who administered day-to-day care to Mme. L. and who made important clinical judgments about bleeding and the transfer of fluid.

Finally, Mme. L. evidenced a feature of catalepsy that would ultimately lead to its downfall as a diagnosis: the ease with which one could swing in and out of it, a plasticity that suggested it was a mannerism rather than an underlying second state.

In Paris, the psychodrama of catalepsy unfolded itself regularly among the fashionable. The case of young Caroline, a seventeen-year-old patient in Alexandre Brierre de Boismont's private asylum in the mid-1850s, must have caused many a medical eyebrow to rise. Her problems had begun with pain in her left neck and shoulder three years ago, segueing into aphonia, to refusing food, and then to the typical phenomena of catalepsy. Now in Brierre's establishment, she might begin the day at 6:30 by suddenly ceasing to talk, lying on her left side and sighing repeatedly "hou-hou," all the while insensible to external impressions, her eyes fixed. This cataleptic state might suddenly, however, give way to bounding about the room or to ecstasy.

Brierre described the case to the editors of a medical weekly. Several of its editorial board came to inspect. When, for example, Laurent Cerise, a well-known psychiatrist, came for an interview, Caroline first received him normally, then began producing *"ses petites exstases,"* meaning suddenly throwing her head back with her mouth open and the like. Cerise attempted to calm her "with a few magnetic passes," producing on the spot "electric jolts and complete insensibility to the outside world." In this condition she started bouncing back and forth from her bed to the carpet, "rolling in every direction and jumping into the air a number of times, meanwhile engaged in prolonged whistling. Sobs gave way to bursts of laughter. Then these symptoms were replaced by the exhausting convulsive cough characteristic of hysterics. After going on for half an hour, these symptoms stopped and Mlle. Caroline fell into an ecstatic pose reminiscent of the seraphic form of Saint Thérèse. Monsieur Cerise and I," wrote Brierre, "we just looked at each other." Both were thinking that if the people of Paris could see this, there would be an epidemic of hysteria.[34]

Wilhelm Schlesinger, a Viennese physician visiting Paris in 1857, gave a scathing account of Baron Jules Dupotet's stage magnetism in the Salon Vauxhall:

> We see cataleptics by the dozen. The magnetizers put the limbs of the magnetized in positions and directions that defy all laws of gravity and mechanics. The hands and feet of a child's doll could not remain longer and stiffer in a given position. . . . On another side of the stage we see some magnetized person following with unbreakable magnetic force her magnetizer. He goes up to her and away, turns to the right and left, runs and stands still, the magnetized person follows him like an automaton with no sign of expression, like the shadow of his own body.

144

A thirteen-year-old girl, "dressed up like an Easter lamb," caught Schlesinger's eye in particular. She reminded him of a wax figure in Mme. Tussaud's in London. Under the magnetizer's commands, she kept flipping back and forth from cataleptic insensibility (not moving an eyelash at the approaching candle) to the preternatural cheerfulness of ecstasy.[35] Reports such as these caused catalepsy to become a medical embarrassment. A previously legitimate second state now seemed little more than a magician's stage trick.

Physicians stopped reporting catalepsy and stopped diagnosing it. Articles on catalepsy in the international medical press declined from a high point of forty-four in 1870–79 to five in 1880–89. Thereafter the *Index-Catalogue* of the surgeon general's office abandoned the rubric as a category for reporting.[36] And once doctors stopped believing in catalepsy, patients seeking symptoms of dissociation would stop becoming stiff as a board with all consciousness apparently abolished—another reminder of the unconscious mind's reluctance to make itself ridiculous.

Yet several core physical phenomena in catalepsy remained. The Bordeaux surgeon Étienne Eugène Azam, whose work, beginning in 1860, is generally viewed as anticipating the second wave of hypnotism rather than harking back to the first, defined catalepsy as muscular contractility instead of death spells and the like. Patients might hold poses for fifteen to twenty minutes, noted Azam (rather than "forever"), without getting tired.[37] In retrospect, this kind of heightened contractility can perhaps be understood as a result of hyperventilation, for people who breathe rapidly reduce the amount of carbon dioxide in their blood, so that their muscles may go into spasm among other consequences. It is clear that many of the patients producing these phenomena were hyperventilating.

Some unspecified proportion of previous catalepsy would turn out to be the catatonia of such major mental diseases as schizophrenia. For a while the two words were used interchangeably. Claude-Étienne Bourdin, for example, director of a private psychiatric clinic in Paris, commented on the presence of catalepsy in a patient with "chronic mania" (an old-fashioned term for psychosis generally rather than for mania in the modern sense): "Sometimes he struck the most bizarre and difficult poses and remained in them for a long time."[38] In 1876 George Savage, the London psychiatrist, described catalepsy in several young insane male patients. "All will pass into dementia and cease to be cataleptic," said Savage with the voice of experience.[39] These were in all likelihood schizophrenic young men (the term had not yet been coined) whose bodily postures would later be described as catatonia.

Finally, in the late 1920s and early 1930s, the term catalepsy experienced a brief revival as Henri Claude and Henri Baruk used it to draw together a variety of psychogenic and neurogenic symptoms.[40] But by then it had been shorn of the elements of circus.

The whole story of catalepsy illustrates the ability of doctors to impose a set of symptoms on patients. We began with trancelike second states stemming from "physical" magnetic energy in the body and ended with circus-style performers putting suggestible individuals into catalepsy on stage. Millions of people came to believe implicitly in, and reproduce the symptoms of, medical ideas that had no more foundation in science than did astrology. Yet catalepsy was sold to the public as scientific doctrine, and because people believed in science, their unconscious minds manufactured symptoms appropriate to keep them abreast of the march of progress.

Induced Somnambulism

Just as with catalepsy, in which patients assumed extraordinary powers over their motor systems, even to the point of bringing on death, somnambulism, too, changed its characteristics during the first wave of hypnotism. It became seen as a disease condition that could be artificially induced or abolished with hypnosis. It also acquired the feature of clairvoyance, being able to see or hear conversations taking place in other parts of town, other cities, to see one's own internal organs or those of others, and to see into the future.

An early instance of the new, hypnotic somnambulism occurred in May 1803 as Doctor Fischer of Halle treated a young man of twenty who had a yearlong history of fits associated with emotional upset. As a prodrome, or foreshadowing, of the attacks the patient noticed an increased repugnance toward everything made out of metal, especially copper. But if he took sulfur he might abort the attacks. The patient also reported a history of natural somnambulism. His friends had treated him with animal magnetism for some previous attacks, and the young man now requested that Doctor Fischer magnetize him.

During a typical magnetic session, the patient felt a kind of welcome fog envelop him. This fog, he said, protected him from disagreeable persons, but if such persons (namely all women and children) came within ten to fifteen paces of him, he would begin convulsing. The patient explained this phenomenon as a "violation of his fog." But if older and stronger men penetrated the fog and touched him, the patient found this agreeable. Even in waking, he preferred the company of strong individuals and avoided persons "who were weakly organized."

Among other phenomena accompanying the young man's fog was a terrible burning sensation whenever the doctor placed his own head against the patient's spine. There were also many sensations surrounding water: regular water was cold, magnetized water lukewarm.

In this phase of a magnetic session he would see his own internal organs. He described, for example, his spinal column, also what Doctor Fischer interpreted as "the sympathetic trunk," a bundle of nerves running down the back of the body.[41] Herewith Fischer echoed a most interesting note, one struck already by the marquis de Puységur's patients: the ability to see one's internal organs under induced somnambulism. If one could see one's own organs, one could also see those of others. From there it was a quick step to diagnosis and treatment, all of which had the result of taking the management of somnambulistic patients who were clairvoyant from the hands of the magnetizing physician, who himself lacked this X-ray vision, and placing it in the hands of the patient.

The best known of such patients who become "physicians" is a classic of literature—the twenty-one-year-old Friedrike Hauffe, from the village of Prevorst in Württemberg. She was born in 1801, the daughter of a local forester. At some point after her engagement at nineteen, she became depressed. It was after her marriage in 1822 that she had the first of her clairvoyant dreams, initiating a whole "magnetic life." Soon after the dream she came down with a fever and within two weeks of the wedding had gone into an apparent coma. A peasant woman appeared to her with the message "Trust no doctor." (It should be said at this point that Friedrike would die seven years later of what might well have been tuberculosis, and that throughout these episodes she had a major organic illness. So her symptoms may not be reduced to somatization alone but seen additionally as perhaps a febrile delirium or even the result of the spread of TB to the brain. However, this gets ahead of the story.)

The months ahead were filled with "nervous" symptoms, abnormal internal perceptions, and histrionic behavior. In her clairvoyance she foresaw her grandfather's death. The psychological and the physical were clearly interwoven in her illness, as is true of most illnesses.

Four years later, on November 25, 1826, she was brought to see Dr. Justinus Kerner in the nearby town of Weinsberg. Kerner, forty at the time, was extremely interested in animal magnetism, having two years previously published a small work on two somnambulists. Sensing in Friedrike an opportunity to deepen his knowledge of the phenomenon, he took her on as a boarder in his home. Thus some of her subsequent behavior was possibly the result of medical shaping, given Kerner's ardent expectations of what somnambulism should be. That very evening at seven o'clock she fell into a "magnetic sleep." She got steadily worse under the standard medical treatments of the time and, a picture of death, pleaded for Kerner to magnetize her. On December 22 a colleague of Kerner's arrived and administered "seven magnetic passes." From this point her remission began. Kerner now took to magnetizing her himself.

She believed herself highly sensitive to various metals and to glass. "Protracted staring at a glass window would produce cataleptic rigidity," Kerner noted. She reacted to substances in different ways:

> The sight of a diamond affected the eyes of the clairvoyant [die Seherin] in the most remarkable way. If I put a small, almost weightless, unset stone into her hand, her eyes involuntarily flew wide open, and the eyeballs stared forth immovably, whereby simultaneously the left hand and the right foot became rigid. As the diamond was replaced by barite, the eyeballs began to roll uncontrollably. Rubies aroused a feeling initially of arm pain, then a restless, involuntary movement, finally a feeling of cold and heaviness in the tongue, permitting only mumbling speech.[42]

One gets the feeling of a climate of suggestion in the Kerner home.

Most striking in the young clairvoyant, however, was her ability to see spirits, to have prophetic dreams, to step out of her own body and see it as though from afar, and to see the inner parts of the body as well. Because she could see into bodies, she also made medical diagnoses and prescribed therapy for Kerner's other patients. A man in Weinsberg, for example, a heavy drinker, was currently in his third episode of delirium tremens and could not be quieted with opium. "Therefore Frau H. prescribed for him in her somnambulic state: an infusion of five spoonfuls of linden blossoms in seventeen spoonfuls of boiling water, added to which while still warm a drachm of castoreum with five spoonfuls of birch sap. The entirety must be taken from seven in the morning to seven in the evening.

"Then she gave in her pythic manner the following rhyme," said Kerner, reproducing it in his account:

> He is no longer master
> of
> His hands and feet,
> They tremble and
> stumble

His brain's all a
mumble.
But let him not yelp,
I'll give him some help:
I say, drink this right up!
Then he'll feel a treat,
He'll sleep and he'll eat
And get out of the
house!

"Thus it came to pass," continued Kerner. "After the confused man drank this infusion he fell into a long and ardently desired sleep, which no opium could have elicited, woke up a day later, and was well again."[43]

The young clairvoyant performed numerous other such feats of diagnosis and prescription, acquiring for these and for her apparent ability to see far away and predict the future, a great local following. However, her career as clairvoyant was cut short by her death in 1829.

The ability of somnambulists to diagnose and prescribe for each other's complaints encouraged a whole subculture of somnambulism in places where the sick congregated. Salomon Stiebel, a physician in Frankfurt and advocate of animal magnetism, ran a small clinic in the years after the Napoleonic Wars that seems to have been filled with young women who believed themselves somnambulic. Marianne S., age twenty, from Würzburg, whom Stiebel magnetized twice daily, was terribly sensitive to metal. One night she found a needle sticking in her nightdress:

> She sprang angrily from bed, ran to the window, smashed in the pane, and would surely have jumped out if [her roommate] Fanny had not had sufficient presence of mind—or the magnetic instinct—to save her. Fanny ran quickly up to her, grabbed her about the body and blew some of the good [magnetic] energy into her mouth which I had blown into [Fanny's] mouth. Thus Marianne calmed herself, found the needle and hurled it away. Fanny however collapsed in a faint to the floor and recovered fully only the next morning when I magnetized her.[44]

Both Marianne and Fanny, with their long lists of nervous symptoms, found themselves plunged not just into a medical climate of suggestion, but into a whole ready-made patients' subculture of somnambulism.

Among Dr. Charles Despine's patients at Aix-en-Savoie in the 1820s or 1830s was a Russian officer, Count D., whose very glance electrified the young women, including a certain Mlle. Isaure. He then began making systematic magnetic maneuvers with his hands: ". . . A few *passes calmantes* about Mlle. Isaure's epigastrium and precordial region, from the distance of five or six inches, sufficed to assuage her atrocious pains . . . pains which ordinarily were suspended only during catalepsy or ecstasy." In fact Count D., himself a patient, took over entirely from Doctor Despine the medical management of Mlle. Isaure.[45]

In 1859 Maurice Macario, describing the patients in his clinic *(institut hydrothérapeutique)* at Serin near Lyon, told the story of Mme. C., age twenty-six, subject to faintings and paralyses since childhood. Having come in paralyzed, she was cured in his clinic after twelve days of hydrotherapy. "It might be remarked," he said, "that from the beginning of her admission to the clinic, this lady was magnetized by one of our male patients, and that under the influence of his *passes magnétiques,* her legs, which customarily were cold, became warm again, feeling returned, and from the next day on she walked better." Mme. C. herself attributed her recovery to being magnetized.[46]

Patients may have found the subculture of somnambulism so appealing, and the assumption of its symptoms so congenial, because in the very nature of induced somnambulism lay the possibility for patients and other nonphysicians to control diagnosis and treatment. And this, in turn, may be one reason why physicians themselves turned against hypnosis in the years after 1900.

The Second Wave of Hypnosis

In the first wave of hypnosis, catalepsy and somnambulism were seen as underlying conditions that could be liberated by animal magnetism, and not as products of suggestion. The first wave therefore augmented considerably the number of motor symptoms, for catalepsy was primarily a motor phenomenon, and even somnambulism—with its inward inspection of the body and the like—generated large numbers of fits and paralyses. The logic of the second wave, however, was entirely different.[47] In the second wave, catalepsy and somnambulism would be shunned as phenomena more appropriate to the circus than to the sickroom. Instead the patient was seen as a kind of empty vessel into which the physician could inject "suggestions" of choice. Rather than there being underlying behavior, such as death spells, ready to explode to the surface, in the second wave the patient was the passive recipient of whatever the doctor deemed medically appropriate. The second wave therefore downplayed motor phenomena and upgraded symptoms on the sensory side. This valorization of sensory symptoms reached its apex with the work of Jean-Martin Charcot. But before turning to Charcot, it is interesting to look at the revival of medical hypnotism in Central Europe and among the "Nancy school" after 1880, and at its impact on the occurrence of psychosomatic symptoms.

Hypnotism underwent an enormous expansion between 1880 and 1900. The number of publications on animal magnetism, somnambulism, and hypnotism listed in the *Index-Catalogue* of the surgeon general rose tenfold, from 54 in 1870–79 to 542 in 1880–89, and then a further 28 percent to 694 in 1890–99. In 1880–89 appeared as well another 116 articles on "suggestion"—a category that had not been used previously— by which was meant mainly hypnotism. If the expansion of the literature is any indication of medical interest, doctors' increased use of hypnotism in the 1880s and after does indeed justify the notion of a second wave.

This second wave burst on Central Europe in the year 1880, in a curious juxtaposition of old and new.[48] The "old" impetus was a series of lecture tours in 1879 and in 1880 by a nonphysician named Carl Hansen, a Danish stage magnetizer.[49] The format was always the same: Hansen would invite a number of men from the audience up to the podium, "put them on chairs with their backs to the audience, and place in the hand of each a glass ball. The subject was then to hold the glass ball up to his forehead and stare fixedly at it. Hansen himself would go from one to the other, making a few gestures and passes in the faces of the subjects. As a rule, after five to ten minutes, the subjects, assured by Hansen that this would happen, began to experience a convulsive kind of clenching of the jaw muscles. This then led to the actual hypnotic state, which Hansen would use for further experiments.

"He would lift the subject's arm and make passes over it with his hand; thereupon immediately all [arm] muscles would become rigid. No amount of force could press down the arm or flex it." Thus Hansen, like all the stage magnetizers, put his subjects first into catalepsy and then started doing tricks with them for the audience's benefit: for example, laying the subjects, who were rigid as boards, between two chairs and sitting on them as though on a bench, without the subjects moving in the slightest. Then with a few more passes he would abolish the cataleptic rigidity and induce hallucinations: "Now he would give a potato to one of the gentlemen with the solid assurance that it was an apple, and tell him to eat it. To the great amusement of the audience the unfortunate victim would bite into the potato and relish it with all evidence of contentment." There were other wondrous experiments: telling one man that he was a lady and should act accordingly, making someone else forget his name, and so forth.[50] This was the act that Hansen brought to Germany and Austria.

In 1879 Hansen toured Chemnitz, among other places, and several of the physicians in the audience became quite impressed by these phenomena, trying to investigate them further.[51] The ice was truly broken, however, toward New Year's Day, 1880, as Hansen returned to the Silesian capital of Breslau for a repeat performance. The populace of Breslau was already swept by enthusiasm for animal magnetism, and schoolchildren were going around making passes and throwing each other into hysterical fits. So great was the mania that a local physician, Sanitätsrat (an honorary title meaning health counselor) Doctor Eger, published a brief article in a local newspaper denouncing Hansen as a charlatan. After the appearance of this article Hansen invited all the local physicians to a special "magnetic matinée."

"Among the first, Hansen asked old Sanitätsrat Eger to climb onto the podium, and he became one of the first to fall into complete hypnosis. Before the eyes of his astonished colleagues, he ate the famous potato, became a nanny and lovingly rocked to sleep in his arms a block of wood. In short, he abandoned himself totally to the will of the hypnotizer."[52] Twenty physicians had climbed onto the podium. Dr. Traugott Kroner, on the staff of the university's gynecology clinic, was unable to open his eyes or his jaw after being hypnotized. Thereupon told to open his jaw, he was no longer able to close it. His colleague Dr. Ernst Fränkel had no better luck.[53]

The sight of old Sanitätsrat Eger rocking to sleep a piece of wood or Doctor Fränkel struggling with his jaw convinced the assembled physicians that hypnosis was something extraordinary. As a consequence, several members of the medical faculty began doing their own hypnotic experiments. For example Professor Oskar Berger, the neurologist, was conducting experiments one day when Professor Hermann Cohn, his assistants trailing behind him, strode into the room and demanded that Berger hypnotize him too. "[Cohn] stared only briefly at the glass ball that Berger gave him, then fell over backwards with all his muscles rigidly extended. Quickly pulled up by the bystanders, Cohn was awakened when Berger blew into his face [the customary method at that time] and immediately regained his feet smiling. He had not hurt himself, and had no idea what had happened."[54] On March 6, 1880, Berger published an article on his research in one of the main German medical weeklies, including the transference of symptoms from one side of the body to the other.[55] Already on January 19 Berger's colleague, physiologist Rudolf Heidenhain, had lectured to a local group on the result of his own researches.[56] The professoriate was coming out in favor of hypnotism as a genuine scientific phenomenon that would permit further understanding of the nervous system. The second wave had been launched.

In early February 1880 Hansen appeared in Vienna. The performance did not go well, as one of the subjects, a chemist, refused to be hypnotized and denounced Hansen as a swindler. Other experiments also failed, and the evening ended in tumult among the audience.[57] Perhaps it was on this evening that Sigmund Freud was present, for he later wrote, "While still a student I attended a public performance of the 'magnetizer' Hansen and noted that one of the subjects became pale as death as she went into cataleptic rigidity and remained so throughout the episode. Therewith I became firmly convinced of the genuineness of hypnotic phenomena."[58] Although the initial reception of hypnotism in Vienna was much cooler than in Breslau,[59] Hansen's seeds did not fall on infertile soil. In the 1840s the medical faculty had been wild for hypnotism, and in the 1860s and 1870s hypnotism still had an avid representative in the form of Moritz Benedikt. Benedikt himself had started doing hypnosis in 1867 when he, a young neurologist from Eisenstadt, was only thirty-two. Over the years he had magnetized many patients, including the mother of the psychoanalyst Rudolf von Urbantschitsch (whom he sometime in the 1870s unsuccessfully tried to cure of sleepwalking with a real magnet). Thus, in the spring of 1880 Benedikt greeted Hansen's arrival with some satisfaction. What did it matter that we do not understand the exact mechanism of the phenomenon? he said. If we insisted on knowing mechanisms, we would have to rule out most drugs.[60] Benedikt always had a taste for the florid phenomena of old-style hypnotism and had told Hansen, perhaps on the 1880 visit, "I have the gift of communication at great distances, and I can easily reach South Africa."[61] But now in 1880 he downplayed the dramatic excesses of catalepsy and wished to see his colleagues adopt hypnotism.

Benedikt was only an honorary member of the professoriate, but by 1885 a real professor, psychiatrist Heinrich Obersteiner, was addressing Vienna's "Scientific Club" on the subject of hypnotism. Obersteiner was evidently using it therapeutically in his private nervous clinic in the Viennese suburb of Ober-Döbling.[62] Six years later Obersteiner said that the staff of his clinic had been doing some hypnotism and suggestion but that psychotic patients were accessible to neither. Nervous patients, however, responded to some extent to hypnotism.[63] (Freud was briefly an assistant physician at the clinic during this time.) Obersteiner also believed in thought reading.[64]

Richard von Krafft-Ebing, Vienna's other famous psychiatrist, said he had used hypnotism only a few times, mainly for hysteria and morphinism.[65] Perhaps it was more than just a few, for Krafft-Ebing had founded in 1886 in Graz-Kroisbach a private clinic named Mariagrün. Some of the "psychic therapy" used there was probably hypnotism. Two of his students, who had taken over the direction of the clinic after Krafft-Ebing's departure for Vienna in 1889, said that the clinic employed "psychic influencing," "psychic treatment," and the like in disorders as diverse as depression and constipation.[66] All those terms meant psychotherapy but at the time had the flavor of hypnotism about them.[67] Thus hypnotism implanted itself solidly in Austria in the 1880s.

Many of the big names in Central European psychiatry now became associated with hypnotism. In 1887 Albert Moll, who had just witnessed Jean-Martin Charcot's demonstrations of hypnotism at the Salpêtrière in Paris as well as those of the "Nancy school," beat the drums for hypnosis in Germany and could take credit for introducing it to Berlin at least, if not all of Germany as he claimed.[68] Among other influential figures using hypnotism late in the 1880s were the German psychiatrist Emil Kraepelin, while still at the University of Tartu (Dorpat), Estonia (a German-speaking university at the time), psychiatrist Paul Julius Möbius in Leipzig, and even the previously skeptical internist Karl Anton Ewald in Berlin.[69] And there was August Forel, the Zurich professor of psychiatry who had always counted as the grand old man of the movement.[70]

Once the professors had lined up on behalf of hypnotism, it became stripped of the parapsychological and the mystical, becoming reduced instead to a form of suggestion little different from persuasive conversation. The psychic phenomena that previously had accompanied catalepsy and somnambulism were hived off into a nonmedical subculture of "Societies for Psychical Research" and the like, whose enthusiasts would ultimately end up knocking on tables at séances and playing the Ouija board.[71] "Somnambulism" itself took on the narrow technical meaning of hypnotic sleep with amnesia. A "somnambulist" became, rather than a young woman who could predict the future, someone who was unable to recall what had happened under hypnosis.[72] Therewith the capacity of hypnotism to induce dramatic second states involving motor symptoms came to an end.

In fact, the "Nancy school," a group of family doctors and professors of medicine in Nancy who flourished in the 1880s and 1890s, saw hypnotism merely as another form of suggestion. The members of this school invoked no dissociations within the human brain as the mechanism of action of suggestion, treating suggestion as some kind of universal and self-understood psychological principle.[73] After 1890 the doctrines of the Nancy school won out over the competing theories of Charcot at the Salpêtrière.

Hypnosis itself would become steadily eroded by other competing forms of psychotherapy. In the surgeon general's *Index-Catalogue*, publications dealing with hypnosis declined from a high point of almost 700 in 1890–99 to 202 in 1900–1909, and 82 in 1910–19. Publications on psychotherapy, by contrast, rose from 38 in 1890–99 to 231 in 1900–1909.[74] And while some of this psychotherapy might still have been hypnosis, physicians were not shouting it from the rooftops. Whereas in the 1890s a number of Central European private clinics announced that they offered hypnotherapy, by 1913 barely a single one did. These highly competitive private sanatoriums no longer saw hypnosis as a card that would draw the public or interest the medical colleagues making referrals.[75]

After 1880 hypnosis, though greatly popular, ceased to be of much importance in shaping psychosomatic symptoms. Once the fits, paralyses, total body tremors, and beliefs about seeing inner organs were sheared away, little remained as a source of suggestion in and of itself. After the doctrine had become neutralized, physicians could use it to implant whatever suggestions they wished, and most of those would be therapeutic ones, entailing the abolition of preexisting paralyses and the like. There was, however, one big exception—hypnotism as practiced by Charcot at the Salpêtrière.

"Permanently Benumbed" and the Climate of Suggestion

The decline of medical hypnosis in the *belle époque* did not mean that patients had lost the belief that they were in second states, but merely that the form of dissociation took on guises other than motor symptoms. Two might briefly be mentioned: the belief that one is "going through life hypnotized" and multiple personality disorder. In the former, one is "permanently benumbed," a sensory complaint. The experience of "multiple personalities," by contrast, represents the kind of fixed, quasi-delusional belief about interior states that has come to characterize psychosomatic illness generally at the end of the twentieth century.

The heightened climate of suggestion that prevailed during the second wave of hypnotism, in particular, makes it easier to understand how individuals might acquire either of these beliefs. So much was hypnosis in the air that becoming hypnotized required little more than a bit of experience: One learned what was expected and then unconsciously did it. The experience of Marguérite M. at the Hôtel-Dieu Hospital in Marseilles illustrates the point about hypnotism as a product of suggestion. Born in Italy, she had moved to Marseilles at the age of fourteen to work as a servant. Six years later she experienced emotional distress surrounding a broken engagement and developed chronic vomiting and "hysterical crises" in the form of a ball rising from her abdomen into her throat. In November 1887 she was admitted to a local hospital, then transferred to the Hôtel-Dieu in January 1888. There, in keeping with her new environment, she displayed some muscular spasms, fits and the like, but they soon receded to permit the vomiting once again to dominate the picture.

Her doctors had treated the vomiting with standard remedies but to no avail. "Finally, tired of the struggle, we tried to hypnotize her but without success."

Now, at this point (in May 1888), another young woman was admitted to the ward, "a hysteric having major crises with delusions and hallucinations. Our patient was profoundly impressed by the tableau which she now had before her eyes. Her own 'crises d'hystérie,' which had almost entirely ceased in order to let the vomiting occupy center stage, returned, and she produced the whole range of convulsive hysteria, sometimes in just the standard form, sometimes in the epileptic form."

Within two weeks the staff were able to hypnotize this second patient. Marguérite at this point became hypnotizable as well. What is more, she loved it, developed florid kinds of nervous pathology, and further, began requesting her own hypnotization. Inserted into a hospital culture where one received medical attention as a reward for learning the proper roles, she learned her role vis-à-vis hypnosis. She also learned what was expected of her when a clinician approached with a magnet: When the magnet was held against her skull at the approximate location of Broca's motor speech area, she stopped talking.[76]

In the years after 1880 European culture as a whole was a bit like this microcosm of a hospital ward. The spirit of second states was in the air, and individuals easily acquired the belief that they were walking around in a more or less permanent state of hypnosis, to which they attributed their problems. This belief emerged often with delusional force among patients in psychiatric hospitals. At Holloway House, a private clinic for nervous diseases in Virginia Water near London, among sixty-five female patients admitted in 1889 to the closed wing, at least four had the fixed delusional belief that other people were galvanizing or electrifying them, synonyms in this context for magnetizing. Miss Clementine C., for example, fifty-three, "complains that she is galvanized by people, and that she is often made to shrink into a shape no bigger than her little finger. . . . She makes rambling accusations against a policeman, against a man named D. and other people whom she accuses of galvanizing and in other ways annoying her." On admission to hospital Mrs. Mary J., age forty-five, informed Dr. Francis Pearse, who signed the second certificate of admission, that "she was electrified every afternoon and that the doctor sent her up Otto [sic] of Roses every night." Mrs. Emily L., no age given, stated that, "she is galvanized by a society of the masonic type, and there is a league against her by means of which she has been locked up." Fanny H., a single woman of forty-six, had a history of erotomania, believing in an imaginary engagement to a Doctor D. She thought "the League" had prevented Doctor D. from marrying her, and that somebody, possibly the League, had electrified her and was using her as a medium.[77]

Nor were such beliefs the province of middle-class Englishwomen alone. Professor X, a world-renowned Viennese medical specialist in his field, was admitted in 1919 with a psychotic depression to the private-payment clinic of the Steinhof psychiatric hospital in Vienna. A sample of his rambling speech from the records of June 26: "The patient asserts that he has been hypnotized for a long time now. There is a consortium causing a buzzing and whirring in his head. Often, calling out 'Parmel' helps against the hypnotizing but gets rid of it only for a few minutes."[78] Thus European culture in these years was sufficiently filled with the doctrine of hypnosis for patients with major psychiatric disorders to seize it as an illness attribution.

For less seriously ill psychoneurotic patients as well, the conviction of being in an enduring second state was common. Perhaps Paul Sollier, chief physician at a private clinic for nervous diseases at Boulogne-sur-Seine, had a reputation for doing well with such cases, or perhaps the condition was merely widespread, but many of the young female patients he admitted to the clinic in the 1890s were convinced that they were going through life hypnotized, *engourdie* (benumbed) being the adjective they used. The case of Marguérite C., age twenty-six, who was admitted in 1892, conveys the flavor of this. She had a long history of generalized contractures, fits, and mutism, as well as of some hallucinations, and conformed generally to the profile of hysteria of the day.

Doctor Sollier interviewed her on November 13, 1893. A partial transcript follows:

Q: Do you feel your organs, do you feel your insides?

A: No, I don't feel anything at all.

Q: Do you feel you're alive?

A: I tell myself that if I died I wouldn't feel any different than right now. That wouldn't bother me. That's the reason you should just let me die.

Q: So nothing matters to you?

A: Absolutely nothing.

Q: And if I told you your brother had died?

A: Wouldn't bother me. Not at all. I don't know what's happened that I've become like this. There was a time when that would have bothered me, but not now.

(Sollier interjected for the reader: "She told me that whenever she injured herself it did not hurt. At sixteen she fell off a ladder, but despite having a large bruise, she did not feel anything.")

Q: When you aren't doing anything, what do you think about?

A: Nothing at all.

Q: What do you feel?

A: I think that I'm not alive at all, that I'm not on earth.

Q: What do you think about the objects around you?

A: They're very small. I see everyone very small. Sometimes one half is one color and the other half another. I don't know why that is. It's just like, when I work, I get things all turned around. [skipping a few questions]

Q: What do you feel in your head when you're talking?

A: It's almost a kind of buzzing.

Q: And what I'm saying, does that really register?

A: No, not at all.

Two weeks later Sollier hypnotized her, during which she told him that for a number of years now "she doesn't really know what she's doing. She doesn't feel any of her internal functions. She doesn't know if her heart beats or if she's breathing. She doesn't feel her stomach or her abdomen. Everything around her seems unfamiliar, she has no sense of time, nor things, nor persons. . . . She has no sense of the reality of things and 'lives as though in a dream.'"

Sollier awakened her and asked her point-blank: "During the day, when you're coming and going and working, are you asleep or are you awake?"

She hesitated and then answered, "I don't know. I always feel numb [*engourdie*]."

158

"Well, well," said Sollier, "since you don't know we're going to find out."

Sollier hypnotized her again, and told her that this time when she awakened it would be completely. He awakened her by blowing on her eyes.

She sat up, rubbed her eyes, and looked around, "Goodness, everything is so big!"

Her face lit up, said Sollier, instead of having that vague, fugitive look. She looked at everything close up, and then turned to Sollier, "Where am I? How long have I been here? It's funny, it's as if I were waking up. I can feel my heart beating, I can feel myself breathe."

She was bursting with questions. She did not recognize either the clinic or any of her friends, said Sollier. "She asked me my name and to explain how she had come here. She was astonished to see that she had her own room, a napkin with her name, that everyone knew her. I think she had been taken back to the time before her illness began, and I asked her today's date."

"But it's November 1890," she told him. It was, of course, 1893.

If this case were unusual among Sollier's patients, one might dismiss it as a bizarre anomaly. But he had numerous young female patients who believed themselves *engourdie*, or in a second state, and whom he awakened through hypnosis to their true selves. Sollier used for this condition the term (which Charcot had popularized) *vigilambulism*, meaning a fugue state in which, Sollier said, *"les grandes hystériques are plunged into generalized and profound anesthesia."*[79] In retrospect, these patients were plunged into a climate of suggestion in which believing oneself "benumbed," or *engourdie*, was considered a legitimate medical symptom. The surrounding culture had suggested Marguérite C. into the particular second state in which, she was persuaded, she found herself. She and her comrades were still physically symptomatic, but experienced the symptoms on the sensory side of the nervous system, a forward-looking sign, and not on the motor side as before.

Multiple Personality Disorder

It was from a similar brew of suggestibility that the diagnosis "multiple personality disorder" came. Although the diagnosis today is controversial—some authorities still consider it an independent disease entity—evidence is mounting that the production of multiple personalities is the result of medical shaping by the physician, or by the culture, of inchoate symptoms the patient is unable otherwise to make sense of.[80] For patients who see themselves in a second state, it is a relatively simple matter to give that state a name, and then perhaps to produce other states as well, each of which has a name and a distinctive "personality" of its own.

According to Henri Ellenberger, a believer in the reality of multiple personality disorder (MPD), the first well-documented case goes back to Estelle L'Hardy, one of Dr. Charles Despine's patients in Aix-en-Savoie.[81] Estelle, age eleven, came to the spa in Aix from her home in Neuchâtel in July 1836, complaining of a complete paraplegia. She had apparently always been a quick learner and had become very impressionable after her father's death in the Paris cholera epidemic of 1832. Two years after he died, she had suffered a minor fall on her back, thereupon developing a riot of psychosomatic symptoms. She was brought to Aix very dramatically, in a basket. The first five months of hydrotherapy produced little improvement, but when Despine began to magnetize her, the whole spectrum of catalepsy and ecstasy began to emerge. Now she alternated between her second state (état de crise) and her ordinary state. In the latter she was paralyzed and felt chilly, her spine highly sensitive. She was unable to arise from bed or change her diet without suffering horribly. In her second state, however, far from being chilly, she demanded ice-water baths. Indeed, snow bathing restored mobility to her "paralyzed limbs."

After her eighth magnetic session she became able, under hypnosis, to get out of bed, dress herself easily, and leap about in perfect health. She could eat everything except meat. But as soon as the hypnotic trance ended, she would return to her old state.

Like so many of the other cataleptics, Estelle was subject to extraordinary psychic phenomena. The ticking of clocks, for example, would put her in catalepsy. She felt her skin "burning" at the sight of a cat even far away. The same would occur if she were to touch silk or fur (this refers to cataleptic theories about "isoelectric bodies" and the circumstances under which they insulate magnetic forces). Her various senses were transposed to the area of her stomach and fingertips and to her elbow and shoulder. She was also able to read a printed text (Despine believed) with her fingers. Most fascinating for Pierre Janet, who resurrected the case from Despine's book (and later for such observers as Ellenberger), a second personality named "Angeline" emerged during her états de crise to direct the cure.[82] Said Despine, "Estelle is indeed a new type in the schema of neuralgias [névralgies], her disorder having neither been classified nor described."[83]

But Despine was referring more to Estelle's demanding manner and bizarrely changing symptoms than to her second personality (which was of more interest to her mother than to Despine personally). He alluded to having seen other patients produce "double existences." In a report on the spa he had issued to the Italian government in 1822 (Savoy belonged to Italy from 1815 until 1860), Despine recognized six distinctive states in a patient named Mlle. Annette De R., one of which was "an incomplete magnetic state which gave the patient an interior feeling of a second existence."[84] The context of Estelle's multiple personality disorder was therefore the theater of florid magnetism and catalepsy then prevailing at Aix. Many of the other patients were producing bizarre symptoms: it must have seemed to an intelligent young girl rather the order of the day that she bring forth some of her own.

Nor was Despine by any means the first to describe cataleptic or magnetized patients who had given names to their second states. One of the first on record dates from 1789. On November 2 of that year, Eberhard Gmelin, physician and celebrated magnetizer in Heilbronn, was called to Stuttgart to see a twenty-one-year-old woman who for several days had been experiencing attacks "in which she believes that, from the age of two on, she has been raised in a monastery in Paris and that she has recently fled to Stuttgart since the unrest there [the French Revolution]." Her family doctors in Stuttgart told Gmelin that for the last two weeks she had been experiencing curious little "crises," in which she would suddenly stop talking, remain unresponsive to questions, but ask people of both sexes to come and sit on her knee, "without considering this improper." When these attacks began, she complained of various physical symptoms, expressing her suffering with much deep staring into others' eyes and asking people, in French, "Can you not bear my look?"

She greeted Gmelin in French upon his arrival. Gmelin, without actually touching her, began making "magnetic" passes over her whole body with the flat of his palms. Now she came out of her second state and, "looking about with pleasant astonishment," began a "where-am-I" routine. She was again a simple German girl. Two minutes later Gmelin touched her lightly, returning her to the trance, and she turned back into a Frenchwoman. Not only were the doctors able to evoke one personality while awake and the other while in a trance, but during her hypnotically induced trances an additional personality emerged, that of "Monsieur Charpentier." Monsieur Charpentier then ceded to the personality of "a little boy." All this occurred in the presence of the three well-known physicians (Gmelin and her family doctors) and crowds of people.

When Gmelin departed Stuttgart the following day, he left instructions for further "magnetization" with the family doctors, who were able to bring her away from the idea that she was French, so that by November 6 she became completely normal and remained so thereafter. This episode, also celebrated as the first case of multiple personality on record, clearly owes more to the climate of suggestion surrounding animal magnetism than to a medical disorder.[85]

Men were not to be left out. In 1805, Dr. F. Fischer of Halle reported the case of a natural somnambulist, "whose personality becomes completely altered [*vertauscht*], he plays a totally different role as he does in the period of being awake." During somnambulism, this second personality was able to see the future, predict the course of attacks, and give instructions on treatment. This second personality "demonstrates in all physical and mental activity an agility and strength which the patient does not possess when awake."[86]

The subsequent nineteenth-century cases of multiple personality disorder on which the pedigree of the diagnosis rests today are well known. In June 1858 the Bordeaux surgeon Étienne Azam met a young woman named Félida X, who went on to have a long and possibly factitious career of multiple personalities. Azam had systematically attempted to replicate on Félida the hypnosis experiments of James Braid, and what she thereafter demonstrated in the way of catalepsy had the strong imprint of medical shaping.[87]

Pierre Janet saw his first case of multiple personality in a woman of nineteen named "L." who had *grande hystérie*. After four sessions of hypnosis, she began talking in a deep voice and brought forth "a sort of catalepsy" with waxy rigidity of the limbs. If Janet closed L.'s fingers into a fist while she was in this cataleptic state, her face would take on an air of rage and her arm would strike out. Then Janet actually did suggest L. into having a "different" personality. She had been put under hypnosis, and in her cataleptic condition could not hear or speak but she could write. The following exchange occurred:

Q: From Janet: Do you hear me?
A: [She wrote]: No.
Q: But in order to answer you have to be able to hear.
A: Yes, absolutely.
Q: So somebody's got to be hearing me, right?
A: Yes.
Q: Who's that?
A: Somebody other than L.
Q: Good! Another person. Shall we call her Blanche?
A: OK, Blanche.

162

Q: Well then, Blanche, do you hear me?
A: Yes.[88]

Doctors also deliberately suggested patients into having multiple personalities. New York neurologist Joseph Collins—the distilled essence of a society nerve doctor who treated Henry James among other well-known patients—intentionally induced multiple personalities in one chronic invalid so that he could cure her. In 1910 Collins saw a twenty-seven-year-old woman who had been ill since early adolescence. At thirteen, "blinding" headaches had come on, together with disturbances of vision. At fourteen, after a tumultuous rage on her father's part, she began to experience twitching, as well as daylong crying attacks. "It was around this time that she had first experienced difficulty in walking; her legs tired easily and she got tired all over." She could no longer do homework and fought with her mother. Failing a grade at school and now very disappointed in herself, at twenty she began her career of invalidism, involving attacks of pain and a motionless right leg. When she was twenty-three her medical attendants removed her right ovary, presumably to cure her hysteria. Now her left leg became involved. Before the ovarian operation she had been in bed two weeks out of four. Now she was constantly in bed and remained there for the next four years.

The patient began taking on the characteristics of a chronic valetudinarian. Her mother devoted herself full-time to the patient's care. The patient had once been in a private clinic for nervous diseases and was said to have "worn out two special nurses."

"No one understands her, and every one who attempts to cure her does so by force," said Collins, in summing up her attitude. "Nurses are cruel to her, doctors are mandatory, heartless, and obtuse. If she could only make them realize how important it is that everything should be done in the way that she is convinced is right," summarized Collins.

She said in one of the notes she began sending Collins daily, "I am so afraid of people who have hard, cross voices, and who speak as though it were a great burden to do anything for me, as though I were a great trouble to them."

Collins commenced a kind of deep psychotherapy, reaching back for memories of early childhood. Over the days, he gave her careful explanations of hysteria, which he defined as a "split personality." He told her that her problem was a warring of these personalities. As soon as they were all "welded together," she would get better. These principles were explained to her many times. He used diagrams and even a skeleton.

She now came to believe that she had "four persons that . . . constitute herself":

- Person no. 1: childish and weak
- Person no. 2: older, with fine character qualities
- Person no. 3: an all-knowing, all-seeing "Mona Lisa"-like personality
- Person no. 4: a "glorious creature" who was supposed to "overcome the faults of all the other personalities"

In a long series of interviews, Collins slowly began reinforcing personality number 4 at the cost of the others. She made steady progress, at first to a "rolling crutch." But then during the menses, "at which time she appeared to suffer insupportable pain," her knees would collapse. They therefore removed her uterus. Four months later her emotional health had improved enough to permit her to leave hospital, and a year later she wrote Collins that she was completely well. "The townsfolk look upon her as a miracle."[89] Presumably "personality no. 4" had now conquered the others.

We hear in this account distant echoes of reflex theory. As reflex theories declined, catalepsy and the other phenomena of motor hysteria declined with them. Multiple personality disorder thus arose in that whole cauldron of illness beliefs surrounding magnetism and catalepsy, and apparently declined with it in frequency as well, becoming less common by 1950 than it had been in 1900.[90] Then in 1957 Corbett H. Thigpen and Hervey M. Cleckley published *The Three Faces of Eve*,[91] and the diagnosis underwent a rebirth, becoming by the end of the twentieth century a common form of dissociation, supposedly resulting from "child abuse."

For students of psychosomatic illness, the point about multiple personality disorder is that a climate of suggestion can elicit not merely physical symptoms such as paralysis, but fashionable mental symptoms as well. What particular mental and physical symptoms appear in a given period depends not at all on the underlying characteristics of a purportedly immutable "disease entity," but on the climate of suggestion prevailing at the time.

In the case of catalepsy and somnambulism, it is doctors who create the climate of suggestion. But why do the doctors change their minds, discarding old theories and introducing new ones? Is it merely the advance of science, or do cultural and social factors play a role as well, as for example in physicians' initial embrace of "magnetic" second states late in the eighteenth century and their rejection of them at the beginning of the twentieth? The notions of magnetism and catalepsy fitted well with the ideas of the Enlightenment, for animal magnetism expanded with a stroke the range of nervous phenomena that could be understood with reference to apparently scientific concepts of physics.

But the rejection of catalepsy and somnambulism as real phenomena may have possessed as much a social basis as a scientific one. Precisely at the turn of the twentieth century, as jubilation about the discovery of second states was ceding to embarrassment over the whole Charcot fiasco, the nature of the doctor-patient relationship was becoming more intimate.[92] These years saw the blossoming of the patient-as-a-person movement. It was at this time that doctors started to be seen as their patients' "best friends," as the emotional confidants of women in particular. This was the foundation of success of the "society nerve-doctor."

How did this new intimacy militate against reductionist medical theories? Doctrines of animal magnetism, like reflex theory generally, saw the patient as a kind of automaton driven by physiological forces, the pelvic neuroses in the case of reflex theory, invisible magnetic fluids in the case of catalepsy. As the doctor-patient relationship closened late in the nineteenth century, this automaton view of patients became psychologically untenable for physicians. Although doctors were still able to reduce their patients' humanity to invisible irregularities in the nervous system, these new nerve theories did not have the deterministic power of animal magnetism or reflex theory. Perhaps it was this new psychological rapport between doctors and patients that permitted doctors to banish theories insisting that patients' minds were held in the vise grip of their bodies.

CHAPTER
7

Charcot's Hysteria

Jean-Martin Charcot, the Parisian internist and neurologist who flourished in the last four decades of the nineteenth century, occupies a
major position in the history of psychosomatic illness because the particular form of hysteria he described became, by virtue of his great medical
authority, an article of belief among doctors and patients. The story of
Charcot demonstrates the enormous capacity of doctors to frame and
shape symptoms which their patients then experience. He was the first
important physician to call attention to the sensory side of the nervous
system in somatization. Toward the end of his life Charcot dwelt briefly
upon psychological theories of nervous illness, helping to legitimate
them. He would have achieved none of these feats in the history of hysteria had he not been, alongside William Osler, the best-known clinician
of the second half of the nineteenth century.

The Paris medical world of the 1880s and 1890s saw Charcot at its very
center. Léon Daudet, son of novelist Alphonse Daudet and just finishing
medical school in 1890, captures the scene. Given that his father Alphonse
was one of Charcot's close friends, Léon was especially well situated as a
commentator. "Towards 1890," he wrote:

> Professor Charcot was at the apogee of his reputation and his power.
> He held the Faculty [of Medicine] bent to his grindstone. His doc-
> trines, whose fundamentals had not yet been overturned, gave an im-
> pression of solidity and even of majesty. . . . No one anywhere in the
> civilized world could publish a book on diseases of the nervous system
> without seeking his approval, his *imprimatur,* in advance. The struc-
> ture of the liver and the kidney obeyed him, as well as that of the spinal
> cord. Physicians sent him patients with ataxia [a form of neurosyphilis]

166

and cases of paralysis agitans [Parkinson's disease] from North America, the Caucasus, and even China.[1]

Charcot had become one of the great public figures of his time. Letters would reach him, even if addressed only, "Charcot . . . Doctor in Europe."[2] And when he died in 1893, the news traveled as though he were a head of state. Such a man had great power to mold opinion.

Charcot's Life

Born in 1825 in Paris, Charcot was a man who grew up in the school of academic hard knocks. Unlike most of the physicians of his day, he came from a working-class family, the son of a wagonmaker who turned out fine, beautifully ornamented carriages. The family determined that Charcot would study, sending him to the Lycée Bonaparte. Charcot then began medical studies in 1844. While all French medical students acquired some clinical experience, only a few of them received formal posts as *externes* and *internes,* which required passing a highly competitive exam. The numerous examinations (*concours*) of this kind that characterize university life in France were supposed to ensure rigorous competition. But passing the exam near the top of a ranked list was often more a matter of whom one knew.[3] Charcot, the son of an artisan, knew no one, and in 1847 failed his first competitive exam for an internship. He passed the following year and would shortly remedy his lack of *piston* (or influence), as the French say, by attracting the attention of Pierre Rayer, one of the faculty giants. It was Rayer who arranged for Charcot to board with a well-to-do family.

Charcot spent his internship at the Salpêtrière, founded in eastern Paris in the seventeenth century. The Salpêtrière—which was not actually a hospital but a combination of poorhouse and home for the aged, with a division for insane women as well—housed some five thousand women. There Charcot accumulated enough data on his elderly female patients to be able to write in 1853 a thesis on gout, receiving his M.D. that year as well.

Obviously a rising star, Charcot did well in the next four years, in what were, essentially, the stages of a residency. The next hurdle in the system, however, was the competitive exam (*agrégation*), which one had to pass to be eligible for a teaching post in the Faculty of Medicine. This involved preparing a thesis in advance, writing for three hours on an assigned topic, and then defending one's writings against an opponent. In 1857

Charcot failed this exam on his first try. On his second try in 1860 he almost failed again, nervous and rambling in explaining his ideas. Only the intervention of his mentor Rayer, a member of the jury, saved him.[4]

These setbacks were not the result of intellectual shortcomings, for Charcot in these years was trailed by a reputation for brilliance. In all probability they owed more to the faculty's disdain for his relatively humble origins, or to Charcot's own unease over his background. (In later years he would fetishize his hobnobbing with the rich and famous in the form of weekly receptions.) In retrospect, it is likely that by 1860 Charcot had learned a lesson: Loyalty to a *patron* was a prerequisite of success in academic life in Paris. Now that he had succeeded, he would make sure his own protégés were loyal to him. His pupil Pierre Marie said many years later, apropos the help Rayer had given to Charcot, "We would all have similar memories of him helping us."[5] Yet splendid though such unswerving loyalty may be, it has a shadow side. One's students may also remain mute at the wrong time.

Now that Charcot had qualified for a teaching post, he requested a curious assignment: to return to the Salpêtrière. Although several major figures in the history of psychiatry in France, such as Philippe Pinel and Jean Esquirol, had previously taught there, the medical division of the Salpêtrière had the reputation of being a graveyard for careers and was shunned by ambitious young researchers. In 1862 Charcot became chief physician of the Salpêtrière's infirmary. Why this choice?

As someone with a commitment to research, Charcot wanted to employ the "anatomical-clinical" method, a means of separating out distinctive diseases that was introduced early in the nineteenth century, notably by physicians at the Faculty of Medicine in Paris. In this method one established at autopsy what a patient had died of, then went back and reviewed the chart to see exactly what antemortem signs and symptoms of disease were associated with the postmortem pathological findings. In this manner, pneumonia became differentiated from tuberculosis, liver disease from heart disease, and so forth. The major organic diseases all have distinctive clinical signs (what is seen antemortem) and of course distinctive postmortem findings as well. Putting the two together was called the "anatomical-clinical method," and until Charcot, it had been little employed in neurology. The whole world of organically caused tremors, chorea, paralysis, loss of sensation, and so forth was more or less an anatomical-clinical mystery in 1862, when Charcot returned to the Salpêtrière.

Charcot saw a major scientific opportunity: using the large population of sick and insane female patients to make fundamental distinctions among organic diseases of the nervous system. As a chronic-care facility, the Salpêtrière offered Charcot the great advantage of permitting him to follow patients until they died, instead of seeing their signs and symptoms at one stage and then not being able to do an autopsy because they had vanished from sight. "Among the five thousand female inhabitants of this great institution called the hospice of the Salpêtrière," said Charcot in 1880:

> were a large number admitted for life as incurable, patients of every age with every kind of chronic disease, in particular disorders having the nervous system as their seat.
>
> It was this large patient population, with this distinctive stamp, that formed what one might call the reservoir of material [ancien fonds], the only one that until recently was available to me for my research in pathology and my clinical teaching.

(Charcot had just opened an outpatient clinic, and "clinical teaching" meant demonstrating patients at lectures.) He went on to explain the utility of such a vast reservoir of material in the study of disease: One can see how a given disease appears in a variety of patients, and how the disease appears at each step of its evolution. "These various types of patients were present here under our eyes in a more or less permanent manner, for the gaps that appear from time to time [with death] in a certain disease category are soon filled anew. We found ourselves, in other words, in possession of a kind of living pathology museum whose holdings were virtually inexhaustible."[6] Thus Charcot encountered at the Salpêtrière a kind of scientific gold mine.

Of his fundamental commitment to scientific research there can be no doubt, which gives his story a tragicomic quality as, in search of science, Charcot blundered into the swamp of suggestion. Sigmund Freud, who knew Charcot for a five-month period in 1885–86 while visiting at the Salpêtrière, told the following story of Charcot's scientific relentlessness: Even before 1860 Charcot was trying to differentiate multiple sclerosis from Parkinson's disease. Both have a tremor. Sometime in the 1850s when he was trying to engage a servant, by chance he came across an applicant with a distinctive tremor who, "on account of her clumsiness, could not get a post. Charcot recognized her condition as the 'choreiform paralysis' that [Guillaume] Duchenne had already described but whose origin was still unknown. He kept on this interesting servant, although she cost him a small fortune in bowls and plates, and when she finally died, he was able to demonstrate on her that this 'choreiform paralysis' was really the clinical expression of multiple sclerosis."[7]

Using this anatomical-clinical method in the 1860s, Charcot was able to describe several major disease entities in the hitherto undifferentiated fog of spinal pathology. In 1864 he and his student Victor Cornil, an intern at the Salpêtrière, described the changes in the anterior part of the spinal cord characteristic of poliomyelitis. Between 1863 and 1866 Charcot and his close friend Félix Vulpian put together the whole anatomical-clinical picture of multiple sclerosis. Although previous researchers had described the spinal lesions of MS—the disease had been considered very rare—Charcot and Vulpian established that these lesions were responsible for the characteristic tremor and other symptoms of MS, symptoms that were similar to the hysteria of the day but different from Parkinson's disease. In 1869 Charcot described the injuries to knee joints in particular that accompany the spinal ("tabetic") form of neurosyphilis, showing that they were not the result of a distinctive spinal lesion but of trauma: The patients, whose sensory spinal tracts were impaired, did not know exactly where their legs were and put their feet down too hard, injuring the joints. In 1869 Charcot also described the characteristic spinal pathology of amyotrophic lateral sclerosis, or motor system disease (now popularly known as Lou Gehrig's disease).[8] Any of these discoveries would have been a major feat in and of itself. That Charcot had such a string of them—and not just in neurology but in internal medicine as well—gave him a towering scientific status. That is the point: If Charcot had a brilliant international reputation, it was because of important, genuinely scientific discoveries: creating a map of the spinal cord and its diseases. Of course the analogy was irresistible to Charcot: If he could map the spinal cord, perhaps he could map hysteria as well.

To understand how Charcot went badly astray on hysteria, one should have a sense of how he proceeded in his research. To utilize the resources of the living pathology museum at the Salpêtrière, he employed both components of the anatomical-clinical method: close observation of the patients while alive and laboratory research on tissues collected postmortem.

In the Paris medical world Charcot was known as a close, silent, observer. Rather than simply doing rounds among the patients in bed in the manner of his predecessors, he had them brought to his office. "He would sit at a bare table," recalled two former students in 1939:

and have the patient come in. The patient undresses completely. The intern reads the history. The chief listens attentively. There follows a long, very long, silence, during which he watches and watches the patient, tapping one hand on the table. The residents who are standing about silently await anxiously some word that might enlighten them. Charcot is still silent. Now he asks the patient to move a limb, has the patient walk and talk, orders that the patient's reflexes be tested, that a sensory exam be conducted. Again there is silence, the mysterious silence of Charcot. Finally, he has a second patient brought in, whom he examines like the previous one, then asks for a third and begins to compare them, still without saying a word.[9]

Nor did Charcot always leave the hands-on part to his residents while remaining seated himself. He was quite skillful at the physical examination of patients, and happened to receive as a patient his old friend Alphonse Daudet. This was in the late 1880s. Daudet was already symptomatic from neurosyphilis, the spread of the bacteria causing syphilis to the nervous system, when he went to see Charcot.

"I was very anxious about this consultation," said his son Léon, "for I had just started my medical studies. I heard my fellow students and the residents of the Salpêtrière talking about it and I understood that it must be something serious. I went home and found my father in his study. He had his little pipe that Flaubert had given him, an inheritance from the author of *Madame Bovary*, in his hand when he began talking."

"Well, here it is," said Alphonse:

Charcot told me the truth, what I'm going to tell you. But don't worry. I have tabes, no question, the classic kind of tabes [spinal neurosyphilis]. Charcot checked my reflexes with a little hammer, and he did it with such skill! But slow tabes. The way it is now I'll make it to ninety [Daudet, around fifty at the time, died seven years later]. That gives me a bit of breathing space. The pains are localized in the legs and at the waist, sometimes in the bladder. My gait is defective. I have a little high-stepping. [With the sensory spinal centers for the legs destroyed, the patients literally did not know where their feet were and so stepped high to clear the sidewalk.] It's very possible it'll stop there. Maybe go away entirely. That often happens.[10]

Of course Charcot had lied to his old friend about the prognosis to make him feel better. It never went away. But Charcot had observed and examined Daudet minutely, unlike normal practice in the clinical medicine of the time. The problem with such close attentiveness to physical signs and symptoms was that Charcot ignored completely the psychological side of illness, risking being led astray by symptoms resulting from the unconscious mind instead of from organic lesions of the spinal cord.

A second, eminently scientific feature of Charcot's approach—but

171

which would stand him ill when confronting somatizing patients—was his introduction to the Salpêtrière of a little pathology laboratory with chemical stains for tissues and a microscope. "Poorly lighted and [located] in the kitchen of a nurse's apartment, next to the cancer ward, it was there that, with [Charles] Bouchard, [Victor] Cornil, and [Alix] Joffroy, began" all the important research on spinal-cord pathology in the 1860s.[11] Thus in these inadequate surroundings, a pathology laboratory in a corner of a nurse's kitchen, Charcot started to do major scientific work.

Word quickly spread. In the early 1860s he started publishing his findings in one of the Paris medical weeklies. These attracted medical students to his rounds, and so in 1866 "a small room in the hospital was set aside for the purpose of instruction and he began to hold clinics and to lecture."[12] The lectures soon became very popular. By the middle of the 1880s the Salpêtrière was in the full course of conversion into a hospital. Charcot had added in 1877 a chemistry laboratory—the first in a Paris hospital—in 1879 a lecture hall with seating for six hundred; there were rooms for electrotherapy and hydrotherapy. There was a photographic laboratory.[13] An outpatient department had been opened in 1881 and a forty-bed neurological inpatient unit for both men and women in 1882 (which made possible the direct admission of interesting cases, rather than having to rely on the *bureau central,* which normally assigned patients to the Paris teaching hospitals).[14]

By the late 1870s the Salpêtrière, with three thousand beds for the elderly and six hundred for the insane, had a teaching staff of six that included, in addition to Charcot, who was the chief physician of the infirmary, Jules-Bernard Luys, the second physician in the infirmary. Luys had come to the Salpêtrière in 1863. Having a special interest in mental illness and in hypnotism, he was responsible for 156 beds of acutely ill patients. There was an otherwise undistinguished surgeon named Charles Périer, and three psychiatrists: Louis Delasiauve, who at seventy-three was being pushed out of the way, his hysteria patients grabbed by Charcot; the equally aged Jacques-Joseph Moreau (de Tours), a well-known figure in mid-century psychiatry; finally, Auguste-Félix Voisin, grandson of the famous psychiatrist Félix Voisin. In 1867 Voisin had founded his own clinic in the Salpêtrière and did experiments on hypnosis.[15] Charcot himself was responsible for 91 beds in the infirmary (Luys having the others), 316 beds for "incurable" patients, above all younger women with cancer who did not have the right to enter the geriatric hospice (known as the *caput mortum* of the Paris hospital system, with its elderly cancerous and rheumatic patients), 86 beds for epileptic patients and 30 more beds for "non-insane" hysterical patients in the infirmary.[16]

One notes from this description of the Salpêtrière that patient-physician ratio was enormously high, which means that the professors using these patients as teaching material would have very little actual sense of the case. Of course there were numerous interns and other medical staff alongside the six professors to provide medical care. But at the Salpêtrière it was not the junior staff that analyzed cases and drew up general "laws of hysteria." It was *le patron* himself, as Charcot was universally known, the great professor.[17] And the professor would have relatively little knowledge of what was actually going on in the cases that were thought to illustrate his doctrines.

One of the ironies of this story is that although the Salpêtrière was bathed in organicity, the vast majority of patients having something seriously wrong with them, the concerns of the physicians were primarily neuropsychiatric. Luys's interests, to say nothing of those of a complement of three staff psychiatrists, were basically in hypnosis and "neuroses." In a world of overwhelming organic disease, Charcot would thus find himself pulled by the climate of medical opinion toward the more spectacular side of nervous illness: the "functional" neuroses. "Functional" in this sense means those supposedly neurological illnesses such as hysteria or hypochondria in which the Salpêtrière's little microscope laboratory had been unable to find a lesion, but in which a lesion was nonetheless assumed to be present. This whole domain of illness without disease, the real essence of "functional," has always been a sandbox for theory builders. The Salpêtrière would be no exception.

What kind of man was Charcot? With his massive, leonine head, deep-set eyes, and brooding expression, he could not exactly be characterized as a jolly man. He loved the recognition that went with being, after 1872, the professor of pathology in the faculty, and after 1882 being the professor of nervous diseases, a chair created especially for him. Regularly on Tuesday evenings he and Madame Charcot, a woman of independent wealth, would have an open house in their grand dwelling on the Boulevard St. Germain. Here France's medical elite, foreign physicians who had come to the Salpêtrière to observe, and important figures from journalism and politics would rub shoulders.[18] This seemed the most natural thing to Charcot, greatness from other fields of endeavor ascending to meet medical greatness. He fancied himself a connoisseur of art and something of an artist as well, and traveled widely in Europe as a pilgrim in search of the lustrous. Unfortunately this interest in art led him to search for representations of hysteria in times past, drawings and statues that, he believed, merely confirmed the correctness of his views about the "laws of hysteria."[19]

Was Charcot more scornful of women than the typical middle-class man of his day? His former student Axel Munthe, with whom Charcot had had a falling-out, said that like all nerve specialists, Charcot "was surrounded by a bodyguard of neurotic ladies, hero-worshippers at all costs. Luckily for him he was absolutely indifferent to women."[20] The malicious Léon Daudet, who is the source for much of Charcot's life outside, found *le patron* lacking here as in many other domains: "It was quite singular that [Charcot] was timid, and his brusqueness in front of women, whom he affected to despise, owed much to this timidity. I noticed this on many occasions, and I would have given I don't know how much to ask him about his sentimental and sex life."[21] On another occasion Daudet evilly but not necessarily incorrectly speculated that Charcot might have had some affairs with his patients.[22]

Perhaps it was not so much that Charcot was misogynist but that he was misanthropic. Looking back ten years after Charcot's death novelist Jules Claretie—who had once written about the Salpêtrière and visited there extensively said: "I do not think any man better personified, indeed incarnated, those years than Charcot. The century of the neuroses found in him its physician. *Le Paris neurasthénique* of those latter years, given over to pessimism, was at the feet of this great Parisian, his sharp eyes buried deeply inside [their] orbits."[23] Léon Daudet commented that Charcot's affection for animals was characteristic of his misanthropy.[24] This love of animals made him in fact quite incapable of experimental physiology (which is why studies of cerebral localization in France lagged behind those in Germany).[25] Thus Charcot, something of a misanthrope, did seem to lack some dimension of empathy. If he had ever attempted to put himself in the shoes of his patients or to see the world through their eyes, he might have found them less bizarre.

Charcot was highly authoritarian, showing an *esprit de domination* in dealing with his associates. According to Edmond de Goncourt, a Parisian *littérateur,* Charcot and his wife had wanted young Léon Daudet to marry their daughter Jeanne. The Charcots became malevolent toward Léon when he married another Jeanne instead, Victor Hugo's daughter. Goncourt commented in his diary, "Someday someone should make public the tyrannical empire that [Charcot] has carved out for himself in the domain of medicine, and his corrupt maneuvers upon the poor souls of his colleagues, the physicians."[26] (Léon Daudet in turn became embittered toward Charcot for having hastened his father's end with a kind of "suspension" therapy, a misguided effort to relieve the pain of tabes by suspending the patients by the neck, thus "lengthening" the nerves.)[27]

It was risky to cross Charcot, which helps explain why few of the people about him tried to blow the whistle on hysteria. He humiliated both Joseph Babinski and Jules-Joseph Dejerine, two gifted young neurologists, by forcing them to adhere to his theories. After Charcot's death in 1893, Babinski must have looked back with embarrassment upon his own earlier publications on how to shift symptoms from person to person with a magnet![28] Babinski's *agrégation* had been torpedoed because of hostility between Charcot and another former student, Charles Bouchard, Charcot supposedly being jealous of Bouchard's rise to prominence. Since Bouchard was on Babinski's jury, Bouchard is said to have revenged himself by sending Babinski to the bottom. Thus Babinski, who discovered a certain physical sign that represented the greatest contribution of his generation to neurological knowledge, never became a professor.[29]

Dejerine had never been directly a student of Charcot's, yet nonetheless in the Parisian medical world he felt he had to appease the master. Just after Charcot's death in 1893, Augusta Dejerine-Klumpke, Dejerine's American wife and a formidable neurologist in her own right, wrote to psychiatrist August Forel in Zurich:

> This winter is going to give us a lot of *grande neurasthénie*. I trust you know that my husband is going to apply for the Charcot chair. But here in Paris people pay much less attention to scientific work, personal merit and unanimous opinion than to seniority. Emotional questions also play a big role in this campaign. Some people reproach my husband for his attitude to Charcot, neglecting the fact that for twenty years my husband was a *victim* of Charcot and not an enemy.[30]

These anecdotes give a sense of the Faculty of Medicine in Paris as a nest of vipers in which it would be extremely dangerous to oppose Charcot's theories.

Charcot's Doctrine of Hysteria

Charcot's doctrine held that hysteria was an inherited functional disease of the nervous system in which such lifelong "stigmata" as hemianesthesia (loss of sensation on one side of the body), constricted visual fields, or headache (*le clou hystérique*) alternated with convulsive fits called *la grande hystérie*. The theory presupposed hidden organicity: Hysteria was an inherited neurological illness, not a psychiatric one, for indeed Charcot was a neurologist and internist, not a psychiatrist. The main stigmata were sensory, including chronic pain, visual disturbances, creepy-crawly sensations in the skin, and hemianesthesia. One stigma the patient was not necessarily aware of—but which could be elicited—was "ovarie," the ability to stop or start hysterical fits by pressing on the lower abdomen, over the point where Charcot believed the ovaries to be.[31]

These enduring sensory stigmata would occasionally be interrupted by motor fits, or *grande hystérie,* just as physicians in earlier decades had believed a spell of catalepsy could interrupt the ordinary symptoms of hysteria. It was on the fits in particular that Charcot unleashed his mania for classification. They could be subdivided into stages, through which patients would inevitably progress.

As for therapy, hysteria was an inherited (or "constitutional") disease that had no cure, though its symptoms could be palliated with the standard therapies. Hypnotism too might abolish some symptoms of hysteria, but the ability to be hypnotized was in and of itself a sign of hysteria. Hypnotizing nonhysterical individuals was, by definition, impossible. Given that hysteria was a functional disease of the central nervous system (and not reflexly caused by uterus or ovaries), men were as much at risk of it as women.

Charcot's encounter with hysteria began when he entered the Salpêtrière in 1862, for he found, sandwiched in between the ward for incurables and the ward for epileptics, a ward for "hystero-epilepsy" in which female patients with different kinds of fits were mingled together. Some of these women were epileptic and insane, others epileptic and noninsane. Still others were problematical young females, dumped by their exhausted families, who had merely hysterical fits, which they often developed on arrival in imitation of the epileptics.[32] This hystero-epilepsy ward was among the saddest at the Salpêtrière, and, as Gilles de la Tourette later wrote, Dante's phrase, "Abandon hope all ye who enter here," might well have been written above the door.[33]

At this point in the 1860s, in Pierre Marie's recollection of events, Charcot succumbed to his desire to classify everything and started classifying the various forms of hysteria. He first set out to differentiate the hysterics from the epileptics. As he observed the patients, it struck him that the two attacks were quite different, that hysteria and epilepsy were in fact different diseases. Retaining the name of the historic ward, he described convulsive attacks in noninsane women as "hystero-epilepsy." Now, maybe some of these noninsane women did in fact have epilepsy, Charcot thought. One could not be sure. By "hystero-epilepsy" he therefore originally meant hysterical fits in a person with epilepsy. Later it meant hysterical fits in the absence of epilepsy as well. Because the term *hystero-epilepsy* itself was hopelessly confusing (did the patients have epilepsy or not?), Charcot later abandoned it in favor of the phrase *la grande hystérie* or *hysteria major*.[34] All three terms referred to attacks of nonepileptic fits. Charcot also noted, apparently in the 1860s as well, that these convulsing women carried about certain neurological "stigmata."

Then in 1870 there was another development. The elderly Delasiauve had been the head of the hystero-epilepsy ward as well as other wards, but the "Sainte Laure" building in which they were housed was collapsing. The administration therefore decided to put the insane hysterics and epileptics in the section of psychiatrist Jules-Gabriel Baillarger and to put the noninsane hysterics and epileptics somewhere else. But where? One possibility would be to create a new service with a new supervising physician, but this was rejected as too expensive for a mere thirty patients. Charcot, however, had indicated an interest in them, and as the senior physician at the infirmary, he got them.[35]

From the time of his acquisition in 1870 of Delasiauve's hystero-epilepsy patients, Charcot busied himself with the study of hysteria, drawn increasingly toward "the great neurosis" and away from the study of organic nervous disease he had undertaken in the 1860s. In the early 1870s he took up the sensory symptoms of hysteria—what ultimately would be the "stigmata."

In the wake of half a century of reflex theory, Charcot occupied himself from the very beginning with the ovaries. As early as June 1872, demonstrating before the interns and residents a forty-year-old woman named Justine from the south of France who had developed a hysterical paralysis, Charcot was searching for any sensory signs of hysteria that might simultaneously be present. As he examined her before the group he found (or induced by suggestion), a complete loss of feeling on the left side of her body, including the mucous membranes and internal organs. She manifested as well an apparent "hemiopia," or loss of vision on one side of the retina and an inability to distinguish colors (achromatopsia). But most interesting of all, she had pain in the lower left quadrant. "M. Briquet gave the name coelialgia to this pain, and assigned it to the muscles. But as far as I am concerned—and in agreement with Négrier, Schützenberger and Piorry [all reflex theorists interested in the ovary], I would call this pain ovarian hyperesthesia, and I believe it to a certain degree pathognomonic [diagnostic of hysteria]."[36] Here Charcot established continuity with the past, invoking other authorities on ovarian tenderness and general loss of sensation, but beginning at the same time to weld these components, available for fifty years in the literature, into a new doctrine of hysteria: a disease in which sensory deficits would always be present, deficits that were indeed diagnostic of the very disorder itself.

In the years between 1872 and 1877 Charcot's doctrine of sensory deficits in hysteria came to include several kinds of inability to feel or perceive that were less well represented in the medical literature than was ovarian tenderness. As early as 1875 Charcot assigned to the category "local hysteria" (in addition to hemianesthesia) certain fixed painful points at various sites of the body (*points douloureux fixes*), spinal pain, and chest pain (pleuralgia), and on the motor side paralysis and contracture. Pressure on the ovaries could unclench or brake all of these symptoms of "local hysteria."[37]

The empirical evidence for such assertions? Charcot cited in a lecture given in 1875 Geneviève, a twenty-eight-year-old woman born, of all places, in Loudun, a village that had witnessed mass outbreaks of hysteria in the past. "Hysterical" since puberty, she now had a complete loss of sensation on her left side, left ovarian pain, and "a bizarre state of mind." "With Geneviève," said Charcot, "compressing the ovary causes the immediate cessation of an attack. She herself is clearly aware of this effect, for she tries on her own to compress the ovarian region from which the aura [presaging the attack] radiates, and when she is unable to do it, she calls upon the medical staff for assistance."[38]

One other interesting feature of Geneviève's fits might be mentioned. They seemed clearly demarcated into three phases. Phase 1 was epileptiform convulsions, foaming at the mouth, and sonorous breathing—a familiar enough kind of fit. Phase 2 was strikingly new: "large movements of the limbs and whole body," a gymnastic kind of jerking and leaping about. Phase 3 was a psychosis. a *période de délire*, the French word *délire* meaning delusions and hallucinations rather than delirium. (The incorporation of this phase indicates either that Charcot had diagnosed a number of psychotic patients as hysterical, or that some of his patients were playacting for his benefit.) "In this period [Geneviève] recounts all the events of her life up to the onset of fits. Sometimes the patient, in this latter phase, has hallucinations: she sees snakes in baskets; she also engages in a kind of dance, giving us a prototypical specimen of what was described in the middle ages as epidemic writhing [*épidémies saltatoires*]."[39]

In 1875 Charcot was edging toward a unified theory of hysteria in which patients like Geneviève would exhibit enduring, unchanging traits such as loss of sensation or headache, and periodically undergo attacks of fits clearly delineated into phases, each phase more bizarre than the one preceding. Hysteria was becoming a disease that called for its victims regularly to fling themselves about the room and then to have delusions and hallucinations.

By 1879 Charcot's doctrine of hysteria had become fully developed: The attacks of hystero-epilepsy—now called *hysteria major* or *la grande hystérie*—were now seen as occurring in patients who did not have epilepsy, and were clearly demarcated not into three phases but four: (1) the epileptoid period (which in turn could be subdivided into tonic, clonic, and so on subphases); (2) the "period of contortions and *grands mouvements*," otherwise known as "clownism," in which the patients flung themselves about the bed, emitted piercing cries, or took improbable positions such as *arc-de-cercle* (also called *arc-en-ciel*), only the back of the head and heels resting on the ground; (3) the period of impassioned poses (*attitudes passionnelles*), in which patients deliberately struck postures of prayer, crucifixion, accusation, and the like; and (4) a "terminal period" in which anything could happen. Charcot then admitted of atypical forms, or variations, of these standard phases. Perhaps an attack would be entirely dominated by the first period, not progressing further. In another variety, "demonic behavior," such as tearing one's blouse from one's breast, might characterize the clownism of the second period. In still another variation, attitudes of ecstasy might preempt all the impassioned poses in the third period. Or hallucinations and delusions might be the chief events of the terminal period.[40]

Although Charcot later developed a theory of male hysteria that called for identical symptoms in men, he remained fascinated with the ovaries. In practice this gave his theories a tropism toward women. At autopsy, for example, he was often uninterested in inspecting the brain but would subject the ovaries to an exact microscopic investigation.[41] In 1878 one of his interns devised an "ovarian compressor belt" to exert continual pressure on an ovary on either side and thus avert hysterical fits.[42] (There was some question as to whether such external pressure compressed the ovaries at all.) Then in 1881 another student perfected an improved and more comfortable version that could simultaneously exert pressure on both ovaries. The Parisian firm Aubry made them.[43]

Throughout Charcot's days at the Salpêtrière, manipulating the ovaries took on a large clinical importance. Fatigued by continually pressing down on the belly of one patient, Desiré-Magloire Bourneville discovered that a series of short ovarian compressions would work just as well.[44] In demonstrating "ovarie" at rounds, Charcot asked his assistants to press on the left "ovarian" region of one patient, a sixteen-year-old girl:

> Immediately an attack of rhythmic chorea breaks out. The patient remains sitting and consciousness is preserved. Her head begins suddenly to turn from right to left and then from left to right, in rhythmic alteration with equal pauses between the individual movements. Simultaneously the right arm begins going up and down, as a result of which her hand beats regularly on her knee as though on a drum. The movements of the hand are synchronized with those of the head. Meanwhile the right foot is noisily stamping on the floor. There are approximately 100 beats of the foot and three times as many of the hand in a minute.

A friend of this patient's who was to be demonstrated next at rounds was also in the hall:

> At the mere sight of the condition of her friend, [this second patient] also has an attack which manifests the same peculiarities and is distinctive only through the rhythmic beating of all extremities. In this patient the attack is terminated by pressing continuously on her left ovarian region. Then attention returns to the first patient, whose attack is still continuing. Charcot calls the attention of the listeners to the fact that, despite the extended duration of the attack, her paralyzed left arm has still not moved.

He then terminated her attack in a similar manner.[45] Such phenomena had previously been seen on the stages of the magnetizers. Now the world's most distinguished neurologist was presenting them as a disease whose "laws" he had discovered.

By 1879 Charcot's doctrine of somatoform symptoms in hysteria was virtually complete.[46] He had assembled, from the bits and pieces of individual hysterical symptoms long represented in the symptom pool, an overarching unitary theory of hysteria, similar to Darwin's theory of evolution or to Claude Bernard's unitary theories of body physiology that also were being constructed in these years. Hysteria was an inherited, lifelong, functional nervous disease whose underlying existence was signposted by sensory and motor stigmata; it was a disease that could erupt at any time in fits, which themselves would march through well-defined phases. Charcot returned time and again to the "laws of hysteria" and saw himself as a kind of Napoleon of the central nervous system. "What I want to emphasize here," he told his listeners in 1882, "is that in the [hysterical] fit, nothing is left to chance, that to the contrary everything

unfolds according to the rules, which are always the same and characterize what we see in outpatients as well as inpatients; they are valid for all
countries, for all epochs, for all races, and are, in short, universal." These
névroses, he concluded, resembled organic nervous diseases in so
many respects that the clinician must continue to hunt for the anatomy
and physiology behind them.[47] Thus Charcot would not be surprised to
discover the stigmata and the successive phases of the hysterical attack
at places far distant from the Salpêtrière.

The Hospital as Circus

But the laws of hysteria acted most visibly in *le patron's* own domain,
the Salpêtrière. The extraordinary behavior occurring in its wards from
1870 until Charcot's death in 1893 transfixed both *le tout Paris* and the
international community. At the Salpêtrière the definitive passage of the
spotlight from organic neurology to circuslike events, although hinted at
in the hysterical patients of the early 1870s, occurred in 1876. In that
year an old-style magnetizer, fifty-four-year-old Victor-Jean-Marie Burq,
who in the manner of the early Mesmer used metallic plates and magnets
therapeutically, asked the Paris Biological Society to confirm the validity
of his "metallotherapy" on female patients with hysterical anesthesias.
Claude Bernard, the president of the society, appointed a commission to
investigate Burq's work, and on the commission sat Jean-Martin Charcot. Charcot therefore invited Burq to demonstrate metallotherapy on
the hysterics of the Salpêtrière.[48] It was like inviting the fox into the
chicken coop. In the climate of suggestibility of the Salpêtrière, what
could have seemed more plausible than "transferring" anesthesias and
paralyses with metals and magnets from one side of the body to the other,
or transferring them from patient to patient? "A number of important
discoveries" flowed from this summer of 1876, said former Salpêtrière
staff member Bourneville, including "the modifications that achromatopsia manifests under the influence of metallic applications, the *transfert*
[dragging symptoms from side to side], metallic anesthesia, and so forth.
These discoveries in turn were the point of departure of some curious
research on the action of magnetized rods, on electro-magnets, on solenoids [electric coils], static electricity . . . etc."[49] Charcot himself demonstrated the *transfert* at least as early as 1878 and probably before.[50] The
circus had begun.

Another act was added to the circus in 1878 when Charcot, to the
"general stupefaction of the learned world," imported hypnotism to the

Salpêtrière. Having realized that metals were among a wide range of agents that could induce hypnotism, he systematically began to experiment on the age-old hypnotic phenomena of catalepsy and somnambulism, phenomena that also seemed to occur during attacks of *grande hystérie*.[51] Arthur Gamgee, a professor of medical physiology at Manchester, came to Paris in August of that year to watch the performance, along with a row of other scientific dignitaries. Charcot would extend a finger of his right hand for the patient to stare at, or ask her to stare fixedly into his eyes, and in a minute or two, hypnotized, she would be instructed to reproduce all the symptoms of hysteria that Charcot wanted to study.[52]

In the crucible of suggestion that existed at the Salpêtrière, this research on hypnotism was doomed from the start. Although Charcot himself occasionally hypnotized patients at rounds for the benefit of visitors, usually he left this to the house staff, who would bring the prehypnotized patients to the morning lectures:

> Thus the patients passed from hand to hand during the morning; in the afternoon the interns and frequently as well the externs, begged by their colleagues from other hospitals or by friends, would again repeat once or several times the experiments from the morning, without thinking anything of it. The result of all these attempts is easy to imagine: at Charcot's behest, a series of suggestions were produced in these patients, unconsciously resulting in actual coaching [*un véritable dressage*] of which Charcot was entirely unaware. In consequence, all of his research on hypnotism was vitiated from the beginning.[53]

Unmindful of the backdrop of coaching, Charcot went on to develop the iron laws of "grand hypnotism" in a manner analogous to the iron laws of hysteria. That such laws might exist seemed credible, given that hypnotizability was one of the hysterical stigmata. An episode of hypnosis, said Charcot, might be divided into three distinct stages—catalepsy, lethargy, and somnambulism—each having distinctive characteristics and clearly demarcated from the others, although they would not necessarily follow in unaltered progression, as did the stages of an hysterical attack.[54]

The most extraordinary phenomena were witnessed. Joseph Delboeuf, a Belgian physician who had come to visit, observed that, "In divided states" [*les états dimidiés*], the young girl is, so to speak, cut in half, one half of her body in lethargy, the other in catalepsy." Further, that in "mixed states [*les états composés*], when her eyes are opened, love is put into her left eye and hate into the right one." "One side of her face smiles, the other is threatening."[55] Because Auguste-Félix Voisin and Jules-Bernard Luys also made much of hypnotism, the Salpêtrière reverberated to the ringing of gongs, as the hypnotized patients were suddenly put into group "catalepsy," or fled in alarm the dangerous "north" pole of a magnet.[56] Daudet commented on how Luys, later at the Charité, was taken in by every "simulatrice nerveuse" in Paris; Daudet had personally observed the patients agreeing on their roles with each other a week in advance.[57] Thus the production of extraordinary symptoms under hypnotism would become a second ring of the circus.

Charcot's lectures every Tuesday and Friday morning took on a circus-like atmosphere as the patients actually bathed in a spotlight in front of the amphitheater. The Tuesday lectures in particular counted as highly innovative in the context of French medical education of the day. On Tuesdays Charcot would know the general subject on which he wished to speak and prepare some notes, but he would not have seen the patients previously, merely picking them from a list of those present in the waiting room of the outpatient clinic that morning. Then he would thrill the audience by quickly identifying in each patient the exact signs and symptoms confirming the diagnosis. What gave both the impromptu Tuesday lectures and the more didactic Friday lectures—written out word for word—their quality of spectacle was the presence in the audience of considerable numbers of nonphysicians who had come there basically to be entertained. Furious at the skeptical reception of his teachings on hypnosis among physicians, Charcot had decided to throw open his lectures to the public, and let them decide the question on the basis of the evidence before their eyes. But in addition to the journalists and other opinion-makers he hoped would come, victims of other hypnotists started turning up as well.[58] The audience thus contributed its part to the spectacle.

In Charcot's hands virtually any patient in these Tuesday lectures could be made into a hysteric. Here we see Charcot demonstrating a female patient of seventeen whose chief complaint was compulsive yawning. Four or five months ago, just after coming into the Salpêtrière, she had yawned at the rate of around eight per minute. Now it was only four yawns per minute, and each yawn lasted now only three to four seconds, as opposed to five to seven seconds earlier. Because Charcot saw it as "hysterical yawning," she must have had other signs of hysteria. Indeed she did. Charcot asked her about her family: Her father was unknown, which Charcot found pathological to begin with; a father does not abandon his child. And a sister had experienced protracted sobbing at the age of eighteen. Clearly her heredity was poisoned.

As for the patient herself, between the ages of three and eight she had had attacks of fainting and fits, probably an aggravated form of hystero-epilepsy, according to Charcot. From age nine until after her admission to the Salpêtrière the fits had vanished. Since last May, however, the patient had reported hoarseness, incessant coughing, and then, after a series of sleepless nights, the yawning had become regular. Since her admission to the Salpêtrière, there had been some fits, with an aura rising to globus in her throat. As soon as these attacks began, the yawning would vanish. (Charcot believed that attacks of hysteria major, a form of which these clearly seemed to him, temporarily suspended the stigmata.) During the attacks, her limbs would go rigid and she would faint. In this interview Charcot discovered, moreover, other hysterical stigmata of which the patient had until then been unaware: patches of anesthesia stretching from the skin of her right arm to the buttocks; the loss of taste and smell; a diminution in the sensibility of the nasal mucosa, a diminution in her ability to distinguish colors, and a bilateral contraction of her visual fields. All were, in Charcot's view, the classic stigmata of hysteria. She had them all, therefore the yawning was manifestly hysterical, evidence that the young woman had inherited an organic condition of her nervous system that would last all her life, for which there was no cure, and that she would doubtlessly pass on to her children. Hospitalization at the Salpêtrière had thus converted a tired young woman into an "hysteric."[59]

At the end of this demonstration, the staff brought another young woman who had already been hypnotized into the room and placed her next to the yawner. This second patient promptly began yawning, and continued to do so even after she had been awakened from the hypnosis. Charcot said they would have to rehypnotize her to abolish the yawning.

It was Charcot's overweening confidence in his own brilliance—a confidence confirmed by a decade of success in organic neurology—plus his ignorance of what was actually occurring on the wards and his complete lack of empathy with his young female patients, that caused him to misinterpret these products of medical suggestion as an independent disease entity called hysteria.

In interviews, not unlike Freud probing for some evidence of "sexual etiology," Charcot would dig ceaselessly until he found stigmata or "heredity." Hysteria was an inheritable disease. Therefore in the family trees of patients with stigmata there must be some evidence of neuropathology, an aunt perhaps who had once been in an asylum or an uncle who had died insane.[60] On other occasions, going "cold" into these spontaneous Tuesday-morning interviews with unfamiliar patients, he would rummage for stigmata in order to show that, for example, a terribly mischievous young woman of fifteen who broke everything in the household and plagued her parents with tricks really had hysteria. (He managed to establish that she had a choking sensation in the throat.)[61] Perhaps the associates of a less powerful man than Charcot would have buzzed in the chief's ear a warning about suggestion or raised the possibility of simulation. Not that Charcot was unaware of these alternative explanations of his findings, but he simply denied them.[62]

To many other observers it was clear that the Salpêtrière was a carnival of unconscious suggestion and conscious simulation from which had emerged a "hysteria" sui generis that was the product of one man's desire to classify run amok. Axel Munthe said of Charcot's hypnotism:

These stage performances of the Salpêtrière before the public of Tout Paris were nothing but an absurd farce, a hopeless muddle of truth and cheating. Some of these subjects were no doubt real somnambulists faithfully carrying out in a waking state the various suggestions made to them during sleep—posthypnotic suggestions. Many of them were mere frauds, knowing quite well what they were expected to do, delighted to perform their various tricks in public, cheating both doctors and audience with the amazing cunning of the hystériques. They were always eager to 'piquer une attaque' of Charcot's classic grande hystérie, arc-en-ciel and all, or to exhibit his famous three stages of hypnotism: lethargy, catalepsy, somnambulism, all invented by the Master and hardly ever observed outside the Salpêtrière. Some of them smelt with delight a bottle of ammonia when told it was rose water, others would eat a piece of charcoal when presented to them as chocolate. Another would crawl on all fours on the floor, barking furiously when told she was a dog, flap her arms as if trying to fly when turned into a pigeon, lift her skirts with a shriek of terror when a glove was thrown at her feet with a suggestion [that it was] a snake.[63]

The Swiss neurologist Paul Dubois, who via his friend Jules-Joseph Dejerine had a good knowledge of Parisian hospital life, found Charcot's hysteria to be a complete medical artifact:

Endowed with the spirit of authority, [Charcot] handled his subjects as he would; and without, perhaps, taking them sufficiently into account, he suggested to them their attitudes and their gestures. Example is contagious even in sickness, and in the great hospitals of Paris, at La Salpêtrière, all cases of hysteria resemble each other. At the command of the chief of the staff, or of the interns, they begin to act like marionettes, or like circus horses accustomed to repeat the same evolutions.[64]

Dejerine himself, who had suffered so long under the master's rule, later dismissed the phases of *la grande hystérie*. After becoming in 1911 the incumbent of Charcot's chair, Dejerine said: "It seems now certain, and I have argued this for thirty years, that the crises delineated by this description are nothing other than coaching [*dressage*] and imitation."[65] But of course Dejerine had *not* said so as long as *le patron* was alive. Few who wanted an academic career in medicine in Paris had, because Charcot was so powerful.

The Diffusion of "la Grande Hystérie"

Although Munthe claimed that *la grande hystérie* was seldom seen outside the Salpêtrière, that is quite untrue. Wherever physicians were found who believed in the master's doctrines, or there were patients who had read colorful accounts in the press of the Tuesday lectures, *la grande hystérie* surfaced.

News of *la grande hystérie* was diffused to the French public via the popular press and fiction. This process started around 1878.[66] As early as 1882 the magazine *La Médecine populaire* said that magnetism had become *à la mode*, "in drawing rooms, journals, and reviews. It is practiced in hospitals, scientific societies, theatres, and homes." In that same year the journal *Les Soirées littéraires* assigned the credit for this revival to Charcot, "another of science's princes [who] exclaimed at the Salpêtrière like Archimedes: 'Eureka! Magnetism exists!'"[67] There were detailed descriptions of how patients demonstrating neuromuscular excitability under hypnosis were supposed to behave: "If you press the skin at the two sides of the vertebrae," wrote one journalist in the *Journal des débats*, "the subject jumps in place, sending his two legs forward briskly."[68] Such instructions add up to an operations manual for the unconscious mind.

The psychodrama of the Salpêtrière figured prominently in the fiction of the day. In addition to familiar names in this text such as Alphonse Daudet and Edmond de Goncourt, Emile Zola drew on Salpêtrière-style nervous pathology in his dynastic novels about the tainted "Rougon-Macquart" family. The family skids towards hereditarily determined ruin in a series of *accidents nerveux*. Guy de Maupassant, himself in the early stages of neurosyphilis, mirrored the whole nervous scene of the 1880s in various tales. In a story called "Le Tic," for example, Maupassant, as narrator, is having a conversation at a spa. His interlocutor explains why he and his family have come:

Oh, my daughter has a strange disorder. Nobody knows its seat. She suffers from incomprehensible nervous accidents. Sometimes the doctors think she has heart disease, sometimes it's the liver, sometimes the spinal cord. Right now they're attributing it to the stomach, which is the whole furnace and the whole control center of the body. That's why we're here. I personally think it's the nerves. In any case, it's very sad.

Maupassant thought immediately of the tic in the father's own hand, and asked, "But isn't that just heredity? Aren't your nerves a little bit sick too?"

The man explained that his nerves had always been very calm and that his own problems had another origin entirely, which was the gist of this particular short story. But Maupassant was asking here about stigmata. Readers of the account would ask themselves if they had any stigmata as well.[69]

In Jules Claretie's novel *Les Amours d'un interne* the young Salpêtrière intern Vilandry is explaining to his father in a letter the hereditary nature of nervous disease, "The patients we get are victims of heredity. Heredity, it's an awful thing and causes a mother and father to transmit their own diseases, their hideous physiques, to a poor little baby just come into the world. Let's say the parents are *nerveux* or the father's an alcoholic, and there you've got a poor little baby doomed to hysteria, just awaiting the first attack, this first attack that, I'm telling you, is a real horror most of the time." Vilandry went on to describe to his father a typical attack:

One fine day there's a sharp, nervous, uncontrollable laugh, the attack is beginning! It starts with shaking, with what we call choreiform movements. And then a horrifying spectacle occurs. As if suddenly possessed, the woman emits a prolonged scream, holds out her arms, and falls over backwards almost gently. Then, her mouth closed, her neck rigid and swollen, the noise of swallowing in her throat, she remains lying there, her eyes wide open, her pupils dilated, looking up, her arms rigid and held out in a kind of cross, literally a crucifix, her legs stiff and held together until such a time as her arms relax. There are attacks like this that might last five hours.[70]

An account such as this represented a veritable do-it-yourself guide to a Charcot-style fit: It identified all readers at risk of having such fits (those with nervous and alcoholic relatives) and explained exactly how one acted in a fit.

French patients responded to this massive medical shaping by often producing the symptoms of Charcot-style hysteria. On April 17, 1889, Edmond de Goncourt wrote in his diary:

It is truly a bit unsettling—Léon Daudet would say stupefying—how society women are carrying on right now. They all seem like the *hystériques* of the Salpêtrière, let loose by Charcot upon the world. One simply cannot imagine the ill-bred eccentricities of these lunatics, and today after the Princess ordered in a bouillabaisse from Marseille, Lippmann's wife (who with her funny behavior and bizarre posturing is not entirely graceless) went around blowing garlic into the face of everyone she knows.[71]

In these chic Parisian circles, Charcotian hysteria seemed to be taken on by women, or interpreted by them, as a kind of in-group style. Henri Huchard, on staff at the time at Tenon Hospital, described his hysteria patients:

When *les hystériques* come together, for example in a hospital ward, their behavior presents some notable characteristics: they electively seek each other out, form isolated groups, shunning with a certain pride the company of the epileptic patients, for whom they cannot have too much contempt. But they quickly become jealous of one another, and combine in little conspiracies, behaving like complete tattle-tales against the others. Then the groups break up as quickly as they have come together. . . . In a service which includes epileptics and hysterics, one may recognize the latter by their custom of decorating the foot of their beds with flowers, or dressing up their hair with ribbons (usually red or blue), of wearing scarves with striking colors, and—just as their whole character is a study in contrast—it is interesting to see them with these get-ups, flowers on their heads, marching about barefoot in the driving rain as their hallucinations [*délire*] or their convulsive attacks approach, their clothing in disarray and their hair to the wind.[72]

Clearly then, among Parisian women the message of how one was supposed to behave in Charcot-style hysteria was being received and understood.

In those decades of quickening communication and rapid rail transport, the message of Charcot-style hysteria was being received in the provinces as well. Léonce Bonamaison, medical director of a private clinic for nervous diseases (*établissement hydrothérapeutique*) at Saint-Didier in the South of France, told of a young American woman, Mlle. X, who had come to France at the age of fourteen. Her parents had died after her arrival, causing a great change in her circumstances. In 1883, at nineteen, she began to develop a whole train of nervous symptoms involving somnambulism and catalepsy. Four years later, in March 1887, she was admitted to his clinic with some of the stigmata of Charcot-style hysteria. She had the full complement of sensory complaints: a hemianesthesia on the left side, intense ovarian pain on that side, exacerbated by pressure ("ovarie") and by walking. She also complained of *clou hystérique* (headache) and "a frequent sensation of burning around the head." She was also unable to see from the left eye.

On the motor side, "Her left hand is maladroit and lacking in power; her left leg is weak and some times collapses."

Mlle. X also used massive doses of the sedative chloral hydrate—up to six grams daily—to combat her insomnia, and took morphine in addition to many other medications. "Mlle. X has a horrible fear of cats; the sight of a cat will almost invariably eventuate in a convulsive fit."

Up to this point we have merely some stigmata, plus the standard symptoms of catalepsy and a kind of pan-nervousness. After her admission to the clinic, however, the Charcot-style fit began to emerge, which she had clearly learned about in the clinic and proceeded to reproduce:

[Her convulsions] took on the classic form of the *grande attaque hystérique* which Charcot has described in his magisterial manner. Without any prodromes save a certain irritability and an exacerbation of her left ovarian pain, she begins a phase of generalized contracture with chattering of the teeth, whistling and the like (tonic phase). Then comes a period of *grands mouvements*, a true attack of clownism, during which the patient devotes herself to the most extravagant acrobatics: jumping, somersaults, standing like a crucifix [*arbre droit*], climbing up on her bedframe or on the furniture. . . . During the phase of delusions and hallucinations which now follows, the patient sees cats (which are normally for her objects of an invincible loathing), her dead mother and so forth.

Further: "In addition to the classic features of the *grande attaque hystérique*, the patient also presented more unusual phenomena, including jumping around *les saltations* with her tongue projecting from her mouth, what the patient calls her 'feeling of being hanged' [*crise du pendu*]." Finally, under hypnosis, Mlle. X reproduced all the phases of grand hypnotism predicted by Charcot: lethargy, catalepsy, and somnambulism.[73] Mlle. X had never been at the Salpêtrière, yet such was the climate of suggestion in this provincial sanatorium that she was able to learn and copy perfectly all the characteristics of Charcot's hysteria and hypnotism.

Elsewhere in provincial France even the most grotesque variants of Charcot's hysteria were faithfully reproduced by patients. Part of *le patron's* doctrine called for multiple spasmogenic and -frenic points on the body, not just above the ovaries. Thus Jean-Albert Pitres, a former intern at the Salpêtrière, encountered at the Saint-André Hospital in Bordeaux a patient named Pauline T. Not only did she have clearly demarcated spasmogenic and -frenic zones over her entire body (the small of her back and both armpits, for example, being spasmofrenic zones), she had similarly hypnogenic and hypnofrenic zones on her body, so that by pressing on her left "ovary" (and also at the bottom of her sternum) one could induce hypnosis, and abolish hypnosis by pressing on both her nipples or the tips of her fingers.[74] In a preface to this work, Charcot expressed pleasure that the experience of Bordeaux demonstrated there was nothing artificial about the hysteria seen at the Salpêtrière.[75]

Nor was it merely Charcot's students who were spreading the contagion. The local doctor in a village in the Seine-et-Oise department reported in a twenty-two-year-old local woman fits that included impassioned attitudes (*les attitudes passionnelles*). Beginning her attack with the epileptoid phase, the patient omitted the second phase of *grands mouvements* and moved directly to gestures of supplication with her hands, cherishing objects, and the like. She terminated her fits according to the book with delusions and hallucinations, seeing herself at a shrine in Lyon, praying there to the Virgin, and then going to a Lyon dentist.[76] Thus Charcot's doctrines in France radiated far beyond the Salpêtrière.

The *grande hystérie* was also encountered abroad, though less commonly than in France. German physicians in particular were quite receptive to the sensory side of the doctrine and cultivated such stigmata as "retinal anaesthesia" in order to explain hysterical blindness. "Ovarie" enjoyed a certain popularity as well.[77] In admitting patients to psychiatric hospitals in Vienna in the 1890s, physicians routinely checked for it.[78] To what extent Central European patients reproduced the symptoms of hysteria major and the stigmata is unclear from the fragmentary reports. Yet these phenomena certainly were known in the patients' world. For example, neurologist Valentin Holst in Riga admitted to the local hospital a seventeen-year-old Jewish woman who had been experiencing headaches, back pain, and general tiredness for about a year. She was placed in a room with a hysteria patient who suffered from loud ructus, or belching, and fits. The woman herself began having fits and loud ructus too, which remained even after her neighbor had been discharged. She also developed some anesthesia in her hand and forearm, and a new kind of back pain localized in one of the thoracic vertebrae. This vertebra then turned into a hysterogenic zone, "in which every pressure on the spot produced either an attack of ructus or a fainting fit without convulsions."[79] Patients' gossip had accordingly converted her from a case of chronic fatigue to an atypical form of *grande hystérie.*

Freud himself in the 1890s believed to some extent in Charcot's stigmata and in the *grande hystérie.* In the "Preliminary Communication" about hysteria that he and Breuer wrote in 1893, Freud said that "severe hysteria" might be provoked, among other mechanisms, "by the stimulation of a hysterogenic zone."[80] His patient Fräulein Elisabeth von R. had such a zone, and when Freud touched a "hyperalgesic" skin spot, she "cried out—and I could not help thinking that it was as though she was having a voluptuous tickling sensation; her face flushed, she threw back her head and shut her eyes and her body bent backwards."[81] Another of Freud's patients, Mrs. K., had in 1895 "cramplike pains in her chest." "In her case," Freud told his friend Wilhelm Fliess, "I have invented a strange therapy of my own: I search for sensitive areas, press on them, and thus provoke fits of shaking which free her." His patient's spasmogenic zones, originally in her face, then shifted to two points on her left chest wall, identical, Freud said, to his own spasmogenic points.[82] The following year Freud told Fliess that he still believed in the "clownism" phase of Charcot's schema of attacks.[83]

Charcot was always gladdened to hear reports from Germany of the kind of hysteria that he himself had invented, such as the famous case of the Prussian grenadier who acted out all phases of *la grande hystérie.* Charcot of course did not want hysteria to be considered a French national disease, in the same way that Freud had not wanted psychoanalysis to become a "Jewish national affair."[84] Yet the occurrence of hysteria major in Germany and Austria was entirely predictable. A steady stream of Central European physicians—individuals of such stature as Rudolph Virchow and Moritz Benedikt—came to the Salpêtrière, reported in German journals what they had seen, and thereby legitimated the diagnosis for their colleagues, ensuring that Central European patients would reproduce the symptoms.[85] The judgment that Charcot-style hysteria was rarely seen outside the Salpêtrière is thus wide of the mark.

In view of the scattered nature of the evidence—and of the incomplete nature of my own sampling of the hundreds and hundreds of cases in the literature—international comparisons of the reception of Charcot's hysteria are risky. Yet his doctrines seem, by and large, to have fallen on deaf ears in England. To be sure, there were a few true believers, such as Thomas Dixon Savill, a physician at the West End Hospital for Diseases of the Nervous System in London, who had qualified for medicine in 1882 and had visited Charcot's clinic in 1888. Savill believed that women with an underlying hysterical "diathesis," or constitution, would sooner or later exhibit such hysterical stigmata as patches of anesthesia of which they had been unaware until the doctor called their attention to it, progressing to "some kind of 'nervous attack' ('attaques des nerfs,' as they are termed in France)." Such attacks might be triggered by "pressure on the inguinal [groin] region."[86] Yet in fairness to Savill, he did have patients who reproduced symptoms that seemed to confirm the theory, such as the twenty-two-year-old woman who since puberty had experienced fainting attacks at the menses. "When I press firmly on either of her inguinal regions she says it produces a feeling of faintness, followed by a feeling of 'sinking in the stomach like you get on a switchback railway, only worse,' then as of a ball rising in the throat (globus hystericus)—sometimes bystanders can hear a gurgling sound as the patient attempts to swallow the 'ball'—and finally she goes off into a faint."[87]

The Birmingham reflex advocate Cornelius Suckling had as a patient in 1885 a woman of twenty-seven, who could have come straight from the Salpêtrière: In addition to paraplegia and globus,

There was marked ovarian hyperaesthesia. Firm pressure over either ovary at once produced flushing of the face, a painful sense of fulness in the throat, and choking, quickly followed by rigidity of the hands and feet, the hands assuming the characteristic posture observed in tetany. . . . The rigidity quickly passed off after discontinuance of the pressure. On one occasion catalepsy was present, the limbs maintaining any position in which they were placed for a considerable time.

Suckling cured her by blistering the skin over the "ovaries," and giving her a Weir Mitchell isolation treatment.[88] He might himself have suggested her into these symptoms with his questioning, or she perhaps had read some newspaper article about the Salpêtrière. In any event, such patients do not seem to have been numerous in England. As Charlton Bastian, president of the Neurological Society of London, said in 1893, Charcot's hysteria major "in anything like a complete form is only very rarely met with in this country."[89]

The English medical establishment, bound to a cautious, antidoctrinaire empiricism, resisted the fanciful flights of la grande hystérie.[90] Samuel Wilks, a physician at Guy's Hospital and a major figure in internal medicine and neurology (he had earlier confirmed that typhus and typhoid fever were separate diseases), said that any psychic shock would serve to cure hysteria, and that this was the mechanism of metallother-apy, galvanism, Lourdes, and so forth, the brains of hysterical people being like a cranky watch: Any shock might start it or stop it again. "The French school," he said, had not understood that.[91] Bastian, another dis-believer, felt that many of Charcot's "functional" cases were really undi-agnosed organic nervous disease.[92] Kinnier Wilson (who became one of the most influential British neurologists of the twentieth century) said in 1910, when he was a resident at the National Hospital for the Paralysed and Epileptic at Queen-Square in London, that hysteria had done so well in Germany and France because, "once the didactic descriptions of Char-cot permeated the textbooks of these countries, the disease was more readily diagnosed and, as is always the case, instances of it seemed to multiply." His more cautious British colleagues, in contrast, had resisted Charcot's theories, particularly the extension of the "conglomerate" of hysteria to a whole range of organic pathology. "Here in England hys-teria has never been cultivated," he said. Unlike the clinicians of Paris and Vienna, "the English neurologist has been far more concerned with organic than with so-called functional nervous disease."[93] English physi-cians might also have shied away from Charcot's hysteria in the 1880s and after because they felt they had been badly burned by reflex theory, in the process of demolition in these years. Anything that smacked of the sensational, with symptoms running wildly about the body and popping up after seeing frogs and bolts of lightening, would increasingly be viewed as the proper province of psychiatry.

A Turn Toward the Psychological?

At the end of his life Charcot seemed to accept a more psychological than organic causation of hysteria. Once psychology came into play as an explanation of somatoform symptoms, patients would shed their previous symptoms in hopes of finding new ones that would be dignified with the label "genuinely organic." Charcot is commonly thought of as the founder of psychological explanations of hysteria, and yet this received wisdom really misses the essence of the man's views.

Charcot was initially quite uninterested in psychological matters. Freud, for example, during his visit to the Salpêtrière in 1885–86, dis-cussed with Charcot his plan to compare the distribution of motor and sensory deficits in organic and in hysterical paralysis, in order to see how hysteria differed. "Charcot thought it a good idea, but it was easy to see that he basically had no special interest in a deeper investigation of the psychology of neurosis. He had come [to hysteria] from anatomical pathology."[94] Charcot's experiments with hypnosis from 1878 on had demonstrated, to be sure, that a mental mechanism lay behind symptom formation in hysteria. He said in conjunction with hypnotism: "I would like to return once again to a subject on which I have already lectured [in Italy in 1885]. I would like to talk about those singular paralyses which have been designated under the terms psychic paralyses, paralysis dependent on idea [here he used the English phrase the London physician Russell Reynolds had employed in 1869], paralyses through imagination." Further: "We now know without a doubt that, in certain circumstances a paralysis can be produced by an idea, and also that an idea can cause it to disappear. But what happens in between is still a mystery." Here he introduced the subject of hypnotism.[95] Yet Charcot at this point was far from calling hysteria a disease of the mind. For him, the ability to be hypnotized was merely evidence that the brain was hysterical.

Two events occurred in the mid-1880s to shift Charcot away from organicity and toward the dim glimmer that hysteria might be psychogenic. The first was his discovery around 1885 of the great success of the therapeutic isolation of patients from their family and friends by putting them in private clinics, otherwise known as the "Weir Mitchell rest cure." Isolation had been particularly promising in the treatment of anorexia nervosa. These young women, physically emaciated and apparently in the grip of a profound "functional" neurosis (meaning for Charcot inherited, physical), would begin eating within days or hours of admission to one of these clinics. Thus the new environment had influenced the mind, suggesting that the disease itself might be "une maladie psychique."[96]

Simultaneously in 1885 Charcot became interested in hysterical symptoms following psychic shocks or accidents, which he called "traumatic neurosis," or "hystero-neurosis." Such a neurosis could develop only in those who were hereditarily predisposed to hysteria, and family histories of nervous disease, as well as the stigmata, could almost always be elicited in such patients. But Charcot saw in traumatic neurosis an interesting analogy to hypnotism. By 1886 he had thought through matters enough to see paralyses elicited under hypnotism and paralyses following a psychic shock as identical.[97] Both were paralysis from an "idea," illustrating the power of ideas to affect the mind. But whereas in hypnotism it was suggestion from a hypnotizer that produced the symptoms, in traumatic neurosis it was "auto-suggestion." In both hystero-neuroses and hypnotized patients, the *moi*, or me, was suppressed, so that local trauma could evoke the conception of a paralysis. If the *moi* were intact, the local trauma would carry no further. One thus acquired symptoms as their mental "representation" rushed into a suppressed psyche. In the years after 1886 Charcot became riveted by experiments on patients who had traumatic neuroses, in which he would reproduce the symptoms under hypnosis in a kind of reenactment of the original trauma.[98]

But Charcot had a highly physiological sense of the meaning of "ideas," and did not mean psychogenesis, the independent action of the mind. For example, in a lecture early in 1888 comparing traumatic suggestion and hypnotic suggestion, he told his listeners that certain psychologists explained muscular movement as the result of a strong idea telling the muscles to move:

> You have to remember also that in the absence of movement [in paralysis], or powerlessness, the same thing happens. Here the idea that is being executed evidently corresponds to a modification in certain regions of the cortex. It is clear as day that there is no idea which does not have a basic substratum in the brain [he used the word *esprit*, which is usually translated as "mind"]. When the idea of the absence of movement becomes predominant, a paralysis may be the result.

Charcot concluded that "in the area of nervous diseases, psychology plays a role, and what I call psychology is the rational physiology of the cerebral cortex."[99]

The final moment in Charcot's tapping toward psychogenesis and away from somatogenesis of hysteria occurred shortly before his death in 1893. The main agent seems to have been the young Pierre Janet, a doctorate in psychology already in hand, who was thirty-three when he received his M.D. in 1893.[100] From 1890 onward in Charcot's wards at the Salpêtrière, Janet had been examining patients in connection with his own theories about dissociation. Charcot, who was becoming increasingly interested in psychological matters, had opened a laboratory for experimental psychology that he entrusted to the then medical-student Janet. In June 1893 Janet published an article in one of the Salpêtrière house organs, the *Archives de neurologie,* calling hysteria a "maladie mentale."[101] Charcot wrote the preface for Janet's book on hysteria as a "maladie mentale," published that year.[102] Also in 1893, in an article on "faith healing," Charcot called attention, in these "highly suggestible individuals," to "the influence that the mind possesses upon the body."[103] It is generally agreed that under Janet's influence, Charcot began drifting away from the iron laws of hysteria in 1892 and 1893, saying that it had become necessary to rethink the whole business.[104]

In the last days of Charcot's life his disciple Edouard Brissaud attempted to expropriate Freud's work for this sudden new construct of hysteria. In a review of an article of Freud's and Breuer's on the psychic mechanism of hysteria that had just appeared in a German neurological journal, Brissaud likened the "traumatic memories" of which the two Viennese authors spoke to traumatic hysteria.[105] Thus on the eve of Charcot's death the old hysteria doctrines were just beginning to break up, yet no member of the Salpêtrière school had yet renounced the notions that only those hereditarily predisposed acquired the disease, that *la grande hystérie* progressed through fixed stages, or that hysteria entailed birth-to-death physical stigmata. There was a contradiction between these core concepts and the notion that hysterical symptoms were implanted by suggestion in patients' minds. It was toward this latter notion that Charcot, weak and infirm in his declining years, had been stumbling. Apparently never fully aware of this implicit contradiction, Charcot died in August 1893, having become, as his student Charles Féré is maliciously supposed to have said, "the star pupil of the Nancy school."[106] The Nancy school had called hypnosis a form of suggestion.

It is technically true that Charcot embraced "psychological" theories of hysteria, but his views were really limited to traumatic neurosis. And even in that limited category, only in those patients genetically predisposed to hysteria would trauma produce symptoms. Hypnosis, Charcot said, could abolish some of the coarser symptoms of hysteria, but not the stigmata. As the range of phenomena deemed hysterical expanded ever more broadly to encompass fever and inflammation and virtually every physical symptom conceivable, there was actually no reason why Charcot's hysteria doctrine could not incorporate rival psychological theories as well, thus appearing, once again, to have confirmed *le patron's* wisdom in anticipating every novelty in neuropathology of his time. Yet the argument that Charcot originated psychological interpretations of hysteria appears to be a basic misreading of his thirty years at the Salpêtrière.[107] The originators of the psychic doctrine of somatization must be sought elsewhere.

The Disappearance of Charcot's Hysteria

For students of the history of somatization, nothing could more graphically illustrate the intimate link between medical shaping and the production of symptoms than the disappearance of Charcot's hysteria within a decade of his death. Maintained by *le patron's* authority, it vanished as soon as Charcot himself disappeared from the scene. What is surprising, however, is the rapidity with which the house of cards fell in.

After 1893 hysteria disappeared from the Salpêtrière. Charcot's successor was an organicist named Fulgence Raymond who, in his inaugural lecture on assuming the neuropathology chair, praised Charcot's work on hysteria and hypnotism, then abandoned the subjects for the duration of his tenure, which ended with his death in 1910.[108] Of Charcot's inpatients, the hysterical performers of the Salpêtrière, some stayed on and gradually forgot their symptoms, others were discharged and maintained normal lives in the community.[109] Many years later, looking back on the Salpêtrière of Charcot, Babinski said:

> There was rarely a day when some patient was not in a hysterical crisis, and it frequently occurred that you would see a number of patients struck simultaneously or successively in the same day. And this was not just at the Salpêtrière but in the other hospitals where similar scenes occurred. This is something that the physicians of my generation know well and which perhaps has escaped some of you younger colleagues. Today [la grande attaque] has virtually disappeared. It is no longer seen and other kinds of fits have become much rarer.[110]

Charcot's own status went into a similar posthumous decline. Now there was no shortage of physicians to say the emperor had no clothes. Mocked Clément Simon of the spa of Uriage-les-Bains near Grenoble: If you cannot find a lesion to explain the symptoms (whatever they are), and if the patient shows any stigmata, then the diagnosis is hysteria. "No one would be surprised at diagnoses of hysterical hemoptysis [coughing up blood], hysterical hematemesis [vomiting blood], hysterical cutaneous gangrene, and hysterical meningitis."[111]

Jules-Joseph Dejerine, who had come to the Salpêtrière in 1895, two years after Charcot's death, told the house staff explicitly not to discuss hysteria in front of the patients; it merely suggested them into new symptoms. "The history of hysterics and neurasthenics in hospital is only too rich in phenomena of this kind," he said pointedly.

Dejerine himself was ruthless with hysterics when anything resembling a fit began. One intern who had been on Dejerine's service said that if a patient started to display a classic crisis,

> all hell would break loose. Patients in neighboring beds would interrupt the guilty one, "Come now, little one [Dis donc, ma petite], the chief is going to kick you out. He hates it when people have crises. We used to have them too, but he sure knew how to make us get rid of

them. You do like us!" And all the nurses including the head nurse would back them up.

Next morning at rounds, the clinical clerks, externs and interns would all mix in and grandly indicate their disapproval, to be sure benevolently, but with such irony! And finally the chief himself would pronounce the definitive word, "I'm going to pardon you this time, because you didn't know. But it better not happen again."[112]

"In the eight years I have been at the Salpêtrière," said Dejerine on another occasion, "the symptoms characterizing what one used to call *la grande hystérie* have never lasted more than a week on my service."[113]

Wilhelm Stekel, the Viennese psychoanalyst who had been in Paris just after World War I, said, "Twenty years after Charcot's death one could not find a single case of hysteria in any of the Paris hospitals." "Now no experienced clinician can pronounce the word hysteria without smiling." While Stekel was in Paris, a book dealer had offered him a copy of Charcot's nine-volume collected works for a mere twenty-five francs.[114]

But it was actually Joseph Babinski—who under Charcot's thumb had felt obliged to write scientific articles about transferring symptoms from patient to patient with a magnet—who administered the coup de grâce to Charcot's hysteria doctrine. Under Charcot, all bodily functions had been considered subject to hysteria, including vasomotor reactions (changes in the size of blood vessels, as in blushing), dermatological complaints such as pemphigus, and local edema. This is where things stood when Babinski discovered, three years after Charcot's death, his "toe sign," which made it possible to determine whether many hysterical symptoms were caused by a genuine organic lesion of the central nervous system or not (if one runs a pointed object down the lateral surface of the sole of the foot, the big toe normally turns down; if the toe turns up, in plantar extension, an upper-motor neuron lesion may be present).[115] The toe sign made it possible to do away with all this vague Charcot-style talk about "weakened nervous centers" and actually determine (though not with 100 percent accuracy) if organic pathology was present or not. If not, the case was hysteria.

What was hysteria? Any symptom, said Babinski, that could be induced by suggestion and abolished by persuasion. By "suggestion" Babinski meant, first, medical suggestion: doctors suggesting patients into anesthesias, for example, in the neurological exam. But Babinski was also willing to accept other forms of suggestion such as "cultural," which is roughly coterminous with the idea of the symptom pool. Under "persuasion," Babinski understood hypnosis or some other form of psychotherapy. The implication of Babinski's new definition of hysteria was that it relegated to the dustbin the famous stigmata, supposedly inborn and lifelong. Hysteria became a transitory affliction, like a stomachache, into which one could be suggested and from which one could recover after a good talking-to (persuasion) by a sympathetic physician. Babinski first broached his new definition of hysteria in 1901.[116] Its logic was so ineluctable that by 1908 it had shattered completely the old intellectual edifice of Charcot-style hysteria.[117]

Physicians ceased believing in the stigmata of hysteria, and patients, unwilling to be seen as simulators or as having symptoms that were "all in your head," stopped producing them. (As early as 1910 many German physicians had ceased checking for ovarie.) It was argued that to avoid suggesting patients into sensory symptoms of any kind, one should simply omit the sensory examination of the nervous system.[118] In 1919 Oswald Bumke said in his influential psychiatry textbook: "The so-called hysterical stigmata have now lost almost all credit, symptoms that until recently were unchallengeable evidence of the presence of hysteria and that were never supposed to be lacking in the hysterical. At least the latter part of this claim is false. We know today that these diagnostic signs were earlier so frequently found because the doctor expected them and conferred his own suggestion upon the patient."[119] And what patient now would dare present hysterical stigmata to such hardened veterans as Babinski and Alexandre Souques: Both said in 1928 that it had been years since they had seen a case, especially the once much vaunted "male hysteria."[120]

The idiosyncratic stigmata that Charcot had devised, such as ovarie, loss of color vision, and constriction of the visual fields would vanish. Yet Charcot had also considered other kinds of sensory problems more commonly found in the population, such as headache or pains around the body, as stigmata as well. Not having been invented by the school of the Salpêtrière, these would not go away with the collapse of its patron. In the shift of somatoform symptoms from the motor to the less easily investigatable sensory side of the nervous system, Charcot plays an important role. A German spa physician, Armin Steyerthal, who at his hydrotherapy clinic in Kleinen, in Mecklenburg, was closely attuned to shifts in fashionable symptoms, picked up this theme. Steyerthal said in 1911 that Charcot's main place in the history of medical thinking on hysteria was causing fits to lose their central place as symptoms: "The fit sheds its previous meaning as the essence of the whole disorder [of hysteria]. Up till now hysteria was a *Morbus convulsivus,* and in the absence of the characteristic attacks nobody would even have considered making the diagnosis. That has now changed." The stigmata had taken over as the essence of hysteria, Steyerthal said. Steyerthal meant stigmata such as symptoms of cutaneous hypersensitivity, pain, and chronic fatigue.[121] Though caution is indicated in claiming too much for Charcot, this enormously influential physician nonetheless directed the attention of his colleagues, for the first time in history, to sensory phenomena. This increased medical attention may in some measure help account for the shift.

The rise and fall of Charcot-style hysteria forms an important chapter in the history of psychosomatic illness because it establishes how extraordinarily dependent the presentation of somatoform illness is on medical shaping. That it lay in the power of one man to bring forth this epidemic of fits and sensory stigmata in the 1880s and 1890s is a measure of the rising influence in these years of the medical profession.[122] The power of physicians to shape symptoms in the first half of the twentieth century would be no less. But it would express itself more in advances in the ability to diagnose organic disease, rather than in the ability to impose on the public what were essentially unscientific cultural prejudices about women as being automatons subject to "ovarie."

CHAPTER

8

The Doctors Change Paradigms: Central Nervous Disease

Before 1870 the reflex model offered the dominant medical paradigm for interpreting nervous symptoms. This paradigm tended to encourage motor symptoms, because the whole purpose of the reflex arc was to convert sensory stimulation into muscular movement. After about 1870, this reflex paradigm was challenged by two new paradigms, each incompatible with the other and both inconsistent with the reflex model. Of the two new paradigms, the one stressing invisible but real disease in the central nervous system came first, and it held sway from the last quarter of the nineteenth century until around the time of World War I. A rival paradigm assigning psychological causes to somatization surfaced only a few years later, competed against the central nervous system paradigm, and finally won out in the second half of the twentieth century. Yet the main impact of the psychological paradigm was not at all what one might expect: Not in the least did the triumph of psychological interpretation make the population as a whole more insightful about the psychogenesis of physical symptoms. To the contrary: Insisting on the organicity of their problems, somatizing patients after World War II would seek the help of the neurologist and internist, specifically shunning that of the psychiatrist.

Medical doctrines as well as the larger culture both change patients' behavior. The history of psychosomatic illness in the nineteenth and

201

twentieth centuries may be written in part—but only in part—as a history of changing medical ideas, for these various paradigms greatly influenced the way patients presented psychosomatic illness to their doctors.

The Destruction of the Reflex Paradigm

Reflex theories began to wane in the 1870s because of a combination of a growing disbelief on the part of the professors, and the accumulation of evidence on the part of the researchers. The two processes were not necessarily related.

The dossier against genital reflexes as a cause of hysteria and mental illness had been building for many years. In 1821, Étienne-Jean Georget, on the psychiatric staff of the Salpêtrière, had said, "According to my observations, the action of the uterus is normal in more than three-quarters of the [hysteria] patients, even during the fit itself."[1] In the early 1850s, Robert Carter, a London surgeon and an authority on hysteria, experimented on twenty poor women to test the usefulness of treating the uterus with caustic applications. He had taken the patients on loan from one of London's medical officers of health. The remedies failed to improve nineteen of the twenty borrowed patients (the exception had, in the latter half of the period under observation, gone to the beachside town of Hastings).[2] Yet these early empirical findings were largely ignored by reflex enthusiasts. It is quite striking how long American physicians in particular were mindless of such data: As late as 1909 Clara Dercum's report on an absence of pelvic lesions in patients with hysteria and neurasthenia would still be considered news.[3]

Another kind of empirical disproof of reflex ovarian theory was the placebo operation. The brilliant young surgeon James Israel, who had just become head of surgery at the Jewish Hospital in Berlin, told this story: Bertha Perlmann, alias Kantrowitz, a young hairdresser of twenty-three from a village near Kovno (Kaunas), had a six-year history of terrible headaches, vomiting, and "ovarian" pain surrounding the menses. Doctors in nearby Königsberg, the regional medical center, had advised her to see Professor Hegar in Freiburg about an ovariotomy. Reluctant to give up her fecundity, she unsuccessfully tried a cure in Franzensbad, then went to Berlin, where doctors again urged ovariotomy on her. "In the meantime," said Israel in reconstructing the case, "her condition had become so bad that she started vomiting on the street and was too weak to travel." So she was admitted to a hospital in Berlin where the vaginal portion of her cervix was removed. Still no improvement. She returned to Franzensbad where three more doctors recommended ovariotomy, making by now a total of six. Her symptoms worse than ever, she returned to Berlin, and saw two more physicians, each of whom recommended ovariotomy. In this state, on November 18, 1879, she turned to Doctor Israel, "urgently pleading for the operation." Eight authorities had now seconded her wishes.

On New Year's Eve Day, 1879, Israel performed an operation on her under chloroform narcosis. The improvement was dramatic. Within a week of the operation, all vomiting had ceased. Ovarian pain, both spontaneous and on pressure, had stopped, and "the patient considers herself subjectively to be well."

"Now gentlemen," said Israel, explaining the procedure to a Berlin medical meeting on January 14, 1880:

> This would have been a lovely cure of a difficult case of hysteria with a bilateral ovariotomy, if in fact I had done such an operation. My operative procedure, however, deviates in one essential point from that of Battey and Hegar, in that I did nothing to the patient at all aside from a simple skin incision under narcosis. We are thus dealing with a skilfully staged placebo-operation and aftercare, which sought the purpose of convincing the patient she had truly been castrated. This goal has now been splendidly accomplished.[4]

Under the cumulative impact of practical demonstrations such as this, the reflex house of cards began to totter.

Among other kinds of new evidence was, after 1870, the discovery of the endocrine system, which offered an alternative explanation for apparent reflex phenomena. In 1874 the Strasbourg physiologist Friedrich Goltz cut the spinal cord of a female dog, which nonetheless was able to come into heat and become pregnant. This established that spinal reflexes did not control the uterus and ovaries, that instead "some mysterious connection . . . mediated by the blood" was responsible.[5] From this point on, the unraveling of the endocrine system would inexorably crush reflex theory—a collapse that was partially a scientific phenomenon.

But also entrained in the demise of reflex theory was a simple loss of belief, mediated perhaps by common sense or by some dimly perceived inadequacy of the theories themselves. This dawning sense of inappropriateness belonged to the larger process of medicalization, which affected both physicians and their patients throughout the nineteenth century. "Medicalization" refers to making individuals dependent upon "official" medical care, as opposed to the unofficial village variety of the corncutter, bonesetter, and midwife. How extensively this dependency occurred, and what its consequences were, remain matters of scholarly debate.[6] Yet it is clear that by 1900 a given individual would be more likely to define symptoms as illness and himself as a patient than in 1800.

Medicalization helped doom reflex theory by bringing doctor and patient closer together psychologically. Harley Street gives us an example of this new intimacy in the doctor-patient relationship. The consultant physicians of the West End of London, who supplied primary care to the upper middle classes, established in the second half of the nineteenth century ever closer psychological bonds to their female clientele. As the cynical surgeon Charles Bell Keetley of West London Hospital (a man said to have been held back in advancement only by "his deafness, his unpunctuality and his biting wit") observed in 1878, "The chief value of the letters M.D. is that they produce an undoubted impression on the general public, especially upon the ladies."[7] Physicians of this stratum had in the first half of the century largely been partisans of reflex theory. It is likely that a more personal, or intimate, style of medical practice established psychological ties to patients that simply ruled out the reflex paradigm, a paradigm that saw patients as automatons guided by their ovaries.

A textbook case of the new medical style on Harley Street was Frederick Parkes Weber, who qualified in medicine in 1889 and during his long life of practice among upper-class men and women was said to have been "beloved by his patients." "He had old-fashioned and very beautiful manners," said one obituarist. "He treated patients with grave courtesy and listened intently to everything they had to say. After consulting with the doctor [who had called him in] he always went back to the patient and said something kind and encouraging. He shook them earnestly by the hand and said goodbye in a way that made them feel he was really sorry to go."[8] It is fair to claim that Parkes Weber probably "medicalized" some of his female patients, in that they would return to him time and again over the years, consulting on what spa to visit that season and writing him letters while abroad on how the waters had been helping their constipation. He first saw Miss Y, for example, in September 1895. She was thirty-seven, and complained of arthritic pains for which she occasionally took morphine. The following year her problem was "stomach and intestinal flatulence, usually during evening, especially about one week before menstrual periods and when there is a change in the weather." Her complaints varied over the years. Virtually each year he would send her to a spa: Marienbad in 1895, Nice in 1898, Bath in 1899, and so forth. In May 1912 she wrote him: "I propose to go abroad for a course of waters and I should like to go carefully into the question with you, of whether La Bourboule, or what I should prefer, Marienbad or Carlsbad, is desirable. I have at times a great deal of asthma, I am also too stout, and am very much troubled with neuralgic and gouty symptoms, which appear anywhere, or everywhere." In July 1913 she wrote him from the Waldhaus hotel at Vulpera-Tarasp in the Swiss Engadine:

> *Dear Dr. Parkes Weber,*
> *I know you like to hear how the cure answers, so send you a line*
> *on the eve of departure for England.*
> *I think the place is delightful, full of interest to me, and I was*
> *thankful I obeyed your orders, and came up here, instead of going*
> *to the Kurhaus at Tarasp.*

She discussed with him "the state" she was in. "Last winter has damaged me somehow, and my heart won't work." There had also been problems with Doctor Leva at Tarasp, who insisted on ordering baths.

Year after year, this aging, wealthy, single woman found in Parkes Weber a sympathetic ear.[9] The point is that for the Parkes Webers of this world "uterine reflex theories" simply were not tenable. They were inapplicable to this class of patients. He did not examine his patients vaginally, and evidently found the whole idea that the uterus affected the brain incredible, for even though reflex doctrine still abounded when he began to practice medicine, he never mentioned it in his notes.

Parkes Weber was not a professor, though he was said to look like one. Russell Reynolds and Clifford Allbutt, however, were, and they offer perfect examples of the denunciation of reflex theory from academic heights. Reynolds, full physician in clinical medicine at University College, London, and in 1867 successor to William Jenner in the chair of medicine, thought reflex theory ridiculous. In 1872 he pooh-poohed genital affections as a source of hysteria: "It is, so far as my experience extends, the exception and not the rule to find any definite malady, or indeed definite complaint, in this direction; while in the vast number of cases there has been absolute health in all particulars relating to the reproductive organs."[10] Clifford Allbutt in Leeds, to take another example of a new, antireflex generation of physicians, was forty-eight in 1884 and already one of the most distinguished internists of his day. In 1892 he would become Regius Professor of medicine in Cambridge. Many ears would therefore perk up when Allbutt scorned attentiveness to the pelvis in treating neuroses: "The essence of the malady is not there, and to try to cure such a malady by local means is as wise as to try to cure a syphilis by antiseptic dressing of its ulcers." He criticized the gynecologists for swabbing away at the cervix "with little Partington-mops of cotton wool on the ends of little sticks" and ignoring all else. "The patient and the doctor are fascinated by the local phenomena while Nature herself is performing on a far larger scale."[11]

Allbutt's colleague William S. Playfair was the archetype of a "society gynecologist," with a large London practice and consultation to royalty. Playfair had introduced in 1881 to England the "rest cure" for nervous disease, a cure devised by the American neurologist Weir Mitchell.[12] One could hear the new wind blowing in the 1880s and 1890s when Playfair discouraged local treatments of the pelvis for neurosis. For example, in 1896 he said that, while overlooking local gynecological lesions was a mistake, a far greater blunder was the "needless local treatment of what may be called the 'tinkering' kind." He went into detail:

Both mistakes are serious ones; but I am constrained to say—and the more I see of neurotic women the more convinced I am—that the latter [tinkering] is much the more serious and common of the two. Nothing can be more deplorably bad for a nervous, emotional woman, whose general health is at a low ebb, than to have her attention constantly directed to her reproductive organs by vaginal examinations repeated two or three times a week, pessaries constantly introduced for "a slight displacement," the cervix frequently cauterised, or the endometrium [uterine lining] curetted, and the like; and yet these are things one incessantly sees. . . . No doubt it is generally done in good faith; but the results are often disastrous.[13]

These several English writers illustrate the general point that in the 1880s and 1890s many respected authorities weighed in against reflex theory.

In Germany a whole new cohort of scientifically oriented gynecologists arose in the 1890s, who found reflex theory out of date and campaigned actively against it at professional meetings. In 1891 Rudolf Kaltenbach, a forty-nine-year-old professor of obstetrics at Halle, had already lashed out at those who gave reflex interpretations of the vomiting of pregnancy.[14] Speaking out around 1900 were a younger cohort, such as Adolph Theilhaber in Munich, forty-six that year and chief physician of a widely known private gynecological clinic (he was not a professor: appointing Jews to professorships of gynecology was still frowned on); Bernhard Krönig, thirty-seven in 1900, who in 1903 would become professor of gynecology in Jena; and Franz Windscheid, thirty-eight, who taught in Leipzig and in 1897 wrote a book on neuropathology and gynecology.[15] These men, rising stars in the research firmament, all had allied themselves against doctrines of "genital neurosis," "uterine reflexes," and the like. Either they were interested in the psychogenesis (Theilhaber) or the neurogenesis (Windscheid) of neurotic symptoms.

An episode that highlights just how sweeping the rejection of "gynecological psychiatry" had become was the misadventure encountered by the ideas of the Genoan professor of gynecology Luigi Maria Bossi once they arrived north of the Alps. Known for the invention of a set of instruments for dilating the cervix, Bossi also propagated local treatment of the uterus for insanity, and the sterilization of women who were mentally ill. "At least half of female suicides [are of] gynecological origin," he maintained in 1911 in the main German gynecological journal. Bossi believed suicide was somehow associated with the menses. In 1912 his views were broadcast fully to the profession with the translation into German of his book on "utero-ovarian illness and insanity."[16]

Bossi had, to be sure, a few German supporters, including Gustav Ortenau, a spa doctor (Bad Reichenhall summers, Nervi winters), who had visited Bossi's clinic and reported enthusiastically on what he had seen.[17] But the only prominent gynecologist to support Bossi was the dinosaur Bernhard Schultze, eighty-four in 1911 and an advocate of gynecological operating rooms in asylums.[18]

Bossi was savaged by the majority of German gynecologists and psychiatrists. The Tübingen gynecology professor August Mayer, for example, indicted Bossi and his "ridiculous" theory as "the summit" of needless gynecological surgery. Bossi and his like, charged Mayer, were so "fixated upon the uterus that they often overlook both body and soul."[19] Josef Peretti, professor of psychiatry at the medical school in Düsseldorf and director of a nearby asylum, noted that in Germany Bossi had "found very few unconditional supporters." Not only was the notion scientifically groundless, but it encouraged families to take their mentally ill female relatives first to the gynecologist, in hopes of avoiding the asylum. The "furor operativus passivus," the belief in surgery as a panacea, was further strengthened, Peretti said.[20] Ernst Siemerling, professor of psychiatry in Kiel, observed that men and children had exactly the same kinds of hysteria and neurasthenia as did women, and yet they were not subject to gynecological disease. Unnecessary gynecological operations made mentally ill women worse.[21] The Bossi episode represented the last eruption of gynecological surgery and pelvic-reflex theory into European consciousness. It was time for a new paradigm.

The Rise of Central Nervous Theories of Psychosis and Neurosis

Alongside the reflex paradigm, an entirely different kind of paradigm for explaining mental illness and bodily symptoms had been percolating—theories that stressed organic disease of brain tissue itself. If patients became psychotic or hysterical, it was not because their uteruses were irritated but because they had inherited a kind of "nervous" constitution that affected their "cerebral centers." Invisible under the microscope, such affections of brain tissue were nonetheless thought to be very real and the cause of neurosis and psychosis.

Theories pointing to the central nervous system went right back to Haller, Brown, and the eighteenth-century doctrine of "irritation." Throughout the first half of the nineteenth century within psychiatry, such organic brain theories competed directly with reflex theory.[22] Characteristic of the early brain-disease theorists, for example, was the Bavarian Johannes Friedreich (who lost his post at the University of Würzburg in 1832 for political reasons). In 1836 Friedreich characterized the position of "somaticists" such as himself thus: "Psychic diseases do not originate in the first instance in the mind [*Seele*] but in a material abnormality, which results in abnormal expression of the individual psychic functions." Although peripheral problems such as infections could cause mental abnormalities, he saw as a major cause of mental illness organic disease in the brain itself, resulting perhaps from heredity.[23] In the years before 1860 numerous other medical writers argued along similar lines, stressing the central nervous system as the seat of madness and emphasizing heredity.

The view that mental illness is nothing more than a symptom of brain disease found its most influential proponent in the German psychiatrist Wilhelm Griesinger, whose main period of influence was confined to about seven years, dating from the widely read second edition of his psychiatry textbook in 1861 and ending with his death from appendicitis in 1868 at the age of fifty-one. The story of how a man with so little experience in psychiatry could have had such a vast impact on the field, not just in Germany but in Europe as a whole, shows that Griesinger launched an idea whose time had come.

Born in Stuttgart in 1817, Griesinger graduated in 1838 with an M.D. from nearby Tübingen, studied internal medicine for a year in Paris, then returned to his native Württemberg and spent the brief time from 1840 to 1842 as an assistant physician at the Winnenthal asylum. On the basis of this meager experience, the twenty-eight-year-old Griesinger wrote a psychiatry textbook, incorporating a number of then-fashionable reflex ideas. At this point Griesinger abandoned psychiatry for the next twenty years to devote himself to internal medicine and infectious diseases, receiving several distinguished professorships—first at Tübingen, then later, after various adventures, in Zurich. In 1861 he published a second edition of his textbook. At this time he had been almost twenty years without contact with psychotic illness in adults, and only months previously had accepted the professorship of psychiatry in Zurich. In the revised edition of his textbook, Griesinger played down most of his earlier reflex views—and indeed shunned the term reflex itself for other such postulated mechanisms as "cerebral hyperemia."[24] What, then, did he believe the cause of mental illness to be? "The etiology of mental illnesses in general," he said in 1861, "is none other than the etiology of all other brain and nerve diseases."[25]

In 1865 Griesinger was called from Zurich to become the professor of psychiatry in Berlin. Three years later, in 1868, in the preface to a new journal he had founded, devoted to the study of "psychiatric and neurological diseases," he described the cause of mental illness in a more telegraphic manner: "The so-called 'mental illnesses' [occur in] individuals with brain disease and neurological disease." It was really a matter of indifference whether a doctor labeled someone "mentally ill" (*gemüts-krank*) or "neurologically ill" (*nervenkrank*). In many cases it was all the same thing.[26] As for the mechanism that converted an underlying constitutional anomaly (brain disease) into the symptoms of psychosis and neurosis, Griesinger borrowed the phrase "irritable weakness" (*reizbare Schwäche*) previously used by Romberg and others: The more excited, or irritated, the brain becomes, the less effectively it executes its functions. In individuals born with a "nervous constitution," irritable weakness amplifies sensory impressions into great agitation. On the motor side, irritable weakness means that "the motor nerves are hallmarked by a decrease of power; there is easy exhaustibility, a tendency to quicker and more widespread but simultaneously less energetic movements, and a heightened tendency to convulsions." Mentally, irritable weakness was characterized by "greater psychical sensitivity, an easier susceptibility to psychic pain, the condition wherein every thought causes some emotional agitation [*Gemütsbewegung*]. This in turn causes a rapid and unopposed change of self-image and mood, also weakness and lack of consequence of the will, a lack of energy in all affairs combined with rapidly alternating desires."[27]

Griesinger's work gave the old notion of irritable weakness a whole new impetus, one moreover in the context of an entirely different paradigm than the reflex paradigm in which it was born. Griesinger's "irritable weakness," an underlying, inborn brain condition, could cause almost any symptom conceivable, which is to say, virtually any symptom could be attributed to it. The above-quoted lines had a profound impact on the understanding of the neuroses over the next half century.

Griesinger's work hitched neurology to psychiatry for a certain period of time. Neurology had started out in internal medicine (stroke, tumor, meningitis), and in the tradition of Charcot would continue to be taught by individuals whose background had been in internal medicine, not in psychiatry. But Griesinger, by assimilating mind disease to brain disease, anchored a quite different approach: Neurology belonged to psychiatry, and vice versa. All mental symptoms were reduced to organic disfunction in the nervous system. "The insane asylum became a neurological clinic," said one observer many years later.[28] The temptation for both patients and doctors to see mental disorders and somatization as the result of "organic nervous disease" would thus be overpowering.

Under the impetus given by Griesinger, "organic brain" theories of psychosis and neurosis became standard in psychiatry in Germany and elsewhere in the second half of the nineteenth century. In fact, the scientific prestige of the Germans permitted them to dictate to virtually everyone save the French (who were under Charcot's spell) what constituted cause and effect in mental illness. The years from 1860 to 1900 were later known as the era of "brain mythology" in psychiatry, attempting to explain mental illness on the basis of anatomical anomalies or physiological lesions in the brain.[29] Freud, who himself qualified as a lecturer in neuropathology in Vienna in 1885, characterized the 1880s as an epoch when "the major authorities in Vienna were accustomed to diagnosing neurasthenia as a brain tumor."[30] In Vienna in those years Theodor Meynert taught that, "Psychiatry is the doctrine of the diseases of the forebrain."[31] Paul Flechsig, professor of psychiatry in Leipzig and a major contributor to research in neuroanatomy, once told Oswald Bumke, "You know, I've never been interested in psychiatry. I feel that as a discipline it's a dead end." Bumke observed that Flechsig's clinic looked like one.[32]

So completely had the doctrine of organicity triumphed that the real purpose of research in psychiatry was seen as clarifying brain anatomy, a purpose that shines clearly from the correspondence with his contemporaries of August Forel, a man not uninterested in psychological issues. In 1878, eight years before being dragged to the bottom of the Starnbergersee by the crazed King Ludwig II of Bavaria, Bernhard von Gudden, the professor of psychiatry in Munich, wrote to Forel about common interests. The chat was all neuroanatomy:

> The study on the optic chiasm turned out bigger than I thought and is already in Göttingen. The study on the brain of the newborn "idiot" is finished, and I've just set to work on the study of the Tractus peduncularis transversus and the mamillary bodies. The sections of the oculomotor- and trochlear-nerve nuclei turned out splendidly. There now can be almost no doubt that the oculomotor nerve has a double nucleus. . . . [The foregoing are all structures in the brain.]
>
> [Anton] Bumm is working away on the retina, [Sigbert] Ganser has sectioned some mole brains, Mayser is getting deeper and deeper into fish and has started to use the extirpation method. [Emil] Kraepelin still hasn't finished with his dissertation.[33]

Virtually all the names Gudden mentioned were, or would become, distinguished professors of psychiatry.

How was this paradigm shift communicated to patients, most of whom did not read medical journals? In the setting of the private clinic, chief physicians took pains to explain to well-to-do patients what was wrong with them, so that they would return. (The nerve doctor who treated Hermann Hesse at a spa near Zurich, by reassuring Hesse about the [improbable] organicity of his complaints, turned Hesse's anger and resentment into gratitude for being "understood."[34]) The dominant paradigm in this influential setting was unquestionably that of organic nervous disease. Caspar Max Brosius, director of an expensive private clinic in Bendorf am Rhein (who in 1858 had imported into Germany the fashionable new English technique of "no restraint" of psychiatric patients), cautioned his colleagues not to make the mistake of "psychic treatment," for insanity was a brain disease.[35] That was in 1878. In 1881 he emphasized again: "Insanity is a *brain* disease." "One combats [psychic symptoms] not through the countereffect of psychic and moral agents, but through rest and care of the sick brain."[36] Ewald Hecker—like Forel a hypnotherapist, and chief physician of a private clinic in Johannisberg near Wiesbaden—was also not indifferent to the psychological side of things. Yet in 1881 he rejoiced that under the new paradigm, psychiatry was rejoining medicine after a long period of mysticism. (Some psychiatrists before 1848 had considered mental illness a punishment for sin.) This rapprochement had occurred because of "the rapidly growing recognition that mental illnesses [*Geisteskrankheiten*] are brain diseases [*Gehirnkrankheiten*] and as such represent simply a band of the large spectrum of neurological diseases [*Nervenkrankheiten*]."[37] Karl Kahlbaum, owner and chief physician of a private clinic in Görlitz in Silesia, said that mental illness was really not different from eye or gynecological disease. It was a disorder of a particular organ system—and not, as people tended to think, a special kind of affliction—and could be treated in a specialty clinic.[38]

All this psychiatric talk about brain disease was therefore not just public relations, designed to mollify the patients while doctors laughed up their sleeves (like prescribing antibiotics for colds today). These physicians believed implicitly in the new doctrine and encouraged their patients to do so as well.

Most psychosomatic illness would appear, however, not in tandem with the major mental illnesses but in the forms of hysteria and neurasthenia. Here too the new paradigm implicated organic disease of the nervous system rather than disturbances of mentation or the action of the unconscious mind. Interpreting hysteria as a central nervous disorder reaches right back to the eighteenth century. In 1776 Andrew Wilson, a London physician, called hysteria a "disease of the principle [of] life itself. . . . In the hysterical passion, the accumulated modification of this principle in the theatre of conception is so irritable, that it reacts instantaneously upon that original potential form of life, which stamps it with its procreating virtue." This was a roundabout way of calling hysteria an inherited constitutional disease.[39]

Even after 1820, when reflex theory became the dominant paradigm, central-nervous theory continued to flourish in its shadow as an explanation of hysteria. In 1837 Benjamin Brodie considered hysteria a physical disease of the nervous system, owing to "imperfect development" during childhood and resulting in an "insufficient generation of nervous energy."[40] London gynecologist David Davis, writing at about the same time, ridiculed uterine theories and called hysteria "an idiopathic disease of the brain, common to both sexes . . . not essentially different in kind from epilepsy."[41] Indeed Robert Bentley Todd, cofounder in 1840 of King's College Hospital, felt able in 1847 to situate hysteria precisely in the brain stem. "Hence it is not to be wondered that a highly disturbed state of this centre is capable of deranging all the sensitive as well as the motor phenomena of the body and even the intellect."[42]

In France, implicating the central nervous system in hysteria was by no means an innovation of Charcot. Pierre Briquet, for example, the greatest student of the subject before Charcot, considered hysteria a malady "of that portion of the encephalon where affective functions are located."[43]

Elsewhere in Europe the rival central nervous paradigm was invoked from the beginning of the nineteenth century. In 1816 Doctor Hohnstock said that hysteria was commoner among women because, "Women in general have a more sensitive nervous system than men, and because this disease comes simply from an excessive sensibility or sensitivity of the nerves." He called it "a chronic so-called nervous disease."[44] A whole rash of German writers from the 1840s through the 1860s—spa doctors, gynecologists, and other physicians—affirmed that hysteria resulted from an affliction of the central nervous system and had nothing to do with reflexes or local lesions.[45]

A final point about the origins of this rival paradigm: From the beginning the paradigm insisted that nervous disease was an inheritable constitutional disorder. In 1702, differentiating "hysterick fits" from epilepsy, John Purcell said that "vapours as well as other diseases [were] transmitted to us from our fathers and mothers," while "apoplexies" presumably were not.[46] Dietrich Busch, professor of gynecology in Berlin, spoke in 1840 of the "transference of hysteria from the mother to the daughter" as quite common.[47] The young Heinrich Laehr, still an assistant physician at the Nietleben asylum near Halle under the famous Heinrich Damerow, gave in 1852 an extensive account of the inheritability of mental illness that reflected the conventional wisdom of his time.[48]

The doctrine of heredity in psychosis and neurosis had become commonplace by midcentury. It remained for such French psychiatrists as Benedict-Augustin Morel, director of an asylum in Rouen, and Valentin Magnan at the Sainte Anne asylum in Paris, to condense the assumption of inheritability into that of "degeneration," meaning that nervous disease got worse with each passing generation.[49] (These doctrines lay waiting for Charcot to pick them up.) The writers on degeneration were, in any event, amplifying a belief system whose roots reached back considerably in time.

Nerve Doctors for Nervous Diseases

It is doubtful that the "pace of life" ever really changes. Individuals have always believed they lived in a "speeded-up" or "nervous" society, no less in late-eighteenth-century Europe or early-nineteenth-century America than today. In 1787 the German philanthropist Joachim Heinrich Campe spoke of "our nerve-sick epoch."[50] Historian James Cassedy writes of the United States in the 1830s and 1840s:

Urban editors and physicians pointed to the detrimental effects on the nervous system of the increasing propensity for "fast walking, fast driving, fast eating and drinking, fast bargains, fast business . . . fast everything but *fast-ing!*" In New York, the preacher Henry Ward Beecher found that the "bustle of the street, the ceaseless thunder of the vehicles, the rush to-and-fro of multitudes of people" was more than many of his congregation could bear.[51]

Europeans at the end of the nineteenth century similarly perceived themselves as living hectic lives plagued by nervous illness. In an 1899 guidebook of private clinics directed toward both physicians and rich laity, Paul Berger explained:

In this era of the machine . . . over-irritation and shock of the nerves themselves, above all the nerves of the brain, the central organ of the nervous system, have occurred on a scale that previous generations have never known nor suspected. We live in an era of nervous diseases [*Nervenkrankheiten*], which are increasing progressively on a terrifying scale.[52]

Contemporaries defined these nervous diseases as "modern diseases."[53] Just as people had once believed that the time of the French Revolution had been an "age of heart disease," fin-de-siècle observers thought themselves living in an "age of nervous disease." Viennese novelist Robert Musil described the Vienna of the *belle époque* as "an age of nerves."[54] In 1894 Leopold Löwenfeld, a nerve doctor in Munich, complained:

The ceaseless hurry and disruption of business life, the feverish pace one has to adopt to get anywhere, the clamor of the wagons in the business-streets, the endless variety that strikes the eye everywhere, all the entertainments that exhaust body and soul and continue until late at night: all these circumstances entrain indisputably an excessive use of nervous energy and do not permit the proper restoration of the exhausted system.[55]

In France, Jules Chéron, an advocate of conservative treatment in gynecology, deplored the tendency of "modern life . . . to resemble more and more *la vie américaine*, which is par excellence a life of overwork, a depressing life. The struggle for existence has never been so bitter, people have never been so crippled in their will, physically and morally more weakened, more exhausted by effort." Chéron thought the struggle was also responsible for low blood pressure.[56]

Such a nervous epoch would require "nerve doctors." The concept of nervous disease—and its attribution to organic changes in the brain and nerves—was already established at the beginning of the nineteenth century. What was new in the last third of the nineteenth century was the emergence of a set of specific "nervous" diagnoses and a corps of physicians to make them and manage their treatment—the nerve doctors or *Nervenärzte*.

"Nervous" diseases, meaning organic affections of the physical nerves, had been recognized since at least the time of William Cullen in the 1770s. In the course of the nineteenth century, this amorphous group of nervous diseases split into two groups, a demonstrably organic group in which structural lesions had been identified ("progressive paralysis" [neurosyphilis], multiple sclerosis, and the like), and a presumably organic ("functional") group in which no structural lesion had as yet been identified but was assumed to be present (for example epilepsy, hysteria, hypochondriasis, chorea, and delirium tremens).[57] By the 1840s this second group had become known as the neuroses, or functional nervous diseases, as opposed to the demonstrably organic nervous diseases.[58] A neurosis was therefore a disruption of nervous function in which an anatomical lesion was lacking.[59] Much later these functional nervous illnesses would come to be called psychoneuroses (a term Richard von Krafft-Ebing revived in 1874, meaning major mental illnesses caused by changes in brain function in which no organic lesion could be found[60]). This split between organic and functional was well established when Wilhelm Griesinger in the early 1860s popularized the mechanism of "irritable weakness" for the functional neuroses. In day-to-day diagnostics, the nerve doctors would probably make more use of the notion of irritable weakness than of any other. By the end of the nineteenth century, therefore, the reflex paradigm had been replaced by an organic nervous paradigm: Psychoses and neuroses were organic affections of the nerves. Mania was an example of a psychosis, hysteria that of a neurosis.

Yet the line between psychoses and neuroses was critical. For whereas the former were thought to be inherited, the latter might not be. The knowledge that someone was "nervously ill" was not (outside the Salpêtrière) necessarily a clap of doom for subsequent generations in the way that news of a family member being "mentally ill" was. Daughters of mentally ill parents might not make good marriages, the prospective in-laws all dreading the prospect of inherited insanity; those of nervously ill parents would find their prospects less impaired. In September 1891 August Forel was called to Venice for a consultation with Queen Elisabeth of Rumania, better known by her literary pseudonym Carmen Sylva. The wife of King Carol I of Rumania, she had some kind of psychoneurotic disorder. On September 7, Forel wrote to his wife, Emma:

215

The Queen is not actually mentally ill [*geisteskrank*]. She only has nervous problems [*nervenkrank*] and has been ruined by spiritualism.

If there should be indiscreet questions, or if there is stupid talk in the papers, I ask you please to emphasize that the rumor she's mentally ill is just drivel. That's very important.

Unfortunately I did mention to Herr Kracht something about a mentally-ill famous person. That has to be corrected. Emphasize instead that we're only dealing with a nervous sufferer [*Nervenleidende*]. This is colossally important and also true. Today I had a longer consultation and then talked with the Queen for quite a while. I emphasize again, she is *not mentally ill*, only a *nervous patient* (at least, that's what we tell the others). For you and Honegger let me just add that she is hysterical and under the influence of frivolous spiritistical nonsense.[61]

Accordingly, while psychosis and neurosis were thought to have the same underlying physiological basis, the nerve doctors considered the one far graver than the other.

It was in Central Europe in particular that such physicians were numerous, in private "nervous" and "internal medical" clinics. A "nerve doctor" was really a psychiatrist, but in an era when official psychiatry meant the asylum. Even though the asylum psychiatrists would also take on the sobriquet "nerve doctor," the term was really envisioned for those psychiatrists out of the asylum in private practice.

Any licensed physician could call him- or herself a nerve doctor (*Nervenarzt, Nervenärztin*) even without specialty training, just as any doctor could call himself a urologist or a hydrotherapist without further ado. Before World War I there were no prescribed training programs or particular certification for physicians who wished to practice specialties. Doctors simply pronounced themselves to be specialists.[62] Wilhelm Stekel in Vienna, for example, after several months' apprenticeship with hydrotherapist Wilhelm Winternitz, started out in the practice of medicine calling himself a hydrotherapy specialist. When patients failed to materialize, he reanointed himself a general practitioner and thrived.[63]

But of course it was possible to get specialty training. Psychiatric "clinics," or wards of teaching hospitals, began opening in Central Europe in the late 1860s: Zurich in 1868, Vienna in 1875, Heidelberg in 1878, and so forth.[64] These clinics were directed by the professor of psychiatry of the university, who had under his supervision assistants and assistant chief physicians. Although there were no exams at the end of the three-year-or-so assistantship, being known as a former assistant of such giants as Wilhelm Erb in Heidelberg or Friedrich Jolly in Berlin gave one a great competitive advantage over all those other nerve doctors who had simply hung out their shingles without doing assistantships. In a town like Wiesbaden, filled with nerve doctors and private clinics, Eduard Robert Schütz made much of the fact that he had previously been Wilhelm Erb's, "first assistant," and Ludwig Abend boasted of having served as "longtime assistant" of Wilhelm Olivier Leube, professor of internal medicine at Würzburg.[65] Accordingly, the more upscale nerve doctors would in fact have served residencies in university hospitals.

The whole nerve-doctor concept was a hybrid from two different segments of medicine. Of the nerve doctors who had done postgraduate training, most came from psychiatric clinics and asylums and had specialty skills in the management of psychotic patients. Some of the nerve doctors, however, came from internal medicine, with a background in neurological disease (demonstrable organic disease of the nervous system.)[66] What constituted proper preparation for a nerve doctor was actually the subject of an enormous turf struggle between the psychiatrists and the internists: The psychiatrists insisted that "nerves" meant mental illness, the internists that it meant organic disease of the type previously treated by internal medicine (whence many neurologists believed themselves to come).[67] The confusion of terminology that swept the "nerve" domain occurred because the psychiatrists had deliberately dropped the term *psychiatrist* (*Psychiater*) in order to use *nerve doctor* (*Nervenarzt*). They did this partly from intellectual reasons, seeing mental disease as brain ("nerve") disease, and partly for commercial ones, because the public shunned anything "mental" and preferred the comforting fiction of organic nervous problems.[68]

Nerve doctors had to present distinctions between "nervous" and "mental" to the public most delicately. Hermann Oppenheim, a prominent Berlin nerve doctor, had a female patient with a hysterical paralysis and leg pain. Once, after she had left his office in high dudgeon, he wrote her:

When I tried to explain all this to you verbally, I realize I got into some difficulty, for I soon noted that my account was upsetting you and that it sounded unsympathetic and inadequate. Of course it was the concept of "psychic" that you resisted so energetically, because you considered it equivalent to psychosis, and you found this erroneous interpretation so upsetting because it aroused in you the painful memory of that other physician who once had questioned your mental intactness. So let me say in advance: I consider you completely sane and do not believe that you are at risk of mental illness [*Seelenstörung*].[69]

Clearly, in order to succeed outside asylums, psychiatrists such as Oppenheim had to take on the protective coloration of "nerve doctors" so as not to lose patients such as this woman to the internists.

In their daily practice the nerve doctors saw primarily patients whose problems were psychogenic rather than neurogenic and who would require some kind of treatment that addressed the mind. Freud, who had trained in neuropathology, soon came to rely in his private practice upon informal psychotherapy and hypnosis:

> This meant giving up the treatment of the organic nervous diseases, but little was lost in consequence. On the one hand, the therapy of these conditions offered few positive results, and on the other, the small number of organic patients disappeared in a private urban medical practice midst the mass of nervous patients. These patients became all the more numerous because of their tendency to run unrelieved from doctor to doctor.[70]

Ernest Jones said of the ease with which Freud drew patients, "Material there was in plenty, for like all neurologists he found that his practice would consist largely of psychoneurotics who were under the impression that 'nerve specialists' could cure 'nerves' as well as diseases of the spinal cord."[71] The nerve doctors would thus be willing partners in the implicit conspiracy with somatizing patients that their problems stemmed from nervous disease.

Of any place in Europe, Berlin probably had the greatest concentration of nerve doctors. The very prototype of nerve doctor, the psychiatrist with an extensive outpatient practice, was Emanuel Mendel. Born 1839 in Bunzlau in Silesia (today Bolesławiec, Poland), he qualified for medicine in 1860 after studying in Breslau, Berlin, and Vienna. He then settled in the northern Berlin suburb of Pankow, acquiring a medical practice that included several small psychiatric nursing homes. Seeing potential for growth, in 1868 Mendel began taking nervous patients into his home (himself sleeping on the sofa), enlarging his quarters into what would become ultimately a world-famous private clinic for "Nervous and Psychiatric Patients" (*Nerven- und Gemütskranke*).[72] Simultaneously in the 1870s he immersed himself in the scientific side of nervous disease, studying with Wilhelm Griesinger (psychiatry) and Rudolf Virchow (internal medicine) at the faculty in Berlin. Thus Mendel had really pulled himself up by his own bootstraps. Never having been an "assistant," he nonetheless, by virtue of his indisputable brilliance and hard work, managed to qualify as a university lecturer in 1873, and in 1884 he even received an honorary professorship. (The ability to call oneself professor added enormously to one's practice, as Freud himself discovered in 1902 after becoming an honorary "professor" in Vienna.) In 1881 Mendel gave up the operation of his private inpatient clinic in Pankow, staying on as consulting physician. Instead he opened an outpatient clinic in Berlin, where he acquired a vast consulting practice and took on a number of junior physicians as assistants, training such later lights as Toby Cohen, James Fränkel, Alfred Grotjahn, and Paul Schuster.[73] In the Berlin tradition established by Griesinger, Mendel was more interested in neurology than psychiatry. "Neurology is easy, psychiatry is hard," he used to say.[74] With Mendel, nerve doctors began to move from practice in asylums to lucrative outpatient practice. As psychiatrists slid toward "nerves," they left psychosis and dementia behind in remote state hospitals, a low-prestige kind of country cousin.[75]

Although the term *nerve doctors* itself sounds vaguely meretricious to Anglo-Saxon ears, any imputation that they were mainly quacks or charlatans should be avoided. Even though they did to some extent pull the wool over the patients' eyes with the term *nervous* (except for the numerous neurosyphilitics, who did suffer organic disease of the nerves), men such as Mendel made important scientific contributions. Mendel himself described in 1881 as hypomania the common psychiatric symptoms of nonpsychotic mania.[76] In the early 1870s Karl Kahlbaum and Ewald Hecker, working together in a private clinic in Görlitz, provided the first systematic description of schizophrenia.[77] Yet unlike university professors, nobody paid these private nerve doctors to do research. They simply diagnosed and treated "nervous patients."

Berlin teemed with nerve doctors, especially in the more fashionable western parts of the city such as Charlottenburg and Wilmersdorf. These German doctors were collectively more organically oriented than was the Charcot school. It was really Hermann Oppenheim who spread the gospel of "irritable weakness" within the new paradigm. In the early 1890s Oppenheim, Albert Eulenburg, and other firm organicists stood in contrast to the Salpêtrière school, with its emphasis upon hysteria as a disorder of "ideas" and the "imagination."[78]

It is interesting to note that a majority of the nerve doctors in private practice in Berlin were Jewish, in contrast to the professors of psychiatry—Wilhelm Griesinger, Karl Friedrich Westphal, Friedrich Jolly, and other non-Jewish physicians who held state appointments. In this period, Berlin was quite similar to Vienna, where 66 percent of the neurologists and psychiatrists were Jewish. Although an exact census of the nerve doctors by religion in Berlin is not available, the medical staffs of most of the sixty-odd private clinics for nervous diseases and internal medicine

219

in the Berlin region were Jewish. This may be compared to the medical profession at the end of the nineteenth century in Berlin as a whole, in which only slightly more than a third of physicians were Jewish. By way of illustration, the three nervous clinics in the pleasant Berlin suburb of Schlachtensee-Wannsee may be cited: In 1900 the Kurhaus Hubertus was run by Martin Maass and Siegfried Kalischer; the private clinic Fichtenhof by Justus Bödecker and Otto Juliusburger (who was later involved in a nasty dispute with an anti-Semitic editor about the role of Jews in psychiatry); and the Sanatorium Schlachtensee by Samuel Mankiewitz and Julius Weil. This pattern would apply to most of Berlin's private nervous and "medical" clinics in this period.[79]

Such popular outpatient clinics as those of Emanuel Mendel and Hermann Oppenheim received as consultation patients large numbers of Jews from Eastern Europe.[80] It is relevant that many "hypochondriacal"—as the doctors of the time thought them—Jews from Eastern Europe flocked to Berlin to see these great authorities.

The attachment of the Jewish nerve doctors to the central nervous paradigm is an interesting kind of chicken-egg proposition. Did their Jewish consultation patients from Eastern Europe somatize because they wished to conform to the theories of the doctors? Or did the Berlin nerve doctors publicize their theories so widely—as in the example of Oppenheim's published letters to his patients—because they wanted to attract the business of patients who found "nervous disease" less upsetting than "mental disease"? After all, competition for private middle-class patients was intense, both at the level of private practitioner and sanatorium. Doctors would necessarily represent theories they believed would strike resonance with their patients. Patterns of doctor-patient relationships in Berlin may therefore be a microcosm of the reciprocal relationship between medical shaping of symptoms and patient susceptibility to such suggestion.

Neurasthenia

Before the central nervous paradigm could be successfully conveyed to patients a new diagnostic term would be required, given that "irritable weakness" was too abstract and "hysteria" either too old-fashioned or tainted with the circus of the Salpêtrière. What forty-year-old businessman would want to see himself as hysterical? The new diagnosis that brought home to patients the message of the central nervous paradigm, indicating to them how they were to behave, was "neurasthenia," or tired nerves.

Neurasthenia in the last quarter of the nineteenth century represented a slight narrowing of the concepts of functional neurosis and nervosity, which had been around for a long time. Ever since a flurry of work at midcentury—for instance Claude Sandras's 1851 book—the French had spoken of "nervous states" (les états nerveux).[81] The Germans had possessed in "nervosity" (Nervosität) a similar grab-bag term for low-grade psychiatric symptoms that could not otherwise be classed as hysterical (no fits) or hypochondriac (no fixed ideas about physical illness).[82] The term neurasthenia had occasionally been used in the past as well to describe this kind of undifferentiated nervosity. For example, German medical writers in the 1830s under the influence of "Brunonianism" (Brownism) understood neurasthenia to mean "nervous weakness."[83]

Then in 1869 a thirty-year-old New York electrotherapist named George Beard, a man who was personally something of a hypochondriac, published an article in a leading American medical weekly, "Neurasthenia, or Nervous Exhaustion." The nature of the disorder, he said, was "want of nervous force." As for its mechanism: "My own view is that the central nervous system becomes dephosphorized, or perhaps loses somewhat of its solid constituents; probably also undergoes slight, undetectable, morbid changes in its chemical structure and as a consequence becomes more or less impoverished in the quantity and quality of its nervous force."

Neurasthenia was conceived of as a functional nervous disease. The symptoms of neurasthenia, according to Beard, were mainly somatoform: "dyspepsia, headaches, paralysis, insomnia, anaesthesia, neuralgia, rheumatic gout," also wet dreams and painful periods. Beard and his colleague Alphonso Rockwell had treated a number of cases successfully with electrotherapy.[84] Eleven years later in 1880 Beard planted the diagnosis firmly in the textbooks when he wrote his major work, A Practical Treatise on Nervous Exhaustion (Neurasthenia), in which the diagnosis itself became expanded to accommodate every physical symptom imaginable and a number of mental ones as well.[85]

Neurasthenia traveled quickly to Europe, though shorn of many of Beard's interpretations. Beard's book was translated into German in 1881.[86] Charcot had introduced the diagnosis to France at least by 1887 and possibly earlier.[87] By 1904 Paul Dubois could write, "Since the works of George Beard, a new nervous disease has been imported from America, and seems to be propagated like an epidemic. The name of neurasthenia is on everybody's lips; it is the fashionable new disease."[88]

By the end of the nineteenth century neurasthenia had become the most modish of diagnoses. In 1906 in the fashionable Harley Street practice of Alfred Schofield (who had taken over the rooms of throat specialist Sir Morell Mackenzie and had the stained-glass window that the kaiser had given Mackenzie for treating his son, the crown prince of Germany, in 1887), neurasthenia was six times more common than hysteria.[89] August Kühner, a general practitioner in Coburg, explained in 1901 in a work of medical advice for the laity that the "low point in our nerve barometer" was represented by "nervosity, pathological irritability, irritable weakness, and nerve weakness (neurasthenia)." He dilated further on this weakness theme: There might be a "weakness of the head nerves," or "cerebral weakness" (also known as "brain weakness"), "expressing itself in various degrees of incapacity for intellectual work . . . further in all imaginable and unimaginable sensations in the head.[90] Freud, who considered himself neurasthenic, wrote in 1893 to his friend Wilhelm Fliess in Berlin, "I am now seeing so many neurasthenics that I may well be able to confine [myself to this type of patient] in the course of the next two to three years."[91] Constantin von Monakow, professor of neuropathology in Zurich, remembered the attitude of the visiting Archduke Rainer of Austria toward brain research, "Oh that is very nice and useful, especially these days where everyone is neurasthenic, ha ha ha."[92]

What exactly was neurasthenia? Beard's original definition, with its talk of "exhausted nervous centers" and long lists of possible symptoms, had been so amorphous that authorities could read into the term whatever they wanted. Thus various interpretative traditions established themselves. There were basically four such traditions, or ways of looking at neurasthenia.

The first tradition was to see neurasthenia as a synonym for general nervousness and evolving psychosis, a mixture of mood disorder, anxiety disorder, obsessive-compulsive or character disorder, combined with somatoform symptoms. Some observers asserted that it really meant the same as *psychoneurosis*, a term that merely called attention to psychological symptoms in patients with physical symptoms.[93] Neurasthenia was often ballooned out of shape by including patients with delusions and hallucinations.[94] "Neurasthenia is a diagnostic wastebasket [*diagnostisches Faulheits-Polster*]," said psychiatrist Conrad Rieger in 1896. It may always be replaced by the more precise terms, "hysteric, hypochondriac, paranoid, melancholic, or demented." Rieger said that once one included somatizing patients with headache and so forth in neurasthenia, the term lost its meaning completely.[95]

In this tradition neurasthenia became synonymous with pan-nervousness, a net cast so wide as not to correspond to a distinct disease entity at all. Andrew Clark, full physician at London Hospital and known as a sharp-eyed clinician, called the word "a mob of incoherent symptoms borrowed from the most diverse disorders."[96] Its function was that of a fig leaf to cover the sensibilities of patients and their relatives, or "friends," in British usage. David Drummond, senior physician at the Royal Victoria Hospital in Newcastle, made this point in 1907:

> We employ the term "neurasthenic" in a very loose and certainly most comprehensive way. It is made to include the north and south poles and all the intermediate lattitudes of functional nervous disease. Anything between the highly-strung, interesting, but irritable young lady who abhors the designation "nervous," and is grossly insulted by the slightest hint that she is hysterical when she complains of an abiding cold spot between her shoulders in her spinal column that nothing relieves, and the stupid, depressed, ever-complaining and, indeed heartbreaking "lie-abed," a lifelong trouble to herself and her friends; anything between the intelligent, vivacious business man with a fixed and altogether exaggerated idea of the importance of a certain sensation in his head or stomach, and the distressing state of neurotic *impasse* as represented by the lifelong depressed hypochondriac, we call neurasthenic, and their name is legion.[97]

Drummond struck a mocking note. George Savage, the London psychiatrist who treated so many of the fin-de-siècle prominent, was more sympathetic, probably because he had had greater experience with the real suffering of psychiatric disease. "The word neurasthenia has been a great comfort both to doctors and to the friends of patients. Not unnaturally these friends dread the term insanity, and rejoice to hear that the patient is only suffering from neurasthenia."[98]

In a second tradition, neurasthenia became the male equivalent of hysteria in women (just as hypochondria had once served this purpose before acquiring its modern meaning). Neurasthenia and hysteria were therefore the same disorder. The mechanism of irritability was thought to underlie both, expressing itself as irritable weakness in neurasthenia and enormous irritability (*enorme Reizbarkeit* was the German phrase) in hysteria. Thus doctors could assign those "weakened" by the fast pace of modern life to a male camp of neurasthenics, and those irritated by labile nervous systems to the female camp of hysterics. Mary Jacobi, a physician in New York, made the critical point: "A distinction is often made, based upon the sex and temper of the patient. If this be a female, and notably selfish, the case is pronounced hysteria. If a man, or though a woman amiable and unselfish, the case is called neurasthenia."[99] For William Osler, professor of medicine at Johns Hopkins University, neurasthenia was really male hysteria: "The individual loses the distinction between essentials and non-essentials, trifles cause annoyance, and the entire organism reacts with unnecessary readiness to slight stimuli, and is in a state which the older writers called irritable weakness. . . . In this group may be placed a large proportion of the neurasthenics which we see in this country, particularly among business men." Further on: "It is sometimes difficult to distinguish cases from hysteria, and this is not surprising, as we cannot always differentiate the two conditions. Neurasthenia occurs chiefly in men; in fact, it is in many ways in them the equivalent of hysteria."[100]

Statistically, the diagnosis of neurasthenia was commoner in men. Among 828 neurasthenic patients whom Rudolph von Hösslin had seen in the 1880s and early 1890s at his exclusive nervous clinic in Munich, 73 percent were men.[101] Thomas Savill found that among his mainly working-class patients likewise in the 1880s and 1890s at the Paddington Infirmary in London and later at the West End Hospital for Diseases of the Nervous System, 61 percent of the neurasthenics had been male; 97 percent of the hysterics, female.[102]

Given such a stark gender disproportion, the diagnosis of neurasthenia must have had a social purpose when used in this second tradition. But what was it? Neurasthenia represented a way of bringing into the office of the nerve doctor rather than the internist the lucrative clientele of middle-class businessmen. Many nerve doctors made a straight pitch for this market, becoming authorities on the health problems of men who must face "the ticker and the market fluctuations." For Charles H. Hughes, a prominent nerve doctor in St. Louis: "The strenuous man of business knows well the significance of an overdraft in his bank account, and does not treat it so lightly as an overdraft on his nerve-center balance."[103] Such metaphors might convince a well-heeled business clientele that a nerve doctor could best treat their somatic complaints.

The neurasthenia diagnosis would also direct medical attention to working-class men whose "small-p" psychiatric problems had previously not been treated. This represented a way of "medicalizing" these groups of the population that hitherto had been outside the net of the physician, save in grave illness. Somatoform complaints—often caused by stress and poverty—were presumably just as numerous among peasant and working-class males as among those of the middle class. Yet such psychosomatic consequences of the "social problem" in this group had previously been matters of medical uninterest. In the 1890s and after, physicians interested in social reform began diagnosing neurasthenia among these men. Of the 285 patients in whom Karl Petrén made the diagnosis of neurasthenia in the popular spas of Ronneby and Nybro in Sweden, 198 were peasants or working class. Fifteen percent of the working-class men were "neurasthenic" as opposed to 11 percent of the women.[104] Two young physicians in the men's division of a sanatorium for workers run by an insurance company near Berlin argued that, as proletarianization increased, rates of neurasthenia would climb as well. As former blue-collar aristocrats such as printers and cabinetmakers were pushed down into the ranks of the wage slaves, stress and anger would exact a "neurasthenic" physical cost. After describing the monotonous new working conditions of men in these occupations, the authors concluded, "They live a life without satisfaction, all aspiration in vain, without any true content and also without recreation of any kind. Whoever is not strong and not radiant with vitality must under these circumstances become a neurasthenic."[105]

These earnest physicians, concerned about the impact of industry on working-class people, were not attempting to medicalize them for any pecuniary end. Yet the theme of recruitment does run through some of the discussion about stress-related illness among the working classes: to persuade those who formerly relied upon folk remedies now to seek medical help. Here is Raymond Belbèze, a young physician who, after eight years of practice in the remote French department Lot-et-Garonne, became convinced that many of his peasant patients were neurasthenic. What was neurasthenia? A "special mental pathology consisting of lack of will [aboulie] and exaggeration of phenomena of perception," said Belbèze. He argued that this presumed lack of will made his patients especially fearful. On a social level, conversation might go along until one "makes some point touching the personal life of one's interlocutor . . . who either terminates the conversation" or heartily seconds your point of view, whatever it is. "This habit of pathological approval incontestably finds its source in fear." According to a surprised Doctor Belbèze, the local politicians "have a tendency to say yes to everything that is said to them." The physical symptoms of this neurasthenia were insomnia and exhaustion. Belbèze, who came from Nevers (in central France) was an outsider to the region; he had converted quite typical peasant behavior—deference to outsiders, a face-saving desire to avoid open confrontation—into a psychiatric diagnosis. He was in effect attempting to convince these men that the standard accompaniments of a hard rural life should be treated medically. (He gave them barbiturates.)[106]

This tradition of using neurasthenia as primarily a diagnosis for men under stress thus served some social ends, either the individual one of augmenting the physician's practice or the collective one of ameliorating the lot of the working classes. In both cases, however, "neurasthenia" was innovative because it directed medical attention, which had dwelt so long on psychosomatic symptoms in women, toward such symptoms in men.

A third tradition in the neurasthenia diagnosis was minor depression. Depression was often referred to in turn-of-the century diagnostics as "nervous exhaustion," indicating its resemblance to neurasthenia. Depressed people often have symptoms that suggest "tired nerves," in that they lack energy, feel unrestored after a night's sleep, and are dysphoric. It is probable that a strong minority of "neurasthenic" patients were in fact depressed.[107]

In a fourth tradition, "neurasthenia" meant chronic fatigue in patients who were not obviously depressed. Chronic fatigue, although present in the symptom pool since ancient times, started to become an important symptom only later in the nineteenth century. As one of the main new symptoms in the shift from motor to sensory, chronic fatigue makes a major claim on our attention. "The longer [neurasthenics] stay in bed, the tireder they feel," said Paris society nerve doctor Paul Hartenberg in 1912. "The neurasthenic might stay in bed ten, eleven, twelve hours a day, without feeling guilty." An hour's rest after each meal was essential, continued Hartenberg:

I end this list of how to fight fatigue through rest with some remarks on saving one's energy. Any unnecessary expenditure of energy must be averted, any superfluous task, any wasting of force. In all of our lives there are some acts we must perform owing to the ineluctable demands of our careers or the demands of *la vie sociale*. Then there are other acts that can be avoided and which the neurasthenic must omit.

Thus, I proscribe any unnecessary walking. I always tell them, "If you have to go shopping, take a carriage, don't walk." Also, I tell them never to stand up unnecessarily. They must take a seat at every possible occasion. As for dinners, parties, going to the theater, trips that are supposed to "distract" them: all this has only the effect of exhausting them even more.

Finally, if there must be sex, Doctor Hartenberg advised his patients, "Have sexual intercourse once or even twice a week, but without unnecessary excitation and one orgasm only [*sans récidives*]."[108]

226

Henri Feuillade, director of a Paris sanatorium, singled out tiredness as the core of "simple" (meaning no psychiatric symptoms) neurasthenia, "characterized by fatigue, the exhaustion of the nervous system, and accompanied by psychological instability, fatigability, anxiety and emotionality."[109]

Women with chronic fatigue in the United States had perhaps a special tendency to seek out the gynecologist rather than the nerve doctor. Edward Weiss, whose 1908 remarks on the classic somatizing patient were mentioned in chapter 3, further commented, "In so far as the pelvic phenomena are concerned, the symptoms are usually quite definite. They are always expressive of fatigue so that some writers have proposed the name of fatigue neuroses for neurasthenia."[110] Said neurologist John Garvey, on the staff at Marquette University medical school in Milwaukee, to a gynecological readership in 1935:

The [neurasthenic] patient feels tired and restless, worries considerably about minor difficulties and is unable to face the ordinary problems of the day without fatigue. . . . Patients suffering from varying degrees of neurasthenia frequently refer and explain the extreme mental and physical fatigue on the lack of proper rest. . . . Frequently one hears the remark, "I have not had a good night's sleep for months" [or] "I have not slept a wink in weeks."[111]

Why so many American women used gynecologists for their primary care is unclear. But as a result, American gynecologists were able to participate knowledgeably in the chronic-fatigue discussion.

In this fourth tradition many physicians were really using neurasthenia as a code word for fatigue, a code word implying that one knew the mechanism of the fatigue: irritable weakness or exhausted "nervous centers."

Neurasthenia, as used in any of these four traditions, was a diagnostic term quite popular with patients. Its popularity is known because the private nervous clinics featured it prominently in their indications for admission (unlike neurosyphilis and dementia, which they saw a good deal of too but which they did not feature in their advertisements.) In contrast to "hysteria," "mental disease," and the like, neurasthenia could be acquired in the absence of hereditary taint. Even Charcot admitted that some cases could come on spontaneously later in life, as opposed to hysteria which was inborn. Although some great authorities did think that heredity caused neurasthenia, enough maintained it was acquired to give the disorder a somewhat cheerier prognosis. This created better atmospherics in dealing with middle-aged businessmen; housewives could coolly be deemed chronic.

In France, Beni-Barde considered neurasthenia incompatible with *la grande hystérie* (which was, of course, inheritable): "Neurasthenia cannot arise in the middle of so much commotion," he said.[112] Fernand Levillain said in 1891, "Neurasthenia is the only one of *les grandes névroses* that one may acquire accidentally, independent of heredity."[113] Although German authorities were split on the subject of heredity, some certainly believed that neurasthenia could develop in the absence of any family history of insanity or "neuropathic" disposition.[114] Joseph Collins liked to reassure patients about their prospects for recovery, unlike their prospects in "psychasthenia" (a kind of pan-neurosis described by Janet): "I look upon neurasthenia as an acquisition," he wrote in a consultation note to another doctor, "not an inheritancy. I look upon psychasthenia as an inheritancy, not an acquisition. . . . The chief reason why the physician should distinguish between neurasthenia and psychasthenia, is that one is eminently curable, the other is not. Neurasthenia is a disease that yields almost uniformly to appropriate treatment, and I have no hesitation in saying to you that your patient will recover."[115]

A final point about neurasthenia is that its symptoms clustered primarily on the sensory side of the nervous system. Even before neurasthenia was conceived as a diagnosis, "nervous weakness" was said to cause "hyperesthesia," or feeling everything much too sensitively. The classic hyperesthetic, his nerves collapsing under the barrage of sensory input, was Mr. Fairlie, in Wilkie Collins's novel of 1860, *The Woman in White*. In the novel we first encounter a sixtyish, wealthy Mr. Fairlie as he receives Hartright, the novel's hero. Mr. Fairlie had "a frail, languidly-fretful, over-refined look—something singularly and unpleasantly delicate in its association with a man, and, at the same time, something which could by no possibility have looked natural and appropriate if it had been transferred to the personal appearance of a woman." The story continues:

"Pray sit down," said Mr. Fairlie to Hartright, "And don't trouble yourself to move the chair, please. In the wretched state of my nerves, movement of any kind is exquisitely painful to me."

Hartright made some remark.

"Pray excuse me," said Mr. Fairlie, "But *could* you contrive to speak in a lower key? In the wretched state of my nerves, loud sound of any kind is indescribable torture to me. You will pardon an invalid?"

Mr. Fairlie decided to show Hartright some etchings and summoned

Louis the servant to fetch them. "The portfolio with the red back, Louis. Don't drop it! You have no idea of the tortures I should suffer, Mr. Hartright, if Louis dropped that portfolio."

Mr. Fairlie apologized for the drawings in the portfolio. "They have come from a sale in a shocking state—I thought they smelt of horrid dealers' and brokers' fingers when I looked at them last. *Can* you undertake them?"

Hartright smelled nothing. He ventured an opinion about the drawings.

"I beg your pardon," interposed Mr. Fairlie. "Do you mind my closing my eyes while you speak? Even this light is too much for them. Yes?"

Hartright began again. Mr. Fairlie suddenly opened his eyes again and turned them piteously towards the window.

"I entreat you to excuse me, Mr. Hartright," he fluttered, "But surely I hear some horrid children in the garden—my private garden—below?"

Hartright lifted a corner of the blind, mindful of Mr. Fairlie's entreaties not to let in any sun. There were no children in the garden.

The interview then came to an end. "So glad to possess you at Limmeridge, Mr. Hartright. I am such a sufferer that I hardly dare hope to enjoy much of your society. Would you mind taking great pains not to let the doors bang."[116] This was de facto neurasthenia with overwhelmingly sensory symptoms.

Even before the description of neurasthenia, this kind of extreme sensitivity was said in medicine to be pathological. What the laity call "nervous weakness," wrote Joseph Amann in 1868, director of the university outpatient gynecology clinic in Munich, "is really hyperaesthesia. Such patients experience

> extreme discomfort in the presence of relatively minor stimuli. Loud noises, thoughtless slamming of doors, heavy stomping while walking, sometimes even loud conversations impress hysterical women unfavorably or cut them to the quick. All loud and bright colors, especially red, are repellent to them, the same for bright light, and some cannot even tolerate the normal light of day. One always finds them therefore in darkened rooms. To many, the tiniest amounts of salt or seasoning in the soup tastes unpleasant and they return it to the kitchen.[117]

Although Amann called this condition "hysteria," such hyperesthesias would soon be ranked under neurasthenia.

After neurasthenia became familiar, authorities emphasized the "sensitivity of the cerebral cortex." Berthold Stiller, chief physician of the Jewish Hospital in Budapest, said in 1907, "The nature of neurasthenia consists in a usually inborn, constitutional weakness and irritability of the sensory centers of the cerebral cortex, in which every internal or external sensation is perceived in an exaggerated, inadequate and pronouncedly unpleasant manner."[118] In describing patients' symptoms, doctors with this belief system would dwell on the sensory side. Levillain claimed that neurasthenics "sometimes have neuralgia, sometimes migraine, sometimes slight dizziness, or transitory disorders of sensation, disorders of the musculature, dyspeptic troubles, palpitations or a thousand other nervous things. . . . The patients themselves say moreover that they suffer from nerves."[119]

In this riot of sensory symptoms, patients of Alfred Boettiger, a nerve doctor in Hamburg, might say:

> I feel as though my head is in a vise; or I feel as if someone is trying to bore with a key through my skull; or I feel as though I had a saddle tied about my nose; or I feel as though my arms are being tied down with sandbags; or I feel as though my back is about to wrench loose; or I feel as though the skin is falling off my thighs; or I feel as though a rope is being tied around my throat; or I feel as though a ball is climbing up from my stomach (the famous globus hystericus, which however has nothing specifically hysterical about it); or I feel as though a stone were lying in my stomach; or I feel as though somebody had jumbled my intestines all up or as though there were a blockage somewhere.[120]

The point is that such patients became firmly fixated upon internal sensations, in demonstration of the fact that they were "nervously ill." What a change this represented from a couple of decades earlier, when they were still convulsing, being paralyzed, and having limbs "draw up."

Neurasthenia refocused the discussion of nervous disease firmly upon the central nervous paradigm. A somewhat bemused Oswald Bumke said in 1925 of Beard's neurasthenia that it had given renewed force to somatic explanations of neurosis. Such explanations had been on the way out, driven back by Charcot at the end of his life and by Hippolyte Bernheim, the hypnotherapist in Nancy. Then Beard's neurasthenia appeared. "With a single blow somatic explanatory paradigms won the upper hand again." There was, Bumke said, probably no similar instance of a single label having such an impact in the history of medicine. Of course there had been no real increase in nervous illness; Bumke disbelieved completely in explanations involving the fast pace of city life and such. Neurasthenia became so popular because, "it managed to explain subjective bodily symptoms in terms of objective physical disease, thus removing any suggestion of the patient's own fault in them." Bumke said dryly, "Doubtlessly this has been a great relief for many patients."[121]

Whatever happened to such a useful diagnosis as neurasthenia, which gave doctors the confidence of dealing with "real organic disease" and patients the reassurance that their symptoms were not "all in their head"? That, indeed, was the very problem with the word. It was so useful that by the 1920s it had swollen to embrace virtually the entire range of psychic pathology, and thus had become meaningless. Said Henri Feuillade in 1924:

> It is very convenient, in order to avoid a precise diagnosis or to conceal from the patient and the family the true nature of the presenting problem, to say, "*C'est de la neurasthénie.*" And under this label one finds melancholics, patients with compulsive thoughts [*des scrupuleux*], the anxious, the obsessed, the phobic, the impulsive, the degenerate, even some cases of neurosyphilis in remission. The newspapers, reporting suicides on the local pages, add that the poor unfortunates have committed their acts in a crisis of neurasthenia.[122]

Two events after the 1920s helped to trim down this overblown term. More precise psychiatric diagnoses stripped away much of neurasthenia's content. Schizophrenia, which Heidelberg psychiatrist Emil Kraepelin described in 1893 as a distinct disease entity, removed some patients from the catchall of neurasthenia, particularly those in the early phase of the disease.[123] Laboratory tests on cerebrospinal fluid were introduced in 1913 to diagnose neurosyphilis, which removed a further portion of the "neurasthenic": particularly males whose symptoms were recent.[124] As for shearing away other neuroses, in 1895 Sigmund Freud identified anxiety disorders as a separate disease entity, distinct from neurasthenia.[125] Although a number of scholars had described obsessive-compulsive behavior, in 1903 Pierre Janet introduced the term *psychasthenia,* whose core was obsessive-compulsive states.[126] Psychasthenia became a popular alternative for those neurasthenics who went back to the house nine times to turn off the gas and so forth. After the 1920s "neurotic" depression, meaning nonpsychotic depression, enjoyed ever-greater popularity, thus robbing neurasthenia of a further subgroup of its clientele.

In the first half of the twentieth century Beard's neurasthenia became reduced to a kind of core symptomatology of chronic fatigue. Angelo

Hesnard, a Paris psychiatrist who was an enthusiastic supporter of psychoanalysis, said in 1927 that once all the components of neurasthenia, such as postinfectious fatigue and depression had been peeled away, "neurasthenia itself becomes reduced to quite a rare syndrome . . . characterized by subjective impressions of a mainly physical nature which awaken in the consciousness of the patient the idea of a nervous fatigue, of 'exhaustion.' But no one has established that these impressions are actually caused by a real exhaustion of the nervous system in general."[127] According to two American scholars, this stripping away of other disease entities "left neurasthenia with the symptoms of fatigue and not much more."[128]

Neurasthenia also lost its popularity after 1920 when another paradigm switch occurred. The diagnosis had blossomed under the assumption that somatization was caused by an organic disturbance of the central nervous system. After the 1920s this paradigm would become increasingly challenged by a new one which asserted that somatoform symptoms were, by definition, psychogenic, meaning they arose in the mind and not from disorder in the central nervous system. Neurasthenia was so laden with assumptions of organicity that it became untenable once this new paradigm had triumphed, and somatizing patients—together with supportive physicians—would seek refuge in other diagnoses whose supposed organicity was without question.[129]

Doctors, Patients, and the Psychological Paradigm

Alongside the reflex and central nervous paradigms flourished a third paradigm, one that emphasized the psychological origin of somatoform symptoms, as opposed to "peripheral irritation" or "exhausted nervous centers." The psychological paradigm started to gather supporters in the 1880s, became the predominant explanation of psychosomatic symptoms from the 1920s to the 1970s, and matters to this story in a rather paradoxical way. If insights about psychogenesis had penetrated the public as a whole at the same time as they infiltrated the medical profession, the picture of somatoform illness in the twentieth century would probably have become very different. But this mass acquisition of insights into the psychology of symptom formation never occurred. Instead, the increasing penetration of the psychological paradigm within medicine sent patients scurrying away from psychiatry and into other forms of medical treatment, in which the organicity of one's symptoms was taken for granted. It was the failure of such insights to persuade the general public that opened the door, late in the twentieth century, to a shift from the medical shaping of symptoms to a media-driven wave of somatization.

Forerunners of the Psychological Paradigm

A stomachache before a battle, a paralysis after seeing a bolt of lightning—doctors have always known of psychological factors in the genesis of physical symptoms. But isolated, casual insights do not add up to the

233

construction of a systematic paradigm. Medical references to "ideas," "the mind," and "emotions" in the production of illness reach well back into the eighteenth century (and doubtless before). Authors have long held, for example, that violent emotional shocks could bring on hysterical fits. As Robert Whytt of Edinburgh, who first used the notion of nervous illness, said in 1765, "Violent affections of the mind, as terror, grief, anger, or disappointments, will sometimes so strongly affect the whole nervous system, as to bring on hysteric faintings, with convulsions, although the body be in every respect healthful and sound."[1] Hysteria, for London physician William Rowley, showed "the surprising effects of the mind on the body: for it often happens," he wrote in 1788, "that the compassionate spectators, from surprise, fear, and sensibility, are attacked with these complaints, as happened lately at Paris by animal magnetism; and it is common in families to see a female attendant attacked in the same manner from a perturbed imagination." Do not tell sad stories to hysterics, he admonished, for "The effects of sympathy are astonishing. . . . A great part of the miseries of the nervous are certainly imaginary. Present sorrow, future apprehensions, occupy the mind with an uncontrolled sway. The disorder to the afflicted is as real as any other the human body is subject to, and equally merits a sedulous attention and humane compassion."[2] Rowley was not far from twentieth-century concepts of psychogenesis: The action of the mind produces physical symptoms that the patient takes for genuine organic disease, experiencing pain as real as in any physical disorder.

Rather than seeing Rowley and his contemporaries as somehow innovative, it should be remembered that the whole concept of "psychosomatic" belongs to that category of lore that physicians have "always known": There has always been some realization that body and soul were connected. The term *psychosomatic* itself seems to have been used for the first time in 1818 by the professor of psychiatry in Leipzig, Johann Christian August Heinroth, and popularized much later by the psychoanalysts.[3]

A remarkable example of eighteenth-century insight into psychogenesis is the story of John Haygarth's "tractors," or metallic rods designed to affect the body's magnetic fluid. Haygarth, an authority on smallpox and acute rheumatism who had been physician at the Chester Infirmary, moved in 1798 to Bath, whereupon he proposed an experiment to his good friend William Falconer, physician of the Bath General Hospital: "The tractors [of Mesmer and Elisha Perkins] have obtained such high reputation at Bath, even among persons of rank and understanding, as to require the particular attention of physicians. Let their merit be impartially investigated, in order to support their fame," he wrote in his letter. "Prepare a pair of false tractors," he urged Doctor Falconer, "exactly to resemble the true tractors. Let the secret be kept inviolable, not only from the patient but every other person. Let the efficacy of both be impartially tried, beginning always with the false tractors."

The two conspirators prepared the false tractors:

We contrived two wooden tractors of nearly the same shape as the metallic, and painted to resemble them in color. Five cases were chosen of chronic rheumatism. . . . On the 7th of January, 1799, the wooden tractors were employed. All the five patients, except one, assured us that their pain was relieved, and three much benefitted by the first application of this remedy. One felt his knee warmer, and he could walk much better, as he shewed us with great satisfaction. One was easier for nine hours. . . . One had a tingling sensation for two hours. The wooden tractors were drawn over the skin so as to touch it in the *slightest* manner. Such is the wonderful force of the imagination!

The next day the two physicians repeated the experiment with the true tractors. The patients were benefitted in roughly the same measure, but none more so. The two doctors concluded the tractors to be a valueless fad: "The whole effect undoubtedly depends upon the impression which can be made upon the patient's imagination." On the basis of these and other data, Haygarth concluded that "the imagination can cause, as well as cure, diseases of the body. [The tractors] clearly establish one rule of medical practice which has always appeared to me highly important. . . . A patient ought always to be inspired with confidence in any remedy which is administered."[4] One could as easily claim Haygarth as Charcot as "discovering the role of the imagination," but all such claims mislead because both physicians merely articulated, at different points in time, what has leapt out over the ages at many observers of clinical medicine.

This relative dribble of psychological insight then rose to a steady stream of commentary during the nineteenth century, though shaded by reflex and central-nervous theories. Although conceding some role to the uterus, Edward Seymour, physician at St. George's Hospital in London, said in 1831 that hysteria was "in general caused by some violent emotion of the mind." As for its therapy: "Anything that will powerfully excite the imagination of the patient in this susceptible state [of excessive nervous irritability] will effect a cure. It is in such cases as these that non-educated practitioners, quacks, and charlatans, obtain such great credit to the detriment of our profession."[5] William Roots of St. Thomas's Hospital described in 1836 a young woman he had once treated at St. Pancras's

Infirmary. "I believe there was not a hospital in London in which she had not been two or three times, and in some instances for eight, nine or ten months. She was the subject of the strongest hysterical paroxysms that I think I ever witnessed." Doctor Roots succeeded, however, in stopping them by "ordering a large blanket and a pail of water, dipping the blanket in the water, removing her clothes, and throwing it over the abdomen and thighs. She was instantly relieved of her hysterical paroxysm." To avert a threatened fit Doctor Roots might say to the nurse during ward rounds, looking at the patient meaningfully, "Fetch a pail of water and a blanket. . . . So strong was the influence of the mind upon that particular condition in which an hysterical paroxysm consists, that by merely making a strong impression on the mind, she never had a paroxysm at the moment it was resorted to."[6] To be sure, these writers were not elaborating complex psychological mechanisms, yet they clearly had incorporated the notion of psychogenesis.

A whole generation of London society doctors at mid-nineteenth century believed in hysteria as "arising in the mind." (And each on occasion has been described as the "discoverer" of the psychological causation of hysteria.) "Emotions," said surgeon Robert Carter in 1853, produce "effects upon the physical organism." Hysterical symptoms "are all alike in affording speedy and evident relief to the emotion itself," a doctrine that later would be portentously known as "abreacting."[7] Although his colleague Frederic Skey believed hysteria to involve some "irritation" in the brain ("The subject is a very obscure one," he said), he nonetheless specifically saw in fits an example of hysteria arising in the mind. "There can be no doubt that a malady spread by sympathy and cured by fear has its origin in the mind. . . . Nearly all cases of paroxysmal hysteria originate in some form of mental excitement, and that of a depressing character, such as sorrow or disappointment." Yet it was not "mere emotion." "Possibly some mental emotion in the form of a forgotten dream or some other occult mental operation which escapes cognizance" was involved.[8] Here Skey was groping toward the more specific mechanisms that Freud later proposed.

Although Dennis De Berdt Hovell, another London physician, used such organic-sounding phrases as "defective nerve-power," his treatment of hysteria and fatigue nonetheless presupposed psychogenesis. Hovell was a noted opponent of reflex theory, and set out to mobilize therapeutically the healing power of the doctor-patient relationship. He urged empathy upon his colleagues, taking the patient's side rather than blaming her for the symptoms. "In my opinion, the most frequent and pernicious source of aggravation in simple asthenia [fatigue] and hysteria arises from a state of fretful worry caused by the erroneous and unjust imputation [by the doctor] of fancy and wilfulness with which patients are too often assailed, but which they have not the strength to repel." So Hovell's first step in treatment was to assure patients that he felt their symptoms were real and not all in their heads. Patients would then stop agonizing about their own guilt in the matter. "Divested of worry, the case becomes simply one of depressed nerve-power, is much easier to deal with, and not unfrequently gets rapidly well."

Here a psychologically minded Hovell was interviewing a young woman of twenty-four who complained of "weakness, intercostal [rib] pain, loss of appetite, malaise et cetera." He wrote her a prescription for what was basically a placebo.

"I have taken this for a twelvemonth," she said.
"Never mind; take it a little longer, and you will get well."
"So I have been told before, but I am not well yet."
"Very true; but if you were as fully satisfied on that point as I am, you would soon get well."
"But *they say* my complaints are all fancy."
"Never mind what *they say;* I tell you they are not fancy, and you must be satisfied of the same thing in your own mind."
"Of course I am."
"Then tell them that they are mistaken."

The patient returned in less than a month to tell Hovell she was "much better and stronger, had lost her pain and regained her spirits, and had been up to see the University boat-race."[9] Hovell had the insight to realize that the first step in managing psychogenic illness successfully was establishing a therapeutic alliance between doctor and patient, rather than treating "inflamed" ovaries or counseling hydrotherapy for "irritated" nervous centers.

Among early English advocates of psychogenesis, most widely cited was probably the London physician Russell Reynolds, who in 1869 described "some of the most serious disorders of the nervous system" as "dependent on idea." A young woman was admitted to his service at University College Hospital whose family had recently experienced a sharp decline in circumstances. This forced her to take an unaccustomed new job as a governess and walk back and forth long distances, all the while nursing an ailing father:

Thus she lived and worked on for many dreary weeks, with paralysis constantly upon her mind, her brain overdone with thought and feeling, her limbs wearied with walking, and her heart tired out with the effort to look bright and be so. Her limbs often ached and a horror took hold of her, as the idea again and again crossed her mind, that she might become paralysed like her father. She tried to banish it but it haunted her still, and gradually she had to give up walking, then to stop in the house, then in the room, and then in her bed. Her legs "became heavier day by day" and she at last reached the state in which I found her when she was carried to the hospital.

Given supportive therapy, "at the end of a fortnight she was as strong and capable of exertion as she had ever been in her life."[10]

This same awareness of an alternative psychological paradigm grew in these years in Central Europe. One of Freud's teachers in Vienna, Ernst Wilhelm von Brücke, casually implicated "dreams" in a consultation requested by his colleague Joseph Skoda in 1851. Skoda's young female patient had come into the General Hospital cataleptic, her limbs motionless but retaining the position in which they were placed. "Professor Brücke, who examined the patient a number of times and tested the individual muscles in the various positions in which the limbs were put, was of the opinion that the patient had been motivated by some murky idea, some kind of dream picture [*eine dunkle Vorstellung . . . irgend ein Traumbild*] to retain the positions given to her."[11] Brücke's colleague Moritz Benedikt, though not the most consistent of men (harboring simultaneously reflex and central-nervous theories), argued in 1868 for the existence of psychic moments in hysteria. "How infrequently do ladies go into fits at parties, and how easily do they do so when fits are convenient for them." It was also true, Benedikt said, that women who often had attacks of hysteria when they were well-to-do, experienced no more if poverty struck them. "A good psychologist is often a far better physician for a hysterical woman than the best pharmacologist," Benedikt concluded.[12] Freud, who started medical school in 1873, was thus trained in a climate seasoned with hints of psychogenesis (though the main paradigm of the Viennese medical faculty in those years was central-nervous).

The most widely-cited exponent of the psychological school, in the days before the psychological paradigm triumphed in Central Europe, was probably the Tübingen internist Carl von Liebermeister. Using the semiorganic, semipsychological jargon that Charcot was popularizing, Liebermeister called hysteria "a functional disease of the brain and most precisely of the gray matter. Or in other words, hysteria is a psychic disease." He called it a weakening of volition (*das Wollen*), as higher brain centers lost their control over lower centers responsible for "feelings, moods and drives." This sufficed to put distance between Lieber-meister and the reflex theorists. He then distanced himself from other central-nervous theorists by insisting that the treatment of hysteria must be "a psychological one" [*eine psychische*]. "The physician will be successful only if he is able to undertake sufficient psychological analysis of a given patient and to empathize [*sich hineindenken*] with the patient's affective and cognitive state."[13]

In the United States before 1900, adherents of a psychological paradigm were few. George Beard had an encounter with his retrograde nerve doctor colleagues at a professional meeting in 1876 in which he, although a believer in exhausted nerve centers and such, did see psychology entering into the cause and cure of functional nervous disease. "Fear, terror and anxiety" produced disease; "reason, joy and hope" might relieve it, he said, which was not inconsistent with the views of many central-nervous writers who conceded to external emotional events a role in exhausting those vital nervous centers. What is of interest in this anecdote is the response of his colleagues, who stormed against even such timid psychologizing as this. "Dr. [William] Hammond remarked that, if the doctrine advanced by Dr. Beard was to be accepted, he should feel like throwing his diploma away and joining the theologians." Hammond was the dean of the American reflex theorists. "Dr. [Francis] Miles, of Baltimore, fully recognized the influence of mind over the body, but regarded the handling of it as far more dangerous than handling the most powerful drugs. To assume to possess a virtue when you had it not, was very dangerous." "Dr. Mason objected to the term mental therapeutics, and denied their existence."[14] Here once again, nineteenth-century American physicians maintained the reactionary views that put the United States at the periphery of a European center.

The Psychological Paradigm Becomes a Major Competitor

In the 1890s and after, psychological views of hysteria spread rapidly. Exactly where the takeoff began is a bit difficult to pinpoint. A group of academic nerve doctors in Central Europe appropriated the ideas of Charcot, then left quietly behind all the hereditarian mumbo-jumbo of the Salpêtrière school, effectively converting the French psychological views from an afterthought of "ovarie" into an autonomous doctrine. This transforming of Charcot's notions about "ideas" into a different model entirely began in 1888 with a Leipzig nerve doctor, a bitter, misogynistic man named Paul Julius Möbius. Möbius, having graduated in medicine in 1877 from Leipzig, opened a private practice there in 1879 and qualified as a university lecturer (*Dozent*) in 1883, a post he resigned eight years later after the government repeatedly refused him a professor-ship (evidently because of his difficult personality). In the mid-1880s he also worked in the university's outpatient neurology clinic. Thereafter he was simply in private practice in Leipzig.[15]

Möbius has become notorious in the history of medicine for having had the bad judgment to title a standard late-nineteenth-century account of gender differences in brain physiology, *On the Physiological Weak-Mindedness of Women.*[16] Möbius later explained the title, "*Ach,* that was just to make publicity for the book dealers." Divorced and alone after a childless, ten-year marriage to a "smart and amusing but very garrulous" wife, he later told Adolf Strümpell about women, apropos Strümpell's forthcoming marriage, "*Na,* you'll find out soon enough."[17] For all his doubt about women, however, Möbius was a scientifically oriented physician who had established, beginning in 1884, that a hyperactive thyroid gland was the source of a condition called Basedow's or Graves' disease. This and his many other writings gave him considerable author-ity, despite the fact that he never received a professorship. His announce-ment in 1888, following Charcot, that hysteria was a disease of the imagi-nation could be considered a landmark. The view was emerging, said Möbius, that hysteria is "a psychosis," "a pathological change in mental condition." Yet hysterical patients often demonstrated no particular men-tal changes. The essential feature of their disease, he said, was somatic. "All pathological physical changes that are produced by ideas [*Vorstel-lungen*] may be deemed hysterical." In other words, any change in bodily function wrought by the mind was hysterical, which was more or less what Charcot believed. A light blow on the shoulder could give a patient the idea, or *Vorstellung,* of a paralyzed arm. Möbius found Charcot's hyp-nosis experiments illuminating because they showed that "virtually all hysterical symptoms may be evoked at will." Möbius diverged from Charcot, however, on a major point: Möbius did not consider hysteria hereditary. "Hysteria is only the pathological intensification of a disposi-tion [*Anlage*], which exists in each person. Everyone is, so to say, a little hysterical."[18]

Möbius later described the growth of his own awareness of how "the mind" (*die Seele*) entered into nervous disease:

In medical school I learned nothing about the mind. At most we heard about the insane, but they were locked up in insane asylums, with which we had little to do because in those days there were no courses in psychiatry. Then when I got out into practice I was still thinking basic medical science and saw in the functional nervous diseases objects of this kind of science. What drove me crazy—and then got me on the right track—were not just the therapeutic failures, for those happen in every kind of disease, but the unexpected successes, which occurred in those cases where theoretically they should not have. Then when I looked around I noticed that also other physicians had the most contradictory experience with nervous patients and that the charlatans did not have worse results than we the scientific doctors. Thus the insight grew steadily that basic medical science was useless against nervous disease and that here, where the mental condition [*seelischer Zustand*] is the most important concern, the therapy as well has to be a psychological one [*seelisch*].[19]

Möbius's own views of hysteria were never very different from Charcot's, whom he eulogized.[20] Yet in Central Europe Möbius's prestige legitimated seeing hysteria as a nonhereditary disease of psychological origin.

What elevated psychological thinking to the status of a paradigm, however, was the recruitment of the professors, important in this story because their contributions appeared in the mid-1890s and early 1900s, exactly at the time when the French nerve doctors, overcome with embarrassment about Charcot's hysteria, had fallen silent.[21] Ultimately, Babinski's and Dejerine's psychogenic hysteria would be seen as equally authoritative as those of the Germans and Austrians, but the publications that carried the new paradigm upward were written in German university towns.

This story has a particular center of gravity, Leipzig. Just as Berlin was the epicenter of the organically oriented nerve doctors, so Leipzig in the 1880s became that of the psychologically oriented school. Who was there? Möbius, a somewhat sour, marginal figure, was active in university intellectual life. Adolf Strümpell, a neurologist who like Charcot had a major grounding in internal medicine, had graduated in medicine in Leipzig in 1875, stayed on, and became professor of medicine there in 1883. Wilhelm Wundt, the founder of experimental psychology, had established his laboratory, the first in the world in that subject, in Leipzig in 1879. Around this nucleus of internists and psychologists, the psychological paradigm would blossom. Emil Kraepelin, for example, whose writings overturned the brain paradigm in asylum psychiatry, had come in 1882 to Leipzig to work with Wundt (as well as doing neurology with major organicists such as Paul Flechsig and Wilhelm Erb who were there at the time). Robert Sommer—the man who coined the term *psychogenic*—spent a year at Wundt's laboratory in 1888. Ludwig Edinger, an important neuroanatomist who wanted to break with (what the Heidelberg neuropathologist Franz Nissl called) "brain mythology" and establish clearly the difference between organic neurological disease and psychogenic disorders, had rubbed shoulders with Kraepelin and Strümpell in Leipzig in 1882.[22]

Next after Möbius in promoting the new psychological doctrine of hysteria came Adolf Strümpell, one of the best-known neurologists of his day. Strümpell had left Leipzig in 1886 for Erlangen, occupied several other chairs of internal medicine (including Vienna in 1909), and then returned to Leipzig in 1910. It was Strümpell who hammered home at professional meetings in the 1890s the point that the imagination (*Vorstellung*) can cause and cure illness. For example, he told his colleagues in 1893 at Erlangen, on becoming prorector there: "The number of apparently physical disorders which arise through primary psychological processes [*primäre psychische Vorgänge*] is at least as great as the number of actual organic disease conditions."[23] Freud and Breuer in their *Studies in Hysteria* which appeared two years later, acknowledged Möbius and Strümpell as "having held similar views on hysteria to ours."[24]

In 1894 Robert Sommer, by now on the staff of the psychiatric clinic in Würzburg, made an important innovation in terminology. He wanted to abolish the term hysteria, and call those conditions caused by heightened suggestibility "psychogenic." Drawing on Möbius and on the work of his own chief of the moment, Conrad Rieger, Sommer defined psychogenesis as referring to those disorders "which may be produced by the imagination [*Vorstellungen*] and treated by the imagination." He gave the example of a boy who had fallen on his head at age five, and attributed a headache that he developed six years afterwards to the fall. "We thus see that here, in a purely psychogenic manner, the imagination has conflated the site of a wound with the sensation of pain."[25]

A final figure in constructing the psychogenic paradigm in Central Europe was Emil Kraepelin, who had worked in Leipzig with Wundt and others in the early 1880s. Readers versed in the history of psychiatry may blanch at seeing Kraepelin put in the psychogenic category, for the man had a personal reputation of being psychologically almost totally insensitive. Kraepelin had become in 1890 the professor of psychiatry in Heidelberg, then in 1904 took the chair in Munich, where in 1917 he founded the German Research Center for Psychiatry, probably at that time the most distinguished such research institute in the world. Kraepelin's psychiatry textbook, whose fourth edition in 1893 began to make important innovations in describing the major mental disorders, became world famous. It would be no exaggeration to call him the most distinguished psychiatrist of his day, a man whose reputation would be overshadowed only by that of the neurologist Sigmund Freud.

Kraepelin was extremely interested in psychological matters. In 1882, for example, just after leaving Leipzig, he wrote to August Forel about his excitement at doing experimental work in psychology. "I hope to master the experimental techniques of investigation in about a year," he said, "and intend then to return to work in some kind of asylum." Several months later he spoke of "the necessity of a thorough psychological investigation of mental illness, as opposed to the Berlin spinal-cord section makers [*Rückenmarkschneiderei*]." In 1894, after Kraepelin had become an influential professor in Heidelberg, a mutual friend (Alfred Vogt) wrote Forel about encountering Kraepelin there. Kraepelin had immediately seized the conversation, maintaining that cerebral localization theory (up to that point the jewel in the crown of the organicists) "had only damaged psychology. Brain anatomy for a long time to come is going to be absolutely valueless for psychology. I know motor and sensory centers, but no psychic ones," the great Kraepelin maintained in this spontaneous conversation.[26]

Although Kraepelin believed that hysteria, like most mental affections, was hereditary, he deemed its immediate causes psychic. "What is truly characteristic of all hysterical illnesses," he wrote in the fifth edition of his textbook in 1896, "is the extraordinary ease and rapidity with which psychic conditions [*psychische Zustände*] become manifest in multiple physical complaints, whether anesthesias or paresthesias, expressive gestures, paralysis, fits, or autonomic phenomena."[27]

Kraepelin's clinical work lacked psychological depth only because he himself was so insensitive to that whole dimension of illness, despite his formal insistence upon it. In collegial relations, for example, he was a fanatical workaholic and teetotaler and seemed quite oblivious that at least this latter quality rubbed some of his colleagues the wrong way (his ardor about the evils of drink gave Karl Bonhoeffer a headache).[28] Of Kraepelin's notorious impersonality the following tale was told: One of Kraepelin's assistants in Munich had accompanied him on a trip to the United States, becoming seriously ill while there. After finally returning to Munich, fully recovered, the assistant told the others over coffee, "If I had died on the trip, Kraepelin would probably have collected my ashes in a cigar box and brought them home to my wife with the words, 'He was a real disappointment to me.'"[29]

Kraepelin was the same with most patients (although his gravely serious interviewing style pleased many as well). In presenting a male "psychopath" at rounds in Heidelberg, he asked the patient what the point of marriage was.

The patient answered smartly: "In order to have a life companion."

Kraepelin then turned to his listeners: "You see even from this answer that we're dealing with a psychopath here."[30]

The seat of Kraepelin's problem—aside from his personality—was his adherence to a nineteenth-century tradition of empirical observation as the route to knowledge. He was, in the terms of Heidelberg psychiatrist Hans Gruhle, "a ruthless fanatic of empiricism." "With psychology in the broadest sense he had no empathy at all."[31] For these qualities, and for his opposition to psychoanalysis, Kraepelin paid the posthumous price of being considered some kind of latter-day extension of the brain anatomists. Yet he was anything but. His work put the brakes on the central-nervous paradigm, and legitimated, if in a rather ham-fisted way, the incorporation of psychological insights into psychiatry.

Just as the young gynecologists who overturned reflex theory at the turn of the century formed a cohort, so did the psychiatrists and neurologists who launched the psychological paradigm constitute a kind of cohort, not just in their clustering about Leipzig and Heidelberg, but a cohort in age as well. In 1895, as the psychological paradigm lay on the cusp of general acceptance, Möbius and Strümpell were both forty-two, Kraepelin was thirty-nine, Robert Sommer thirty-one, and Kraepelin's acolytes in Heidelberg, such as Robert Gaupp and Franz Nissl, were all in their late twenties and early thirties.

This post-Griesinger generation of young neuroscientists was the first to distinguish rigorously between mind disease and brain disease.[32] In doing so they gave the psychological paradigm its initial legitimacy within the medical profession. As Oswald Bumke said in 1926, the main trend in neurology over the last fifty years had been "the increasing differentiation between the organic and the functional, and the ever-growing recognition that the functional was psychological."[33] By the end of the 1930s neurology and psychiatry, though joined together in specialist certification, would distinguish themselves from each other on the grounds that neurologists were competent for real organic disease of the nervous system, psychiatrists for organic diseases such as neurosyphilis with florid psychiatric symptoms and for all illnesses arising from the action of the mind, including somatization. The ultimate assignment to psychiatry of somatoform disorders represented a fateful chapter, from the patients' viewpoint, in the history of psychosomatic illness. It meant that classic hysterical and neurasthenic symptoms were no longer medically legitimate, and that patients must instead produce symptoms appropriate for "real" doctors who claimed to treat real organic illnesses.

Patients' Medical Therapy Is Physicians' Psychotherapy

The original rise of the psychological paradigm within medicine was not communicated to patients. Instead, at the turn of the century psychologically oriented physicians continued to let patients believe they were receiving organic therapy. This maintenance of the myth of organicity in the hands of early psychotherapists took the form of using the doctor-patient relationship for a "good chat," called persuasion.

Although psychotherapy can imply a technique of which the patient is fully aware, historically the term has meant the therapeutic manipulation of the doctor-patient relationship: The physician is aware of directing treatment toward the patient's mind; the patient himself believes he is receiving medical therapy. Psychotherapy in this latter sense, the unavowed treatment of the patient's mind, reaches far back in time. In 1753 Antoine Le Camus wrote a book entitled *Medicine of the Mind (La Médecine de l'esprit)*, in which he proposed psychic therapy but contented himself with historic citations without giving much in the way of guidelines.[34] More explicit systems of psychotherapy in dealing with serious mental illness go back to the "moral therapy" of Enlightenment psychiatry, most notably in England Samuel Tuke's Retreat at York (a famous progressive private asylum), or in Germany to Johann Christian Reil's "psychic treatment method" (*psychische Kurmethode*) at Halle.[35] Yet these systems were designed mainly for psychotic patients in asylums, and there is no evidence of their adoption by nerve and internal medicine specialists in the private sector.[36] The first person to use the term *psychotherapy*, as opposed to *moral therapy, psychic treatment,* and the like, was the English psychiatrist Hack Tuke, the youngest son of Samuel Tuke. Hack Tuke started out around 1852 as a physician at the Retreat, then was obliged to give it up for reasons of health and retire to the English seacoast, where he remained for fifteen years before becoming a consultant psychiatrist in London. In 1872 Tuke published his book *Illustrations of the Influence of the Mind upon the Body*, a chapter of which was entitled "Psycho-Therapeutics, Practical Application of the Influence of the Mind on the Body to Medical Practice." Among such applications Tuke envisioned "calming the mind, when the body suffers from its excitement" or "arousing the feelings of joy, hope and faith," perhaps also giving "the most favorable prognosis consistent with truth; by diverting the patient's thoughts from his malady."[37] In 1888 Möbius had insisted that the best therapy for hysteria was a psychological one (*psychische*): instilling in the patient confidence in an early recovery. To this end, anything that would affect the patient's imagination—such as the doctor's personality or placebo-style physical therapies—would work.[38] These formulations are just recastings of what doctors have always known, rather than specific recipes for influencing the mind.

Modern psychotherapy stemmed directly from the second wave of hypnotism, not from Charcot's hysterical variety but from the Nancy school, the group of hypnotherapists centered around Hippolyte Bernheim and Ambroise-Auguste Liébeault at the University of Nancy. Therapeutic hypnotism really came to an end with the Nancy school, going out of style in the decade before World War I. But the story of nonhypnotic psychotherapy began with the Nancy school too, specifically with Bernheim's recognition that hypnotism was really "suggestion." One could have two kinds of suggestion: suggestion under formal hypnotic "sleep" as such and suggestion outside the context of hypnotism (*"la suggestion à l'état de veille"*).[39] The latter procedure really amounted to not much more than a good talking-to, in which the doctor would sit down and discuss with the patient the motivations for his or her actions, urging rational behavior in the future. This concept was the essence of the new psychotherapy.

Two Amsterdam physicians, Frederik van Eeden and Albert Willem van Renterghem, widely publicized hypnosis and nonhypnotic suggestive therapy for use in clinics and office-practices.[40] As Van Eeden explained in 1893, intelligent patients would respond to a non-hypnotic variety of explanation and counselling: "With patients like these, one must not only cure but educate. One has to make them understand, give them a plausible notion of what is going on, play up to their desire for independence." In thus appealing to patients' reason, "one finds oneself on the ideal highroad of psychotherapy."[41]

By 1890 *suggestion* and *psychotherapeutics* had become synonymous terms for appealing to patients "in the wide-awake condition." "There is no doubt a daily use [is] made of this agency by the numerous body of family physicians," wrote Edinburgh psychiatrist George Robertson in 1892,

who have acquired the respect and confidence of their patients. A word from what is called "our own doctor" will often do more good than scientific medicinal treatment by a skilful stranger. Unconsciously and

246

in these indirect ways psycho-therapeutics is probably very greatly made use of by the profession, and I think the success or otherwise of many physicians depends largely on having or not having acquired the power of giving such mental suggestion to their patients.

Robertson concluded optimistically: "I believe that [psycho-therapeutics] may be used to alleviate or remove the symptoms of most diseases; though the instilling of faith and hope is of value in the ultimate recovery, much more immediate and palpable benefit can also be done to the patient by removing unpleasant symptoms."[42] As early as 1892 psychotherapy was being touted for the treatment of patients who were physically symptomatic.

Bernheim's psychotherapy, or nonhypnotic suggestion, was broadcast to the world by two physicians from French-speaking Switzerland who happened to be close friends: Paul Dubois, who after 1902 was professor of neurology in Berne, and Jules-Joseph Dejerine, who became in 1911 holder of the Charcot chair of neuropathology in Paris. Former schoolmates in the 1860s in Geneva, each represented a departure from the previous story of psychotherapy: Neither was a psychiatrist in the technical sense. Dubois became more influential in spreading psychotherapy; Dejerine was much more of a scientist.

In 1891 Dubois began to unfold his psychotherapy of "rational persuasion," which found its most fluent form in his 1904 book *The Psychic Treatment of Nervous Disorders*. (Although persuasion was Babinski's term, he offered few guidelines about how to conduct it.[43]) The key to Dubois's approach was convincing the patient he or she would get better. "In order to reach this end, the physician must know how to get hold of his patient," Dubois said. "It is necessary from the very start that he should establish between them a strong bond of confidence and sympathy." The patient should see the physician as a "friend with no idea but to cure him. We practitioners ought to show our patients such a lively and all-enveloping sympathy that it would be really very ungracious of them not to get well." As practiced on inpatients, Dubois's therapy was really just an updating of Weir Mitchell's rest cure. But in office practice Dubois's emphasis on rational persuasion, as opposed to monotonously repeated suggestion, was genuinely innovative. As part of his moral therapy (that is, improving the patient's morale), the doctor should "sit down beside his patient and listen to his plaints with the greatest patience. Above all he should never be hurried—or, at least, never appear to be." Do not "come in like a gust of wind" and look at your watch, Dubois advised his colleagues. "The patient should have the impression that he is the only person in whom the physician is interested. . . . Let your patient talk; do not interrupt him, even when he becomes prolix and diffuse." Lecture the patient succinctly on the evils of selfishness and such. "Give him on all these subjects, short lessons on rational moral-ity." (It is no wonder that Dejerine, who himself had sought psychother-apy from Dubois after Fulgence Raymond was chosen for Charcot's chair, found his friend's doctrines a bit on the preachy side.[44]) Thus, Dubois said, doctor and patient became implicit partners. "In these treat-ments the patient and the physician seem to work to obtain the same result—the one by his confidence and good sense, the other by his clear and convincing explanation of the matter."[45] Note that this partnership is implicit: Nowhere is it said that the patient is aware of receiving psy-chotherapy. As far as the patient knows, he or she is in a standard medical or neurological consultation for an organic disease.

Here is an example of Dubois in action with his therapy of persuasion: "Mme. W———, after an altercation with her cook, was seized with para-plegia. I found the patient in bed, very much disturbed by what had happened. Her legs were in tetany [cramped] when stretched out, and the patient was incapable of making the slightest movement."

While Dubois examined the patient, she asked, "Is it serious? Shall I have to stay a long time in bed?"

"Serious? Not in the least; it is only a nervous weakness brought on by emotion. In three days you will be on your feet!"

Dubois then took the relatives to one side and said:

You have heard that I have said she will be cured in three days; I could have said three weeks, three months, or more, for I have seen these paraplegias last for years. It all depends upon the idea that the patient gets into her head. Take care, then, to take it for granted that the pa-tient will be cured within the fixed time. Do not make believe to be-lieve it; that will not do; believe it—all of you believe it!

On the third day the patient was up and walking again.[46]

Dubois's therapy combined the enthusiasm of a revival meeting with careful consultation between doctor and patient. Every little sign was commented on as a prognosis of recovery. A patient who was emaciated, tired, and had pains all over her body had not yet recovered after two months of treatment. "I found her in utter despair," said Dubois.

"I want to go away," she said, bursting into tears.

"I understand your discouragement," said Dubois. "But I do not share it, and I will tell you why: you have, it is true, the same pains, but I see that you have made some progress. Not only have you grown stronger but you have lost that trembling of the feet that you had on your arrival."

What trembling? The patient had not even noticed it. She wanted help for her headaches and backaches.

Dubois told her: "To you the trembling of the feet means nothing; to me it is as important as the headaches; it also is one of the symptoms of your disease. These are, I might say, spots of the same ink, and if we have succeeded in effacing the smallest there are chances that we shall succeed in making them all disappear. Stay! Take courage!"

The patient stayed a month more and returned home cured, unaware that she had received "psychotherapy."[47]

To Dubois's basic system of persuasion, Dejerine added only one element, but it was an important one. Finding Dubois's program too intellectualized, Dejerine stressed the power of emotional "sympathy" between doctor and patient. "For me, the foundation stone, the only basis on which all psychotherapy can rest, is the benevolent influence that one human being exercises on another." Hysteria could not be cured with syllogisms, he said. Psychotherapy worked only "when the person you are doing it to has confessed to you his entire life, that is to say, when he puts absolute confidence in you." Sentiment, not persuasion, was the key to psychotherapy. Transposing the sense of Charcot's article about faith healing, Dejerine said: "It is faith that saves, and faith that heals."[48]

This systematic use of the doctor-patient relationship to effect psychotherapy had been elaborated by both Dubois and Dejerine but was known mainly as "the Dubois method." Until perhaps the mid-1920s it was the dominant form of psychotherapy in western society. One may trace its rise, and the concomitant decline of "suggestion," in the *Index-Catalogue* of the U.S. Surgeon General's Office, whose compilers retrospectively found 116 publications on suggestion (mainly nonhypnotic) in 1880–89, 46 in 1890–99, 102 in 1900–1909, 58 in 1910–19, and 31 in 1920–29. Publications on psychotherapy, by contrast, rose from 38 in 1890–99, to 231 in 1900–1909, 76 in 1910–19, and 84 in 1920–29.[49] Thus the decade before World War I was that par excellence of nonpsychoanalytic psychotherapy, most of it related to Dubois's and Dejerine's doctrines. (Psychoanalytic literature was classed under another rubric.)

Descriptions of their psychotherapeutic techniques make it clear that many physicians had incorporated Dubois's *"dialectique sentimentale"* (Hesnard's phrase) into their practice.[50] In England in 1907 the Newcastle internist David Drummond praised this kind of "good chat" therapy. "The best treatment, he said, consists of an honest and straightforward statement to the patient, dealing with the facts of the case . . . a statement that, by its very firmness, disinterestedness, and kindliness, wins the confidence of the patient and encourages him to think better of himself, and to make a real effort to rise above his trouble and ignore himself. . . . The sooner we begin to talk rationally [to our nervous invalids] the sooner will we acquire the art of curing them. Many a patient has returned to a doctor, it may be months or years after his first visit, the chief factor of which was a plain talk, and when asked as to his state and how the prescription suited him, has replied, "Oh, I am much better; but it was not the medicine that did me good, but what you said."[51]

(Note, however, that such patients, filled with confidence in the physician and his words, were not aware of being the objects of psychotherapy.) Edwin Bramwell, son of Byrom Bramwell and a distinguished Edinburgh neurologist and internist, applauded Dubois in 1923 for having broken with the brain-disease ("materialistic") attitude toward the neuroses. He urged family doctors to undertake "suggestion and persuasion." The practitioner "must realize that to dismiss a patient suffering from a neurosis, with the remark that there is nothing the matter with him, is an act of cruelty."[52] The advice that Thomas Arthur Ross, medical director of a private English nervous clinic, gave to family doctors in 1929 about treating the neuroses was pure Dubois: Listen attentively to the histories of chronically neurotic patients, he urged:

The patient will reveal himself as a person who has habitually reacted badly to the calls of life; and a physician who has listened patiently to one of these people has thereby acquired great power over him. The patient feels that here at least is someone who has cared to try to understand. . . . [The patient] will not like it at first, and he will probably need a good deal of guidance; but if these people are taken in hand in this way it is surprising how many will respond.[53]

In the United States, the decade before World War I saw a great growth of Dubois-style psychotherapy. In a meeting of the Boston Society of Psychiatry in 1908, for example, Smith Ely Jelliffe, a New York psychiatrist who had translated Dubois's work into English, conceded that many psychotherapies were flourishing now: "Hypnotism, waking and sleeping suggestion, psycho-analysis by means of Freud's hypnoidal or distraction method [sic: Jelliffe would later end up an enthusiast of psychoanalysis, using a totally different method], Sidis' hypnoidization principle . . . Weir Mitchellism and others." Dubois' "re-education methods," Jelliffe believed, "had offered the most help." There was in the consultation a "special rapport. . . . This is the element in psychotherapy which cannot be taught—the rest is teachable and understandable."[54] The following year Jelliffe's New York colleague Joseph Collins, a member of the central-nervous old guard, scorned the new psychotherapeutic movement and all its work, which he dated from the English translation of Dubois's book (in 1905). After its appearance, he said, the American medical profession "gave heed with frenzy. Soon there began to be heard in medical meetings, papers—by internists as a rule—which set forth the great therapeutic value of psychotherapy. A reference to the current medical literature of the past two years will give an idea of the hold which this subject has obtained on the general practitioner."[55]

Events in Central Europe transpired more or less in the same manner as in England and the United States, and it would be unnecessary to rehearse them in detail were it not for the presence of a particular advocate of psychotherapy who came, not from the ranks of neurologists and psychiatrists as most of those mentioned above, but from the depths, and deeply authoritative ones, of internal medicine: Ottomar Rosenbach. Rosenbach demonstrated the effectiveness of psychotherapy not just on obvious neurotics with hysterical aphonias but on patients who attributed their subjective complaints to "heart" disease and the like, patients whose conviction that they had an organic disease gave them a horror of hypnotism or any other avowed form of psychotherapy. Born into a medical family in a small town in Silesia in 1851, Rosenbach graduated from Breslau University in 1873. For the next four years he worked at the medical outpatient (and inpatient) clinic at the University of Jena, under two internists known for their psychological sensitivity: Wilhelm Leube, who coined the term *nervous dyspepsia*, and Hermann Nothnagel, one of the first internists associated with the philosophy of treating the "patient as a person" (a holistic movement within internal medicine that grew up in reaction to the therapeutic nihilism of such mid-nineteenth-century Viennese internists as Joseph Skoda; Nothnagel himself became professor of medicine in Vienna in 1882).[56] In 1878 Rosenbach returned to Breslau as a hospital physician, also lecturing at the university. Almost twenty years later he left Breslau again, departing university life as well, to acquire a large private practice in Berlin.[57] In 1880 Rosenbach began to write on psychotherapy and continued his interest in the subject right through to a large book on it in 1897.[58]

Aside from hypnotism—to which he had always maintained an uneasy relationship because it "stupidified" the patient—Rosenbach employed two varieties of "rational" psychotherapy. First was "the didactic me-

251

thod." If it was clear that the patient's symptoms came from an "idea" (*Vorstellung*), the physician should give the patient new ideas and convince him with objective clinical findings of the falsity of the old ones. For example, Rosenbach asked imagined heart patients to do muscle exercises and then showed them that pulse and respiration had scarcely changed. Or showed "spinal" patients that their reflexes were normal. As for stomach patients "who suffer from the notion [*Einbildung*] of not being able to eat certain foods, the objective demonstration must be furnished that they digest their food better than they think. The best way to do this is to pump out their stomachs after they eat the supposedly indigestible foods and show them through the inspection of the stomach contents *ad oculos,* that digestion has been proceeding without incident."[59]

Secondly came the "painful method," of suppressing symptoms with unpleasant treatments that the patients considered true organic therapy, such as the "faradic brush" (a fanlike array of wires splaying out of a long handle gave off shocks[60]). Rosenbach had, for example, treated hundreds of children successfully over the years—children who seemed to take some pride in the production of their various vomitings, aphonias, air swallowings and hysterical coughings—with this painful electrical brush.[61]

Rosenbach worked the treatment of "emotional dyspepsia," meaning psychogenic stomach and bowel disturbances, into an entire program. Educate the patient and strengthen his will and his stomach, Rosenbach encouraged. "You have to pressure him as hard as possible to abandon previous [eating] behavior and return to a normal life-style." These patients had generally taken on all manner of bizarre food avoidances and dietary rituals. "It is of the greatest importance to free these sufferers of their previous fixed ideas, namely about imagined 'stomach' enlargement, which has been the fashionable disease of the last decade." The next step was to discuss with the patient the results of palpation, percussion, test meals, stomach washing, and stool analysis, which established that all organs are in order. Then the patient must stare death in the face and resume eating the previously avoided dishes. The psychological element in this therapy, Rosenbach resumed, was "to convince the patient of his erroneous life-style and of the false interpretation of his internal sensations."[62] Rosenbach's work on "emotional dyspepsia" in particular had a great impact upon internists' subsequent management of such complaints as irritable bowel syndrome. While Möbius, Dubois, and Dejerine greatly influenced psychotherapy as understood by psychiatrists and neurologists, Rosenbach established the basis of psychological therapy in internal medicine, from the doctor's viewpoint. Of course there was no question of the patients' realizing they were being treated with psychotherapy.

The Psychoanalysts Hijack Psychotherapy

In the public mind today, psychoanalysis is virtually synonymous with psychotherapy and even psychiatry. References to going to a "shrink," originally meaning depth psychology, or to being "on the couch," the classic piece of psychoanalytic office furniture, are routinely heard. This state of affairs began in the 1920s, as psychoanalysis grabbed control of the other budding psychotherapies. Its major consequence for our story was instilling in patients with somatoform symptoms a horror at the prospect of psychotherapy. For psychoanalysis was the only one of the early psychotherapies in which the patient realized he was *not* receiving standard medical treatments for legitimate organic disease. The origins of the history of psychoanalysis are too well known to require recapitulation here. Suffice it to say that the publication of Sigmund Freud and Josef Breuer's *Studies in Hysteria* in 1895 excited considerable, though somewhat delayed, interest in the cathartic method, getting patients to experience a sudden release of pent-up affect, or catharsis, as they reflected on traumatic moments in their early years. The assumption was that childhood trauma was responsible for the symptoms the patients exhibited in adult life, and if the patients themselves believed this doctrine, the catharsis was often successful.

True psychoanalysis, as developed by Freud after 1895, was not the cathartic method. Freud's psychoanalysis attempted to chart the pathways of the unconscious mind. In suggesting exact models for the genesis of neurotic symptoms Freud differed from, or improved on, if one will, his many predecessors who had written about psychogenesis and psychotherapy. The Bernheims and Möbiuses had offered little more than a "black box" by way of explaining why symptoms arose and why psychotherapy worked. Terms such as *suggestion* or even *exhausted nervous centers*, though sounding scientifically precise, were just black boxes in that they failed to indicate an exact mechanism. Freud suggested, rightly or wrongly, such a mechanism. As his theories unfolded from the late 1890s to the interwar years, the mechanism involved three main doctrines: (1) the principle of the patient's "resistance" to unwelcome truths about the past, truths that had been "repressed" into the unconscious; (2) the causal significance of sexual events, particularly sexual fantasies in early

253

childhood; and (3) the importance of child development in determining the adult personality.[63]

Before 1930 these doctrines were the focus of much controversy. But over the half-century from the publication in 1895 of *Studies in Hysteria* until the end of World War II it is fair to claim that advocates of psychoanalysis grew steadily, while opponents—members of an older generation who had embraced some other part of the psychological paradigm or indeed the central-nervous paradigm—steadily declined. This advance may be traced in three areas: general medical interest in the Breuer-Freud cathartic theory, the adoption of psychoanalysis properly understood, and the elaboration of a psychoanalytic approach to somatization.

The cathartic method won more medical adherents than psychoanalysis proper, even after Freud's true analytic doctrines had become familiar, because it was briefer and required no special training. The Breuer-Freud technique encouraged a wide-ranging rumination about the past that the patients themselves enjoyed, seeing such careful "history taking" as evidence of the doctor's concern for them.

Typical in his application of the cathartic technique was young Felix Gattel, who had graduated in medicine from the University of Würzburg in 1893 and then joined the staff of a private nervous clinic in Berlin. In Vienna in 1897, he was studying with Freud and working at the psychiatric and neurological outpatient clinic of Vienna's General Hospital. Here we see him treating Fräulein Ella E., a twenty-eight-year-old woman whom a colleague had referred for neurasthenia. Her chief complaints were head- and neckache and various other bodily pains dating from two years before. Her father had died when she was twelve. She was in the middle of the birth order between two brothers, and claimed to have no childhood memories, nor ever to have experienced any sexual feeling. She had vivid dreams, sometimes awakening anxiously at night.

In the first interview Gattel instructs her to come back the next day and tell all her memories.

Day Two: She tells a dream, says also that she was very anxious as a child and slept with her mother, occasionally if the mother was unwell with a brother who was three years older than she, whom she forgot to mention yesterday because the brother had later died. Apparently the brother played sexual games with her.

Day Three: She feels much better. She says she has nothing more to tell. Gattel says he thinks she's holding something back. Finally she says that during a trip to Munich she found she could fall asleep only in the position of Titian's *Venus* (with one hand at the pubic area). Also, she

254

forgot to tell him about an officer she was mad about, but nothing happened between them.

Day Four: Last night she had more neck pain. She says she has nothing more to tell. Gattel tells her the pain won't go away until she confesses whatever it is she's hiding.

Day Five: First she reports a nightmare. Then she confesses: "You know, earlier when I was telling you about my brother in bed, I told a lie about how old I was because I was already twelve. Then there was something else. When I was about four or five, before I even went to school, I used to run after a gentleman whom I can't remember much about now and follow him right up to the end of the village where we lived. I got him to do dirty things with me. But that was my own initiative because it made me feel so good. Naturally I was embarrassed about it later and forgot the whole thing, but the day before yesterday, in the evening when I was sitting on a bench, it all occurred to me again."

Day Six: Nothing more comes out. She begs until Gattel finally consents to let her take a phenacetin [an analgesic] powder if she gets another headache.

Day Seven: She cancels the appointment.

Day Eight: She is feeling fine. Another huge memory surfaces: Two years ago she almost became engaged to a man for whom she felt nothing. It was shortly thereafter that the headaches began. When exactly? It turned out that an officer whom she admired had made her an "immoral proposition." Although she liked him a lot and felt excited by him, she "naturally" declined. That evening she greatly strained her eyes sewing. From then on the headaches began.

Day Nine: Her condition continues well. She has to leave town for some reason. Gattel suspects a sexual history even before the age of four, otherwise she would not have run after that man. The follow-up: "After some time I heard again from Fräulein E. that, despite this rather rudimentary analysis, she was doing well."[64]

Gattel thus provides an early and rather caricatural example of the cathartic method. One notes that Fräulein E. was aware of receiving psychotherapy, though she might well have preferred a more medical approach with the phenacetin flowing freely. Whether she had experienced all the events in question or merely reported them to please her physician is impossible to determine. In any event, the closeness of the doctor-patient contact evidently did her some good.

The cathartic technique was often a way station on a nerve doctor's path towards full psychoanalysis. Leonard Seif and Franz Riklin, for example, both of whom later became full-fledged analysts, began with the

Breuer-Freud cathartic technique. Seif used it rather unsuccessfully in Munich, and Riklin in Zurich attempted to link each of his patient's symptoms—for example, those of a young woman who was a long-standing victim of paternal incest—to some specific event in her past.[65] Other psychiatrists who used the term psychoanalysis often had nothing very specific in mind. Jakob Kläsi, on the staff in 1917 of the university psychiatry outpatient clinic in Zurich, practiced "psychoanalysis," as he put it, "not only in the form that we owe to Freud and which he introduced into psychiatry, but in the form of a Freud-like, intense psychological investigation, a seeking after a deeper understanding of connections and of the personality."[66] This amounted, in other words, to taking a very careful history.

Although the psychoanalytic movement was slow to implant itself in England, the jargon became fashionable there already before the First World War. For example in 1906 Alfred Taylor Schofield, a Harley Street nerve doctor, called hysteria "distinctly a disease of the subconscious mind, of unconscious suggestion."[67] And Sir Hermann Weber, a consultant internist and balneologist (a specialist on spas) who, although retired in 1913, still saw patients at his Grosvenor Square home, said he preferred psychoanalysis to suggestive therapy and to Dubois's persuasion in the treatment of nervosity.[68] In 1912 William Stoddart, a staff psychiatrist of the Bethlem Royal Hospital ("Bedlam") in London, considered the popularity which fugue-style "second states" were then enjoying to be evidence that Babinski's doctrine of suggestion was correct. He lamented: "Babinski has rather gone out of fashion in favour of Freud for the moment."[69]

A number of American psychiatrists too understood psychoanalysis as a general grab bag of catharsis and deep chats. By 1909 Robert Edes, now sixty-eight, had retired from his post at the Adams Nervine Asylum and was accepting cases at home. He praised what he understood as psychoanalysis. "Freud's method does not demand the induction of hypnotism, but an attitude of confidential trust evoked by long continued and careful questioning as to the earliest recollections which have given rise, through long trains of association, forcibly repressed or fallen below the threshold of present consciousness, to morbid psychic conditions." This was not every therapist's cup of tea, he added: "It is not every man who can listen sympathetically to a daily rehearsal of imaginary, self-developed woes, or the maudlin details of a self-accuser."[70]

Word of psychoanalysis spread widely in the United States in those years, but what individual practitioners understood by it was often not at all what Freud had preached at his lectures at Clark University in

1909. In 1910 George Parker, director of the psychiatric outpatient clinic of Roosevelt Hospital in New York, tried psychoanalysis on a young woman who had gone into a hysterical fugue after learning that her brother had just been decapitated by a train. (She then discovered that a friend of the brother's had instead been the victim.) "Psychoanalysis began with the production of light hypnosis," said Doctor Parker. He then analyzed her dreams. "This is a clear example of the mechanism described by Janet," he concluded.[71] So much for Doctor Parker and psychoanalysis.

Many physicians referred to this kind of picking and choosing among Freud's doctrines as "psychoanalysis." For example Edward Mayer, a professor of neurology in Pittsburgh, was unsympathetic to Freud's views on sexual etiology but liked the interpretation of dreams ("[it] has proved of great value in our analysis of psychoneurotic patients"):

Time given to [neurotic] patients since I have used Freud's methods has become a pleasure instead of annoyance as formerly and even, although I believe that suggestion is a powerful factor, the delving into their inner life without a complete mastery of or belief in Freud's methods, has given me weapons to use in their treatment which were hitherto concealed from me.[72]

When therefore we speak of the "rapid acceptance of psychoanalysis" in the United States and elsewhere, we are often dealing with physicians who used a simulacrum of this trendy new therapy to achieve closer emotional rapport with their patients. Under the umbrella of the psychological paradigm, this first tradition of psychoanalysis did not diverge sharply from the psychotherapeutic views of a Möbius or a Dubois.

The second tradition within psychoanalysis was represented by those who believed in the real thing. Although not so numerous as those who savored mainly the phrase, the scientific prestige of the true believers dethroned Dubois-style psychotherapy and made psychoanalysis acceptable in university departments. After 1900 the practice of real psychoanalysis entailed (a) embracing a specific model of psychogenesis and (b) employing a technique emphasizing free association and the analysis of dreams.

The battle for psychoanalysis among the professors is well known, its gist being the conversion of the Zurich psychiatrists Eugen Bleuler and Carl Jung before World War I, although neither remained a convert.[73] Spurred on by these Swiss (and lightly anti-Semitic) Christians, true psychoanalysis attracted steadily increasing numbers of adherents in the decade before World War I. In November 1908, Karl Abraham, a nerve doctor in Berlin who had studied in Zurich and was an early enthusiast of psychoanalysis, wrote Freud about a recent meeting of the Berlin Society of Psychiatry and Neurology. Abraham himself had presented a paper. "The audience remained attentive right until the end," Abraham said, "and despite the lateness of the hour wanted to have a discussion." Although several members had vigorously attacked Abraham's views on the sexuality of children and the like, "I have the impression that a whole lot of colleagues went home at least *half* convinced."[74] This *succès d'estime* occurred, it should be noted, in the midst of Europe's most organically oriented assemblage of psychiatrists. By 1914 Karl Bonhoeffer, the professor of psychiatry in Berlin, considered the whole question urgent enough to include in the written examination for aspiring medical officers of health a question on "the significance of psychoanalysis for psychiatry."[75] One of the candidates who had taken the exam, Johann Schultz, later chief physician of a fashionable private sanatorium, said in 1923 that in Central Europe, psychotherapy had become more or less tantamount to psychoanalysis.[76]

Among the Swiss professors there had been great triumphs too. Hans Prinzhorn, in a review of who was who in psychoanalysis in 1923, said that in Switzerland there was "scarcely to be found a psychiatrist, or even a neurologist, who has not had to come openly to grips with psychoanalysis and acquire some experience with it." All this was thanks to Jung and Bleuler. Prinzhorn continued, "After Jung left university life [in 1913] and formed his own circle of supporters, pure Freudian doctrines won even more ground in Switzerland." Recently even Constantin von Monakow, whose assistants were all members of the Zurich psychoanalytic society, had come aboard! To be sure, the university psychiatric clinic at the Burghölzli asylum no longer employed any members of the psychoanalytic society, but the spirit of psychoanalysis, said Prinzhorn, was present there, root and branch.[77]

This story of psychoanalytic success in Central Europe could be repeated for other countries, with only some variation in timing. By the 1920s medical writing on psychotherapy had become dominated by analytically oriented physicians. The *Index-Catalogue* of the U.S. surgeon general began classifying publications on psychoanalysis in the decade that began in 1910. In 1910–19, 148 books and articles on the subject appeared, compared to 76 on psychotherapy generally and 58 on suggestion. In 1920–29 there were 302 publications on psychoanalysis, compared to 84 on psychotherapy and 31 on suggestion.

Within mainline psychoanalysis itself, a separate tradition arose of diagnosing and treating psychosomatic conditions. Surprisingly, this tradition did not arise from Freud. Although at the beginning Freud had meant by hysteria a given set of physical symptoms ("conversion symptoms"), later his understanding of the term became quite different. By the early 1900s Freud had lost interest in treating the pseudoneurological, or hysterical, symptoms seen in neurological practice (Freud was trained as a neuropathologist, not a psychiatrist). Instead he came to see hysteria as a kind of underlying psychic mechanism responsible for all conceivable psychic phenomena, not just somatoform symptoms.[78]

It was rather among Freud's followers that writing on somatization accumulated.[79] One source was the group of analysts in Berlin, who in 1920 founded a psychoanalytic outpatient clinic. The clinic was soon discovered by somatizers. Clinic director Max Eitingon wrote in 1924 that many of their early patients had been chronic doctor shoppers. "[We had] very many chronic, inveterate neurotics, long-standing organic cases and old cases of abnormal illness-behavior built upon the remains of organic disease, patients who for years had run from clinic to clinic, and from one health-plan doctor [*Kassenarzt*] to another and now sought consultations in our new clinic as well."[80] In 1921, after an analysis with Hanns Sachs, Franz Alexander became an assistant physician at this outpatient clinic.[81] We return to him in a moment.

In 1927 this Berlin group founded an inpatient sanatorium in the Berlin suburb of Tegel, the Schloss Tegel, directed by Ernst Simmel.[82] They had leased a large, late-nineteenth-century sanatorium whose previous director, Walter Reinhorst, had apparently been unable to make a go of it. The group now proposed to treat the whole range of psychoneuroses, partly with psychoanalysis, partly with conventional therapies. Given a high priority among the neuroses was somatization. In an advertisement in 1928, the Schloss Tegel insisted that it treated, in addition to hysteria, phobias, obsessive-compulsive disorders, and the like, "organ-neuroses and the psychic component of organic illnesses."[83] Simmel described typical patients at the Schloss Tegel including "a woman with a difficult case of hysteria, who almost perishes of anxiety, meaning cardiac and intestinal complaints, at night in the master bedroom, who then breaks out in the morning in unquenchable crying as the husband goes off to work."[84] The Berlin group of analysts thus acquired extensive experience in dealing with somatoform disorders.

The febrile mind of Viennese analyst Wilhelm Stekel coined the term *somatization*, using it as early as 1924. Stekel, one of the four original members of Freud's circle, wrote on every psychiatric topic imaginable, and so it is not suprising that he glanced at psychosomatic illness as well. In 1932, for example, Stekel described "an interesting somatization": a bank director who had just been fired, became depressed and developed numerous bodily pains:

> He came one day to my office complaining of a terrible pain in the upper thigh, radiating down from the hip. In the course of the analysis he mentioned that the previous night he had been troubled by an obsessive memory. Four years ago he was on a chamois hunt. He and a guide had been tracking game, and discovered a chamois on a peak across the valley. They fired off a shot and the chamois plunged into the abyss that lay between. The hunters climbed rapidly down and found the animal still alive, suffering with its hip shattered. The guide finished the chamois off. The banker's thoughts had remained on that animal all the previous night.

Stekel's analysis: The banker, similarly on the heights of success, had also been shot down by his colleagues.[85] Stekel did not remain on the subject of somatization long enough to make any contribution to it beyond Freud's basic notion, stated in 1905, that repressed neurosis was somehow expressing itself as a physical symptom.[86] But at least Stekel gave the term somatization to the literature.[87]

The next chapter in psychoanalytic efforts to deal with psychosomatic illness commenced in 1930, as Franz Alexander left Berlin for Chicago. In 1932 Alexander founded the Chicago Institute for Psychoanalysis, part of a wave of pre-1933 psychoanalytic migration to the United States. (Two other Berliners, Sándor Rado and Hanns Sachs, founded training institutes in New York and Boston in these years.) Doubtless reflecting the psychosomatic enthusiasms of the Berlin group, in 1933 Alexander began to write about the influence of specific psychic conflicts on specific kinds of somatoform symptoms.[88]

Alexander's research had a major impact on approaches to psychosomatic illness in the United States. It must be remembered that after 1933 the world center of gravity of this kind of research suddenly shifted to the United States. The Jewish scientists who had loomed so prominently in this history were being expelled from Central Europe and after 1939 would be systematically murdered. Although an indigenous American tradition of psychoanalysis existed, it was overwhelmed by the inrush of world-famous Central Europeans in the 1930s. Alexander was among the first of these arrivals and had a decisive influence in setting the research agenda for somatization. In 1943, for example, he wrote:

> The vegetative [visceral] concomitants of various emotional states are as different from each other as laughter from weeping—the physical

expression of merriment from that of sorrow. It is therefore to be expected that just as the nature of the chronic unrelieved emotional state varies, so also will the corresponding vegetative disturbance vary. . . . Gastric neurotic symptoms have a different psychology from those of emotional diarrhea or constipation; cardiac cases differ in their emotional background from asthmatics.[89]

As a result primarily of Alexander's work, such ailments as hypertension, irritable bowel syndrome, asthma, and contact dermatitis would until the 1960s be seen as the main psychosomatic disorders. It might be pointed out that Alexander's ideas on most of these conditions have since fallen into disrepute. Few authorities today consider hypertension to be a psychosomatic ailment, although it may be exacerbated by stress. But as a result of Alexander's work in the United States, a vast segment of mind-body problems became situated squarely in the domain of psychiatry. Other more indigenous American traditions of holistic medicine, such as Helen Flanders Dunbar's interest in the psychoanalytic roots of somatoform illness, were pushed aside. (Dunbar's work, it should be noted, situated the diagnosis and treatment of such disorders in departments of internal medicine.)[90]

With Franz Alexander, and with the general seizing of the psychological paradigm by the analysts, any hope of achieving public enlightenment about somatoform illness came to an end. "Psychosomatic" had now been branded "psychiatric" instead of "neurological." Consultation with a psychiatrist for the symptoms of somatization now became tantamount to "seeing a shrink," lying on a couch attended to by *New Yorker*–style cartoons of little men with pointy beards and thick accents, and learning "it was all in one's head." Psychoanalysis, which had set out to inform the public, correctly or incorrectly, about the unconscious roots of neurosis, thus achieved the paradoxical result of strengthening the public's conviction of organicity.

Patients Reject the Psychological Paradigm

Given the reluctance of the unconscious mind to be made a fool of, patients have always tended to reject psychological interpretations of physical symptoms. They find this kind of attribution unsettling because it seems to make inaccessible to them the remedies of medicine, conferring upon their symptoms a kind of hopelessness. Patients often think, Who after all can control the action of his or her unconscious mind?

As an example of the kind of evidence that inclines me to this sort of generalization, I refer to the several years I spent as an observer in an inpatient clinic for psychosomatic disorders, one situated in a psychiatric hospital. For a patient even to accept admission to such a hospital would require, one would think, some smidgen of self-insight about psychogenesis (indeed many of the chronically somatizing patients referred to this clinic rejected admission on the grounds that they had a "real" organic illness). Nonetheless, among the ninety-two patients whose charts were selected for quite intensive study, only one had any substantial insight into the role of psychological factors in illness. Seventy-six percent had no notion whatsoever of psychological factors, resolutely considering themselves victims of organic disease, and 24 percent demonstrated "some" insight. Fully one quarter of the patients had a fixed belief in a given diagnosis, such as fibrositis.[91] Another such study in the 1980s concluded that "a substantial proportion of psychiatrically-ill patients believe their illness to be physical in origin." Avoiding psychiatrists, "they present to general practitioners or directly to hospital specialists, describing their illness in entirely physical terms." Such patients also refused psychiatric referrals.[92] Thus at the end of the twentieth century, the "century of psychology," somatizing patients tend to shun any psychological explanation of bodily illness.

It would be distorted to suggest that all patients in all times have been resistant to the psychological paradigm. Of course there have been reflective sufferers, such as the "hysterical" but well-educated female patient at Bad Driburg who in the early 1840s told Anton Brück: "Most of the women I know do not understand this need to be loved [besoin d'être aimée]. And who would admit it to herself, even if she suspected it, and what would it help if you knew it or not, because changing things is beyond our reach." She herself had remained childless, and had "run the gamut of all the hysterical passions."[93]

Given the great success of psychoanalysis among the urban upper-middle-classes in the 1920s and after, directors of several of the organic private clinics haunted by this circle did advertise psychoanalysis, in addition to the standard list of physical therapies. For example Doctor Lewald's internal, nervous and psychiatric clinic in the Silesian resort of Obernigk (today Obornïke), once the young doctor Hans Merguet had taken it over in 1924, advertised to medical readers the availability of "psychoanalysis," as did Georg Wanke's nerve clinic for nonpsychotic patients in the Thuringian resort town of Friedrichsroda, to cite two of a handful of examples.[94] These sanatoriums appealed to a small upper crust already drenched in psychoanalytic jargon and therefore not resistant to it.

Yet the public as a whole has always been refractory to any notion of "nerves" smacking of psychology or the action of the mind. Benjamin Travers, senior surgeon at St. Thomas's Hospital in London, spoke in 1835 of the "levity and ridicule extended even to the term [nervous disease]. If the term escapes a medical man in consultation, the patient is offended at such an imputation, and assures him that he or she is far too sensible a person to be nervous."[95] Rudolf Schindler, an internist in Munich in the 1920s (and the inventor of the flexible gastroscope), had seen many such patients,

> who belong to the nerve doctor but do not seek him out! But it is obvious why they do not. They know they have heart pain, stomach pain or menstrual pain. Thus they go to the internist, the gynecologist, or finally in desperation to the surgeon. If that still does not work, they go to the quacks [Kurpfuscher]. . . . They have no idea that they have a nervous or indeed a psychiatric illness, and they refuse to believe it when you say it to them short and sweet. For what is making them ill lies beneath the threshold of their consciousness.[96]

This kind of testimony makes clear that the public saw through the transparency of calling oneself a nerve doctor. Somatizing Central Europeans, to whom the convenient fiction of the Nervenarzt was supposed to appeal, sought out the internist instead.

Similarly in the United States the somatizing public shunned the psychiatrist. Malcolm Bliss, a physician in St. Louis with fifteen years of experience, deplored in 1908 the difficulty in

> get[ting] the patient to realize the mental origin and method of management of his troubles. . . . Most psychics are indefatigable in their search for medicinal remedies and come to offices laden with thirty or forty prescriptions, about half of which call for one or another of the bromide salts [sedatives]. . . . I have had patients with whom I had labored diligently [in psychotherapy], settle themselves rebelliously in a chair and declare they were not going to leave until they got a prescription for some medicine.[97]

This lamentation about the lack of insight in somatizing patients constitutes a steady stream in medical literature. Every decade has its offerings. Here is Herbert Berger in 1956 on the subject of his first few years of medical practice in a small town: "The certainty that I lived in a belt of inbred neurotics became firmly fixed in my mind. Coming from a large urban center myself, I felt fairly certain that the residents of my community had intermarried . . . and that this explained the large number of functionally incompetent individuals whom I met." Later he realized that this was just a typical general practice. "Gradually I have come to recognize that these individuals never wish to be told that they are *just* nervous. The word 'imagination' is anathema to them for they are certain that they are seriously ill, and they expect and demand that the physician treat their disease with considerable respect. It is often necessary to medicate these people." Referral to a psychiatrist, said Berger, was impossible. "The patient is often reluctant to admit even to himself that he is mentally sick, whereas he can continue to believe that he is organically ill as long as he visits the office of a non-psychiatrist." Berger treated these patients with placebo therapy (giving them injections of a muscle relaxant called mephenesin) plus a kind of Dubois-Dejerine-style psychotherapy.[98]

Over the years a kind of informal consensus on the management of the somatizing patient established itself within internal medicine and neurology: Seek out the convenient fiction. "Almost every one is filled with the belief that he is debilitated," wrote Baltimore physician Daniel Cathell in 1882. "Say to the average patient, 'you are weak and need building up,' and you will instantly see by his countenance that you have struck *his* key-note. So much is this the case, that many of the sick, fully impressed with this idea, will want you to treat them with tonics and stimulants, even when their condition is such that these medicines are not at all indicated."[99] In Harley Street it was rather more fashionable to tell patients they had "malnutrition and dyspepsia producing nervous exhaustion" (rather than the reverse). Alfred Schofield warned his colleagues against "treating the case too lightly and making too light a diagnosis. In many cases this is fatal. The patient *knows* she is much worse than you say; she sees you have quite failed to understand her case, and she leaves you uncured and hopeless. I have lost myself more than one promising case by falling into this mistake, and I daresay most of my readers have too."[100]

Axel Munthe, the young Swedish physician who had studied with Charcot and established an upscale nerve practice in Paris in 1881 when he was twenty-four, eventually became quite adept at telling nervous patients what they wanted to hear. In the beginning:

They seemed quite upset when I told them that they looked rather well and their complexion was good, but they rallied rapidly when I added that their tongue looked rather bad—as seemed generally to be the case. My diagnosis in most of these cases was over-eating, too many cakes or sweets during the day or too heavy dinners at night. It was probably the most correct diagnosis I ever made in those days, but it met with no success. Nobody wanted to hear anything more about it, nobody liked it. What they all liked was appendicitis. Appendicitis was just then much in demand among better-class people on the look-out for a complaint. All the nervous ladies had got it on the brain if not in the abdomen, thrived on it beautifully, and so did their medical advisers.

Then, said Munthe, word got around that surgeons had started operating on appendicitis, surgery nobody wanted to undergo:

A new complaint had to be discovered to meet the general demand. The Faculty was up to the mark, a new disease was dumped on the market, a new word was coined, a gold coin indeed, COLITIS! It was a neat complaint, safe from the surgeon's knife, always at hand when wanted, suitable to everybody's taste. Nobody knew when it came, nobody knew when it went away.

(This was not colitis in the modern sense.)

Munthe tried the new diagnosis unsuccessfully on several patients, at which point Charcot referred "the Countess" to him. Munthe proposed appendicitis to her as an explanation of her symptoms. "At first she did not know if she had appendicitis, nor did [I], but soon she was sure that she had it, and I that she had not. When I told her so with unwise abruptness she became very agitated. Professor Charcot had told her I was sure to find out what was the matter with her and that I would help her, and instead of that . . . she burst into tears, and I felt very sorry for her."

"What is the matter with me?" she sobbed, despairingly stretching her hands toward Munthe.

"I will tell you if you promise to be calm."

At once she stopped crying, wiping her eyes and saying bravely, "I can stand anything, I have already stood so much, don't be afraid, I am not going to cry any more. What is the matter with me?"

"Colitis."

Her eyes grew large. "Colitis! That is exactly what I always thought! I am sure you are right! Colitis! Tell me what is colitis?"

Munthe did not himself know, nor did anybody else at that time because the real organic disease called colitis had not yet been discovered.

"The Countess smiled amiably at me. And her husband who said it was nothing but nerves!"[101]

Munthe's account still stands, more than a century later, as one of the classic descriptions of pathoplasticity, or the tendency of illness attribution and presentation to change with fashion. It is impossible to read of his countess's "colitis" without thinking of such fashionable illnesses of our own time as twentieth-century disease, chronic fatigue syndrome, and fibrositis.

The psychotherapy paradigm triumphed because it seemed to offer physicians a sensible explanation of why patients somatize and how to treat them. But the advocates of all of these therapies underestimated the deep terror with which patients contemplate physical symptoms. No therapeutic approach would succeed that did not reassure patients of the reality of their symptoms. No therapy that forthrightly assumed the non-organic nature of the symptoms would be accepted by the patients.

CHAPTER

10

The Patients' Paradigm Changes

When the doctors' idea of "legitimate" disease changes, the patients' idea changes as well. When the doctors shifted their paradigm from reflex neurosis emphasizing motor hysteria to the central-nervous paradigm of sensory symptoms, the patients shifted accordingly: Symptoms of psychosomatic illness passed from the motor side of the nervous system to the sensory. Anxious to present legitimate disease, somatizing patients in the last quarter of the nineteenth century and the first quarter of the twentieth abandoned the classic hysteria of the past and adopted sensory symptoms that would correspond to the new medical paradigms of central-nervous disease and psychogenesis. Pain and fatigue came to the forefront of the consultation as examples of symptoms that "exhausted cerebral centers" would be likely to produce. For what better corresponded to the notion of intrinsic cerebral deficits than the highly subjective sensations of pain and tiredness?

The Decline of Motor Hysteria

In the social history of medicine there is no more striking phenomenon than the disappearance of classic hysteria. Enthroned in the middle of the nineteenth century as the quintessential illness of the "labile" woman, the fits and paralyses that had been summoned from the symptom pool since the Middle Ages—spreading almost epidemically during the nineteenth century—virtually came to an end by the 1930s. Although doubtless caused by many circumstances, this change was in part a consequence of changing medical paradigms. As Kinnier Wilson, the distinguished English neurologist, said in 1931: "Possibly the outstanding feature of hysteria as revealed to us by the records of former generations and the knowledge of our own is the changes which its clinical syndromes have suffered." He quoted Hippolyte Morestin's remark: "Hysterics follow scientific trends and adapt themselves to medical progress." Wilson added that, since the days of witchcraft, "the poor hysteric has done her best, has never failed to respond to the calls made on her." The problem for the hysteric now, he said, was her puzzlement in the face of the psychological paradigm. "Today we seek the clue to the ailment in the unseen psyche, and she is somewhat at a loss accordingly; her elaborate somatic manifestations are rather at a discount. A cold scientific environment besets her instead of a world of emotional extravagance and limitless credulity. . . . The times have changed, and we, both physicians and hysterics, have changed with them."[1] While expressing age-old male prejudices in a particularly malignant tone, Wilson had seized the essence of the paradigm shift among patients.

The major source of information about symptoms is doctors' reports. Undoubtedly these are fragile as objective sources of evidence, given that the physicians reported on what they found of interest. Yet the hysteria of the nineteenth century was so striking that it is inconceivable that doctors suddenly became blind to it. The convulsing housewife, the young woman bedridden with apparent "paralysis": The doctors were saying that they no longer saw these patients. That doctors could have somehow become insensible of them is no more likely than the possibility that fifty years from now, when environmental disease will have ceased to be fashionable, doctors will be oblivious of patients dragging their oxygen tanks around with them. Such patients will have ceased to exist. Just as changing fashions will probably erase "total allergy disease" and its cousins, so around 1900 changing medical paradigms overcame classical hysteria.

At the psychiatric hospital in Florence, for example, grave hysteria declined from 4 percent of all admissions in 1898–1908 to 0.1 percent in 1938–48.[2] Whereas the total number of patients diagnosed as hysterical at Cery Hospital, the university psychiatric clinic of Lausanne, did not change between 1910–29 and 1970–80, the kinds of symptoms that "hysterical" patients presented did alter significantly: Eighty-one percent of all hysteria patients in the former period displayed muscular tetany and agitation; only 27 percent did so in the latter. Fainting declined from 47 to 31 percent of all patients, and globus hystericus (lump in throat) from 13 to 5 percent. The dissociative conditions so popular at the turn of the century also dropped off sharply: "Twilight states" (*états crépusculaires*), which is to say second states, declined from 57 to 24 percent of all hysteria patients; amnesia dropped from 32 to 18 percent. By contrast, general fatigue rose from being present in 4 percent of all hysteria patients to 13 percent, and visceral problems from 8 to 22 percent. Whereas no patients had complained of sexual frigidity in 1910–29, 22 percent (all of them women) did so in 1970–80.[3] Although knowledge of overall changes in hysteria is complicated by variations in how doctors and patients understood the term (surely there were anorgasmic women in 1910!), a shift from motor to sensory forms of somatization is evident from these data.

Walter von Baeyer, a veteran psychiatrist in Nuremberg who looked back in 1948 at hysteria at the municipal hospital in that city, indicated that this shift began before the 1930s: "The old hysteria, the primitive presentation of abnormal reactions to experience, has almost disappeared from this clinic," he said. He considered these changes "neither the result of the economic crisis of the 1930s nor the Nazi propaganda and the War, nor the misery of the post-war period. . . . It seems truly to be the case that the style of reacting abnormally has changed over the years."[4]

In England the old hysteria had vanished by the interwar years. Dr. Patria Asher, a medical officer in the British army writing in 1946, found "frank conversion hysteria [so] rare" that she felt justified in publishing the case of a twenty-year-old female private who had a hysterical paralysis of her right arm.[5] James Halliday, a public health official in Glasgow interested in psychosomatic illness, commented in 1948 on the "downward trend of hysteria between the World Wars. Although no exact statistical data exist the evidence suggests that in the course of the present century there was a decline in the incidence of gross physical manifestations of hysteria in women. It is probable, too, that there was a contemporaneous decline in males."[6]

In France, wrote Angelo Hesnard in 1927, "Hysteria has almost disappeared from the hospitals since the War." What we now see, he said, is *la petite hystérie*, meaning "women who content themselves with a few gesticulatory movements, with a few spasms followed by sobbing . . . grimaces, mannered contortions or excessive emotional gestures, clamped jaws and the like."[7] In fact the French would long retain this curious mix of twitching and psychic disaffiliation, giving it the improbable organic diagnosis of "la spasmophilie," a disorder found in France and nowhere else.[8]

In the United States, doctors commented early on declining hysteria. Israel Wechsler, professor of neurology at Columbia, said in 1929: "Hysteric paralysis has become a comparatively infrequent phenomenon in civil practice." He found one of the classic forms of motor hysteria, called astasia-abasia, the inability to stand upright or walk without falling, "very rare."[9] In 1954 Paul Chodoff, a prominent psychiatrist and psychoanalyst in Washington, D.C., admitted rather unwillingly: "Hysterical conversion phenomena undoubtedly do occur less frequently than formerly, and this decrease can be attributed in part to a change in the cultural climate" (a change in which, according to psychoanalytic theory, obsessive-compulsive behavior would begin binding up the anxiety that had formerly attached itself to hysteria).[10] "Why has the incidence of the major symptoms of conversion hysteria decreased to the point that they are today rather rarely seen in the civilian practice of psychiatry?" asked Washington psychiatrist Henry Laughlin in 1956. Like many observers, he thought it was because the patients were more "educated" and "sophisticated."[11] But it was not that patients had somehow become smarter over a period of thirty years. It was that they were learning from the press about the doctors' new paradigms, and responding accordingly.

On the basis of such medical opinions, it is likely that motor hysteria had indeed declined. In epidemic hysteria, for example, this transition from the motor to the sensory side of the nervous system is evident. François Sirois studied seventy outbreaks of epidemic hysteria between 1872 and 1972, the kind found among young women in factories and schools, the target population of epidemic hysteria. He suggested that a shift occurred from convulsions, globus, laryngismus, abnormal movements, and the like to an increase in reported fainting and in "nausea and abdominal malaise, and headaches."[12] Thus, roughly speaking, a shift from motor to sensory.

Typical of epidemic hysteria in our own times are groups of employees who are suddenly seized by vague, nonspecific complaints. For example, in February 1990, thirty-four toll takers at New York's Triborough Bridge were overcome out of the blue by "nausea, headaches and chest pains," all sensory symptoms. Although the workers and their union stoutly insisted that "toxins" had caused their illness, an extensive investigation turned up no organic causes.

Could their employers, the Triborough Bridge and Tunnel Authority, prove it was hysteria?

"No. I don't think we want to prove it," said a spokeswoman. "These people work very hard, and we don't want to make little of what happens to them."[13]

On the whole, then, symptoms in epidemic hysteria seem to have passed from being more on the motor to more on the sensory side, though the demarcation in these florid outbreaks is not an absolute one.

Similarly, motor hysteria seen in combat diminished greatly from World War I to World War II. Among German troops, the Parkinsonian shaking characteristic of shell shock during World War I had given way to other kinds of symptoms by the time of the 1939–45 war. Oswald Bumke, the professor of psychiatry in Munich who was in charge of psychiatric and neurological services in the Munich military district during World War II, later said: "In contrast to the First World War there were few neuroses. 'Shaking does no good,' one of my assistants on the Eastern Front wrote me. 'People prefer to get wounded.'" Bumke explained that doctors no longer believed the shaking:

> In 1916 almost all German neurologists came to agree upon the purely psychological origin of shell shock. Since then we have trained an entire generation of physicians in this tradition. Shell shock is now nipped in the bud, meaning that we would let the front soldiers rest for a couple of days instead of sending them home as in 1914–18, where their symptoms would become fixated and contagious to others. By 1945 the military district had over 30,000 beds and over 3000 neurological cases; and the neurotic division almost never contained more than 30 or 35 soldiers.[14]

Hans Bürger-Prinz, director of psychiatry at the large municipal hospital in Hamburg, said in his memoirs in 1971, "If one takes both of the great wars as two distinctive periods for comparison, it becomes immediately apparent that in the Second World War, hysterical symptoms disappeared almost entirely. They simply no longer existed, neither at the fighting front nor on the home front. Not even in the terrible trial of the nights of bombing."[15]

The same shift occurred in France. Whereas among French troops, classic conversion hysteria with its paralyses and contractures had dominated shell shock during World War I, by the time of the 1940 conflict cardiac and gastrointestinal forms of somatization had become popular. According to two students of shell shock in France: "Hysterical conversion drifted in the direction of somatic pathology." By World War II anxiety had fled to the internal organs, they concluded, because motor deficits had become too easily diagnosed as hysterical.[16] Numerous other studies of shell shock and combat-fatigue arrived at a similar conclusion: motor hysteria had vanished from the battle front by the time of World War II.[17]

271

Because old-style hysteria was a disease of fashion, one would expect it to disappear first in the most fashionable groups of the population, enduring longest in the least fashionable. There are not many data graded finely by social class or on the basis of urban-rural differences. Yet several casual observations suggest that the most stylish groups were at the leading edge of change. Oswald Bumke, in 1919 still professor of psychiatry in Leipzig, said: "We see the coarsest psychogenic phenomena, such as severe contractures and convulsions, most commonly among young women from the countryside." He attributed this to a lessened ability of the rural population to control "childish" impulses.[18] Giovanni Mingazzini, professor of psychiatry in Rome, said in 1926:

> Whoever compares the noisy, theatrical manifestations of hysteria forty years ago with the very modulated forms of the present day will surely be surprised. The four classic stages of the hysterical fit, which are recorded in all neurological textbooks and which really did appear in the years 1880 to 1900 in epidemic form, not just in France but in all of Europe, are no longer to be seen. The incomplete and atypical kinds of fits are also rare, to be found mainly among nuns and farmwives. What has been said of fits is also true of hysterical paralyses.[19]

In 1954 Stephen Taylor, a London physician with an extensive society practice, said: "In the countryside gross hysterics are still seen. In the slums, too, there are gross hysterics, as well as work-shy psychopaths. In suburban housing estates, whining anxiety hysterics predominate."[20] Thus, according to the later Lord Taylor, "whining anxiety hysteria" was to be the wave of the future.

Several other accounts suggest that by 1900 motor hysteria had long disappeared from middle-class London. Earlier chapters indicated how often such early-nineteenth-century consultants as Benjamin Brodie commented on motor symptoms among middle-class Londoners. Of all that, by the 1880s and 1890s, not a trace was to be seen. The *Lancet's* Paris correspondent said in 1890: "Speaking from an experience of six years' residence, a woman in any form of hysterical fit in the streets of London is a rare occurrence, while a similar exhibition in the streets of Paris is— while short of being an everyday phenomenon—at least not infrequent."[21] And Alfred Schofield, Harley Street nerve doctor par excellence, said in 1906 that among his patients pseudoneurological symptoms ("neuromimesis") in their pure form had ceased to exist. He then tabulated the symptoms of 350 of his recent patients who had "functional nervous disease": Only 2 percent of his 228 female patients had motor problems ("paresis"), and none of his male patients. Forty percent of his female patients (and 36 percent of his male patients) were characterized by "debility only"—in other words, by fatigue.[22] Interestingly, Doctor Schofield's office was at 19 Harley Street. Frederick Parkes Weber's office was also at 19 Harley Street.

The Paradigm Shift on Harley Street

In 1906 Frederick Parkes Weber was forty-three years old. Son of Sir Hermann Weber, himself a distinguished consultant, "Parkes" Weber carried on the family tradition of combining an extensive knowledge of the spas of Europe with a fabled command of internal medicine.[23] Parkes Weber therefore became a magnet for somatizing patients, intent on the belief that they had real organic diseases other physicians had not managed to diagnose. Because some of the records of Parkes Weber's practice, principally in the years 1900–1909, have been preserved,[24] we are able to form a quite accurate impression of the problems that were presented on Harley Street, a microcosmic setting for the transition in the pattern of symptoms. Among the hundreds of patients whom Parkes Weber saw over this period, the records of thirty-nine indicate individuals who seemed retrospectively to manifest some "nervous" element.

The impression derived from these records is that classic hysteria had certainly vanished from this population, for so unusual were references to motor symptoms that a statistical analysis would be superfluous. Very rarely did Parkes Weber encounter a patient such as "Miss X," presented in the chapter on gynecological surgery, who was unable to walk and required a bath chair. The bulk of his patients' complaints were of fatigue, pain, and gastrointestinal distress. True, a number complained of difficulty swallowing and globus, yet it was not the classic kind of globus that began in the pelvis and migrated upward to the throat. Parkes Weber himself considered many of his nervous patients "neurasthenic" because they were fatigued, and treated virtually all of them by finding suitable spas for summer and winter. In these years he had quite an organic bent, accepting most symptoms as evidence of real physical illness.

Only in the 1920s did he begin to believe that some apparently organic cases were in fact psychogenic. In a chart note of September 1940 about one woman who had been in his practice for decades, it dawned on him that she had been hyperventilating and swallowing air, giving rise to a lifetime of symptoms that he had attributed to her thyroid gland and to an overactive sympathetic nervous system. (She had also had several major episodes of depression.)[25] In these later years Parkes Weber showed

himself sympathetic as well to psychotherapy. He complained about patients' relatives, whom he called (after H. G. Wells), the "Gawdsakers,"
meaning as Parkes Weber put it, "dangerous friends and relatives who
say to the doctor: 'For gawd's sake, doctor, cannot something be done to
relieve the patient?' The finding of 'nothing organically wrong' ought
sometimes to save the life of patients by saving them from dangerous and
useless operations leading to their death. Psychotherapy and 'time' may
achieve the true cure."[26]

The practice of this complex and interesting physician gives a sense of
an already accomplished paradigm shift among the English elite. Parkes
Weber's clientele drew from the upper middle class and aristocracy, including a sprinkling of Jews from the East End who, although not well-
to-do, wanted to obtain the best medical care available. Many of the patients, such as Lady X, whom Parkes Weber saw in August 1906, were
chronic somatizers. Coming as a consultation case from Sir Hermann
Weber, Lady X was a thirtyish married woman who was socially prominent among the avant-garde. Her chief complaints were headaches, tiredness, and constipation.

Lady X had been at Bad Kissingen in 1905. Her doctor there, noted
Parkes Weber in the chart, "apparently thought Kissingen did not act
sufficiently on the liver, and did not recommend her to return to Kissingen. (She has literary tastes.). . . . Headaches since childhood. Constipation almost constant since age of 16 years. Stiffness of back last two
years." "In regard to the 'liver' I understand there have often been knife-
like pains in the right hypochondrium shooting to the back."

What to do with Lady X? "I advised a course at Franzensbad if she
goes without husband, and at Carlsbad or Tarasp if she goes with her
husband—afterward Upper Engadine or Tyrol if not too late or too cold."

A week later Lady X started for Tarasp in Switzerland, evidently with
her husband. Four days before Christmas 1906, her family doctor wrote
Parkes Weber that while at Tarasp, "patient suffered from severe constipation and indigestion and goutiness—no albuminuria—she is too thin
still—the knees were not improved by Tarasp treatment, but Dr. V. hopes
the general condition was improved." That was the end of the case of
this otherwise healthy thirtyish woman who was headachy, tired, and
constipated.[27] A century previously she would have had fits and the vapours. It is likely that Lady X had internalized the new symptom paradigm.

A more pronounced nervous element characterized the problems of
Reverend Y, fiftyish and, in June 1907, back in England briefly from

his permanent residence in the South of France. Reverend Y's problem: "morbus asthenicus," or tiredness. Parkes Weber went to work on his new patient. "For his neurasthenic condition (irritable weakness with palpitation etc) I gave him a pill containing [strychnine and arsenic]. In the meantime he must go to the coast till the end of July to escape hay fever and take (up-hill) walking exercise, live in the open air, and live the simple life in regard to diet (dry meals, mastication etc). Then he must see me again regarding course of treatment in Buxton or Harrowgate spas."

For the remainder of the summer Reverend Y complained of minor ills and toyed with his various medications of arsenic, strychnine and bromide pills. He also—shades of nasal reflex theory—had his nose cauterized.

September 30: Reverend Y, at Buxton, complained of "a peculiar temporary sensation of impending death." Parkes Weber suggested all medications be continued.

October 12: "Seems to have had some gastro-intestinal discomfort and tenderness yesterday, but there is no sign of any appendicitis and nothing abnormal to be discovered at present. Tongue natural. No fever. Bowels opened this morning with cascara [a powerful purgative]."

January 17, 1908: "I had a letter from Sir H[ermann] W[eber] from the Grand Hotel at ——— saying that Y was in the Grand Hotel there, and looked depressed. He had had a nervous break-down and was treated during several weeks by Dr. Sanders of Cannes in an establishment with massage (it was a regular Weir Mitchell 'cure')."

Reverend Y's case continued until October 1918, along the above lines. During the war he became somewhat preoccupied with what he called a "gouty throat irritation." Reverend Y's "nervous attacks" had by now come to an end. Life, however, he found trying. Giving up his chaplaincy, he contented himself with traveling with his brother around the Mediterranean. It is abundantly clear from Reverend Y's chart that he did not have an organic illness and was, instead, a garden-variety somatizer such as would be found in any medical practice.[28]

Reverend Y was, however, distinctive in seeing his own symptoms as evidence of "nerves." Most of Parkes Weber's patients resolutely attributed their pain and fatigue to organic illness. Mrs. A, thirty-six, from a small town in Devonshire, was typical of this large group. In September 1904, she and her husband had come up to London and were staying at the Hotel Russell. She had an eight-year-old daughter. Parkes Weber noted she had been an "invalid some years."

September 22, 1904: "Present condition: patient is a thin, active, nervous type of woman. Small veins of face rather obvious. . . . Always much pain at monthly periods. Lately neuralgic pains in head and back."

Mrs. A returned to Harley Street the next day. "She looks rather pale and shriveled." Parkes Weber examined her abdomen, found nothing, and took a blood sample. "I regard the case as one of neurasthenia, and advised abstention from tea and coffee."

Mrs. A now went to a rest home in Worthing, from where her husband wrote Parkes Weber on October 13, "Mrs. A thinks sea air does not agree with her." Could the doctor suggest some other spa? "I suppose," concluded the husband, "that Caux or Les Avants would suit her nerves for the winter as well as anywhere." Parkes Weber wrote back indicating that Mrs. A should have "a Weir Mitchell treatment" (a rest cure).

Therefore Mrs. A entered a convalescent home in Worthing. Six weeks later the operator of the home, Giulia Hawkes, wrote to Parkes Weber about the patient:

> I am writing to you for Mrs. A today, that she has been doing this sort of rest cure for three months [sic], and feels better, and is slightly fatter. She cannot walk more than twenty minutes at a time; her headaches are *just* as bad as ever; particularly just after the period; she gets neuralgia exactly the same, which lasts two or three days, throws her back, undoing the good that has been gained. . . . Last Friday Mrs. A was up *all* night with a racking headache, it could not have been worse; the enclosed prescriptions kindly return, Mrs. A says they give her very little relief, and they rather weaken her, she knows. None of the headache prescriptions does any good.

A local physician, Dr. Frank Hinds in Worthing, had been attending Mrs. A at the home. The representative of the home continued, "Dr. Hinds tells me privately that until the change of life, Mrs. A would never be strong; but he considered her decidedly better; now she looks very thin. Do you think Dr. Deffer's Sanatorium (where Mrs. B went) would benefit her next spring?"

In September 1905 Mrs. A saw Parkes Weber again in Harley Street, after which she underwent another rest cure under Dr. James Taylor's supervision at Miss Stirling's Home in London. "Not improved by six weeks' treatment (tough beef steak etc), lost eight lbs. and could not sleep there."

On April 28, 1906, Parkes Weber saw Mrs. A for the last time. "She looks to me rather shriveled, has some eczema (caused by sitting in the sun?) on backs of hands. She says her general condition is exactly the same as when I saw her in Sept. 1904. She is now staying for a day or two at Hotel York, London. I advised course in June at Schlangenbad with [Heinrich] Mueller—then stay at Axenstein, Axenfels or Salisbury."[29]

These cases indicate what a wonderful symbiosis had established itself between doctor and patient under the central-nervous paradigm, which Parkes Weber then adhered to. The physicians diagnosed "neurasthenia," "nervous exhaustion," "nervous breakdown," and the like, and the patients responded by being unable to walk more than twenty minutes and developing darting pains all over their bodies. Both doctor and patient conspired in courses of what was essentially placebo therapy at these spas. Both kinds of symptoms—chronic fatigue and psychogenic pain—had become more common by Parkes Weber's day than ever before.

Chronic Fatigue

From the viewpoint of the patient, pain and fatigue had the benefits (1) of corresponding to what doctors under the influence of the central-nervous paradigm expected to see, and (2) of being almost impossible to "disprove." Highly subjective sensations, neither pain nor tiredness can be said not "really" to exist, in the way that the Babinski test can "disprove" a hysterical paralysis or an ophthalmic diploscope can "disprove" the presence of achromatopsia (claimed inability to see colors). One could disprove medically many motor symptoms by demonstrating their lack of an anatomical basis. The potential anatomic basis of fatigue and pain was, by contrast, so much more complex and difficult to investigate that patients could retain the symptoms far longer before physicians would start murmuring the word "hysteria." Advancing medical knowledge had the ironical result of driving somatization deep into the nervous system, where a "million-dollar workup" would be required to clarify matters.

Writing the history of chronic fatigue as part of the symptom pool involves disentangling it from the diagnosis of neurasthenia. This is a chicken–egg problem: Did a rise in the frequency of fatigue prompt adoption of the diagnosis neurasthenia? Or did Beard's creation of neurasthenia elicit a rise in the complaint of tiredness among patients who wanted to be taken seriously? Both are likely.

Even before Beard launched neurasthenia, at first tentatively in 1869 and then to massive fanfare in 1880, doctors had been reporting "great exhaustion" and the like in patients. This variety of literature seems to quicken in the 1860s, simultaneously with the new popularity of the central-nervous paradigm. In his 1867 account of "hysterical pain," London surgeon Dennis Hovell described a woman with "great exhaustion." She tried "exercise" (an hour's drive in a carriage) and "was so prostrate on her return home . . . that she was obliged to be carried into the house, much to her annoyance, as the proceeding was rather a public one." "She also said that merely going out in the air produced a feeling of great exhaustion and took away her appetite for food." Hovell treated her psychologically, assuring her that he took the case seriously. Thus "the fretful, irritable, snappish tendency soon passed by, and she was one of the first to laugh at her own *fanciful illness*." Hovell said it was a general characteristic of "asthenia" and "depressed nerve power" that "exercise is followed by exhaustion, pain and other symptoms, and not by that reaction of strength which attends a condition of health."[30]

Joseph Amann, the Munich gynecologist, reported in 1868 the case of a thirty-eight-year-old unmarried woman whose fatigue had piggybacked on catalepsy, the latter still a common condition at that time. Typically, she would lie in bed a week or two because of "general weakness," then experience "a tenseness and bloating out of her abdomen with an urge to defecate, followed by globus hystericus, nausea and dizziness. She then feels herself a whole other person and hears a terrible rushing noise, as though a mountain stream were racing over her head, or as though hundreds of people were simultaneously conversing. Midst these symptoms she would lose consciousness completely, become cold and stiff in her entire body, her eyes completely closed." The catalepsy finally over, her fatigue would resume.[31] This combination of symptoms, the one backward looking, the other forward, is as interesting as the piggybacking of paralysis and anorexia in these years:[32] The unconscious mind was having difficulty discerning the trend of the times.

Weir Mitchell, in his first description of the rest cure in 1875, knew nothing of neurasthenia and assigned profound fatigue to spinal irritation. Nervous cases varied of course, he said, but one of the main symptoms was a "state of painful tire." He added in a note: "This symptom of [in]ordinate sense of fatigue is found in many forms of disorder in women. The worst cases to handle are girls with what is called spinal irritation by some, and spinal anemia by others."[33]

Reports of fatigue and exhaustion then multiplied in the 1880s, coinciding with but not necessarily caused by the dissemination of the diagnosis neurasthenia. Many writers did not even use the term neurasthenia. Josef Schreiber, one of those international spa doctors who divided his time between the South Tirol in winter and the Austrian mountain resorts in the summer (he owned clinics in Merano and Alt-Aussee), described a "highly-educated neurasthenic" he had treated in 1884 at Merano:

He would become so agitated that he would strike his dearly beloved wife, and in his dark hours might also fly at me if we insisted that he leave his bed and get out in the fresh air. Then in better moods he would joke about his behavior and said to me the following: "You cannot imagine what agitation, what egotism, I fall into, when I feel the need not to move my arms or feet and you force me to give up this condition of requiring total rest. I just become crazy, but it's right of you to extract me from this painful condition of psychological entrapment [*moralische Gefangenheit*]."

Schreiber attributed neurasthenics' loss of appetite in general to "the horror they feel at every activity, at every muscle movement."[34]

Chronic fatigue blanketed the world of the private nervous clinic before World War I in Central Europe. August Diehl, a psychiatrist who had come around 1901 from Hermann Oppenheim's outpatient clinic in Berlin to Lübeck, there to manage his own private clinic for the next ten years, mentioned in 1911 some two hundred cases of "nervous exhaustion" he had successfully treated with bromide and the rest cure. The bromide was necessary, he explained, because otherwise one could not get the patients to lie still.[35] Semi Meyer, chief physician of a sanatorium near Danzig, described the "collapse of nervous functions" of his young female patients:

A young woman will come into the clinic who can scarcely move, who neither wants to think nor is able to, who seeks only rest. We might be told that she has overexerted herself, and the clinical investigation gives no indication of hysteria. Following our diagnosis of "exhaustion neurosis," we put her to bed but gain nothing by doing so; she merely becomes weaker and more inert. Then one day the husband comes to visit or there is some trivial upset, and all at once our patient suddenly shows a quite different clinical picture. She is agitated, and stays so. She becomes rude, or has a fit of some kind.[36]

Again, in these fascinating accounts, old-style symptoms such as fits piggyback on new. By World War I, the middle classes of Central Europe would leave fits behind, while reports of fatigue continued to increase in frequency.

In France neurasthenia established itself in the late 1880s after Charcot approved the diagnosis. The accounts of French authors suggest that they must have been seeing patients with such symptoms for some time.

In 1891 Fernand Levillain, a student of Charcot's who divided his time between Nice in the winter and Royat in the summer, described the tiredness of neurasthenic patients as though he were long familiar with it: "It is quite curious that the symptoms of lassitude and exhaustion of the limbs are much more noticeable in the morning. Neurasthenic patients are surprised that, after a long stay in bed and even after a good sleep, they are still tired. They derive benefit from resting their limbs, which feel heavy to them, and they have trouble arising from bed."[37] In 1911 in Paris nerve doctor Paul Hartenberg said that the female neurasthenic was someone "unable to do her hair at a single go; she cannot hold up her arms for the time thus required. In order to get dressed to go out she has to pause and rest several times."[38]

Through the Vichy years and beyond the French would continue to complain about chronic fatigue. As the whole subculture of middle-class valetudinarianism crashed about him in World War II, Charles Fiessinger, eighty-five, advised fellow physicians in 1942 how to treat patients with "chronic asthenia": two to six months of bed rest, with strolls in the garden. "It is rare to see an asthenic recover before three or four years. . . . Psychological treatment is a waste of time for someone who needs rest. Be gentle with the patients, encourage them and let them talk as much as they want. A garrulous nurse is a nightmare for the poor asthenic." As for spas, Doctor Fiessinger thought Divonne, Néris, Plombières, and Salies-de-Béarn indicated.[39] It was clear that over a lifetime Doctor Fiessinger had acquired much experience with chronically fatigued patients.

Drawing on this old tradition of chronic fatigue, in 1967 Raymond Pujol described *"la névrose des téléphonistes"* (receptionists' syndrome). It was characterized by

> maximum and profound asthenia of both physical and psychological nature at the end of the workday, a drop in attentiveness, in interest and in memory; disturbances of mood and personality, nervousness, irritability, episodes of anxious agitation, hypersensitivity to noise, hyperemotivity with tearful moments and moments of depression. . . . Many receptionists say that work makes them nervous [*les énerve*] and that the more nervous they become, the faster they work, but that simply closes a vicious circle which exacerbates their problems. Their sleep is always disturbed; right after work they have an irresistible need to fall asleep then later there is often insomnia.

The list of symptoms of this syndrome, like those of neurasthenia, went on and on, to cover every possibly psychogenic upset.[40] Clearly in Europe, the rise in reporting of chronic fatigue at the end of the nineteenth century opened a wellspring that would swell into a great torrent by the end of the twentieth.

How about the New World? Although the diagnosis neurasthenia itself lasted longer in Europe than in the United States, chronic fatigue joined the mannerisms of middle-class American life as early as the 1870s and figured prominently in the symptom pool right up until the 1960s, when, like anorexia, it started to become epidemic.

George Beard launched neurasthenia in 1880, when the whole notion of nervous exhaustion was already a root-and-branch part of American culture. Augustus Hoppin's novel *A Fashionable Sufferer,* published in 1883, assumed that the reader was familiar enough with the notion to find amusing the heroine, a rich young widow "both lovely and lovable," named NE, or "nervous exhaustionist." Having become "weakly, hypochondriacal, and *exigeante,* she has summoned a handsome young physician to attend her, and lives in a sort of medical bondage. She imagines herself to be the most unfortunate of mortals, even while munching away at royal dainties."

Enter Mr. Cynicus Douce, to pay her court. He helps make her comfortable and gets her a cushion.

Cyn: "And this little bench for your feet, perhaps?"

NE: "Yes, I think so; but please remove those violets; they are too strong this morning!"

Then she asks for her "vinaigrette" and takes a sniff: "Bliss! I'm all arranged now; but don't you even cough while I'm reading [something she's received] I can't bear interruptions."

Cyn: "I'll hold in till the last minute."

Hoppin tells us in an aside, "There is nothing more queerly queer and unnaturally natural than what is called 'the nervous exhaustion of ladies.' It is a deceitful complaint. It generally attacks the handsomest and the richest of the sex. . . . First comes a sharp, wee quirk in the head, then a horrid neuralgic tweak in the 'small' of the back; and then again it 'jangles' up and down the spine with agonizing force. . . . It is undeniable that there is a goodly number of charming women in the world, so many that they may be said to form a class by themselves, whose vocation in life . . . is to trade upon their supposed weakness with the rest of the world. Really nervous, lacking bodily vigor, and at first requiring both the sympathy and the attention of their friends, they end by becoming beautiful tyrants, before whom everybody must make obeisance."

281

In the novel Hoppin allows the "nervous exhaustionist" to go on vacation. "Her maid, Thomas the quiet man-servant, her quinine, her props—her little hair pillow to stuff under her left ear,—and all the other petty paraphernalia of invalidism, had been hauled up from the station by installments."

The NE settles her food with little tablets of quinine before and after meals. Must she be careful with her diet? The NE says that her doctor "lets me eat everything. He says where nervous prostration has taken place, patients are to have their own will."

"I wish my nervous centre was prostrated, then," says Mr. Douce.[41]

Although the "nervous exhaustionist" shades over into the picture of chronic neurosis, her woes suggest that chronic fatigue was already familiar to American culture by the early 1880s.

In 1895 Robert Edes, then at the Adams Nervine Asylum, sketched chronic fatigue into the picture of "the New England invalid." As he described her:

This is the invalid with nothing to do, and who requires a household to help her do it. She has had no hardships, she has studied moderately at school, and perhaps has had a fall or an acute sickness, but she does not convalesce beyond a certain point, and is, or thinks she is, as helpless as [any] other. She is apt to think that all she wants is "rest," when she has never done anything that ought to tire her, and has done nothing but rest for years.[42]

At the turn of the century such women represented not-at-all-bizarre figures in middle-class East Coast culture but rather a kind of archetype of nervosity. Said Philip Knapp, who in 1885 had established neurology services at the Boston City Hospital, "There are a considerable number of neurasthenics who are congenitally weaklings and who go through life with a scanty supply of strength. They are typified by a case, where there was no especial strain or worry, who said, 'I can do just about one thing a day.'"[43]

As in Europe, medical references to chronic fatigue continued in the United States at a kind of low, background level throughout the first half of the twentieth century. In 1911, for example, Lewellys Franklin Barker, an internist at Johns Hopkins, referred a Mrs. J., a woman with literary interests, to the Creighton Sanatorium in Lutherville, Maryland. Gibbons Smart, on staff at the sanatorium, described the case: "Weight 130 pounds but pale, anemic, complaining of general pains; extreme fatigue on least exertion. So extreme was her fatigue, in her own mind, that conversation could not be carried on for more than five minutes;

then must come a long period of rest." After the patient had learned "self-mastery" at the sanatorium, her pain and fatigue vanished and she went on to write a play at her home in Ohio.[44] Among 688 patients seen in the practice of two physicians in Louisville, Kentucky, around the years 1927–28, 19 percent complained of loss of pep or exhaustion. Of the fatigue patients, 37 percent also reported pain and stiffness of the joints.[45]

Many such fatigue patients were men, the archetype being the chronically exhausted businessman.[46] But when the discussion comes round to women and fatigue, one must remember that the situation of female patients in particular was very different before the 1960s. Physicians emphasized how little these middle-class women had to do, whatever the reality of their lives. Far from juggling "two careers" as today, many of the patients were clearly bored and restless at home, developing their symptoms "as weapons," in Abraham Myerson's phrase, to be used against their husbands. Myerson wrote a book in 1920 about *The Nervous Housewife*:

> Every practicing physician, every hospital clinic, finds her a problem, evoking pity, concern, exasperation, and despair. She goes from specialist to specialist,—orthopedic surgeon, gynaecologist, X-ray man, neurologist. By the time she has completed a course of treatment she has tasted all the drugs in the pharmacopeia, wears plates on her feet, spectacles on her nose, has had her teeth tinkered with [extracted for "autointoxication," a supposed abscess "poisoning" the rest of the body], and her insides straightened.

The nervous housewife, in addition to her other symptoms, was also tired. Myerson told a joke:
One man meets another and says, "By the way, I heard that your wife was the champion athlete at college."
"Ah yes," says the husband. "Now she is too weak to wash the dishes."[47]
In 1934 Chicago obstetrician Joseph De Lee spoke of the "immense army of women suffering, if I may coin the phrase, subinvalidism and who say they have never felt well since their first baby was born."[48] He assigned their fatigue to obstetrical damage.

Horace Richardson, who divided his time between a psychiatric practice in Manhattan and a private clinic in Massachusetts, said in 1935 that, "in an analysis of a thousand cases of so-called neurasthenia, it will be found that the outstanding symptom in at least eighty percent of the cases is an overwhelming sense of fatigue." He described, essentially, "receptionists' syndrome":

A young woman of thirty odd years appealed to her doctor for the relief of a constant feeling of muscular weakness and fatigue, and for vague, indefinite sensory symptoms in various parts of her body. She was a stenographer in the office of a busy executive. One morning, following a particularly difficult day, she awoke with the feeling that she had not rested well during the night. Her fatigue worsened. "Finally she resigned from her position, spent most of her time in bed and sat up only occasionally."

Her family doctor was called in. There were no physical findings. The doctor settled (under the influence of the autointoxication theories popular in the 1920s and 1930s) for removing some of her teeth. "Within a month she was back in bed."

Further specialists were called in. There were more procedures: A nasal sinus was drained; her appendix was removed. She had four further abdominal operations within four years. "The sense of fatigue never disappeared; the patient was now confined entirely to her room, and for the greater part of time had special diets and required constant attention."

A rest cure and colonic irrigation proved also in vain.

"At last she was sent to a psychiatrist, boasting of the number of physicians she had seen, talking about the various operations she had undergone and mentioning the strange malady that no one had been able to cure." The psychiatrist, evidently Richardson himself, soon got to what he considered the bottom of the case: problems with her fiancé and the sudden appearance in the office of her female supervisor, who had been wearing an engagement ring.[49] In the nineteenth century such a psychic shock might have produced convulsions or a hysterical paralysis. In Manhattan in the 1930s it produced profound fatigue.

By the 1940s, weakness and fatigue were seen commonly in primary care. Frank Allan, an internist at the Lahey Clinic in Boston, said in 1944: "One of the problems most frequently encountered by the general practitioner and the internist is a complaint variously described as weakness, exhaustion, fatigue, loss of ambition, low vitality or weak spells." Of three hundred cases they had investigated intensively, only 20 percent were caused by a physical disorder, such as a chronic infection, diabetes, anemia, or heart disease. The other 80 percent were "nervous." Of those 239 cases, 18 percent occurred in connection with frank "psychoneuroses," 3 percent were owing to depression, and 79 percent were the result of "benign nervous states," such as nervous exhaustion and nervous fatigue.[50]

As for gender differences, by the 1950s women presented at the doctor's office more often than men with symptoms of fatigue. In a survey of the symptoms of 113,000 patients seen in 106 general practices in 1955–56 in England and Wales, 92 percent more women than men complained of "debility and undue fatigue."[51] Of course not all these patients had chronic fatigue, much less the colorful, unshakable attributions of illness that characterize fatigue today (chronic Epstein-Barr virus infection and myalgic encephalomyelitis). Yet the tiredness of these women patients points to a distinctive gender component in the change of paradigms.[52]

Thus one answer to the question What had become of hysteria? is that the patients had become tired, choosing symptoms on the sensory side of the nervous system that were more difficult to disprove medically.

Psychogenic Pain

It is more difficult to write the history of pain than of chronic fatigue because of the problem in differentiating organic from psychogenic pain, and because pain is a transhistorical, ubiquitous element of the human experience. Clearly the kind of pain caused by lesions has its own history, for how individuals respond to pain is culturally determined to some extent. As Ivan Illich writes: "Culture makes pain tolerable by interpreting its necessity; only pain perceived as curable is intolerable."[53] For example, some cultures accepted the pain of childbirth as tolerable simply because there was no alternative. By contrast, Western civilization in the first half of the twentieth century viewed the pain of childbirth as intolerable, and often obliterated its perception with a general anesthetic.[54]

In the case of psychogenic pain, the culture is responsible for its origin in the first place. For cultural reasons, pain is selected from the symptom pool. Yet how people experience pain, how they describe it to others, and whether they seek help for it are very complex matters, varying in ways that may not be immediately apparent from historical documents and commanding the historian to caution. However it does seem that psychogenic pain, under the tutelage of the central-nervous paradigm, increased in frequency as a symptom presented to medical doctors in the last quarter of the nineteenth century and the first quarter of the twentieth. This increase may well have been the consequence of the growing legitimacy of sensory symptoms, a result of the success of the central-nervous paradigm.

That such an entity as psychogenic pain exists, pain arising from the action of the mind rather than from a peripheral lesion, there can be no doubt. Paul Joire, a psychologically minded family doctor, encountered a case in 1892 in Lille. The story began with the patient's sister. The sister had genuine gallbladder disease, evidently stones in a bile duct, which gave her agonizing, spasmodic pain:

> On August 14 [the sister], who for the last few days had been subject to repeated attacks of hepatic colic on the right side, was hit by a new episode of unprecedented ferocity. The attack lasted seven hours with atrocious pain in the right upper quadrant and on all the right side; there was a painful epigastric point, a point of pain at the scapula, and radiation of the pain to the shoulder and the arm [all characteristic of biliary colic].

The sister writhed in her bed, grasping occasionally at her right side, "as if to tear out the pain, in a characteristic gesture of this violent crisis, a gesture unforgettable for the family." Several days later a large stone was found in her stool, confirming the diagnosis.

The patient's brother, a young man of twenty-three, had been present at much of his sister's agony. Doctor Joire thought him somewhat nervous and hysterical in any event, as the brother demonstrated areas of a Charcot-style hemianesthesia and occasional muscle twitching in the upper limbs. When vexed, he might also take on a nervous tremor that would last for several hours.

> This young man had been powerfully affected by his sister's crisis and in the following days felt ill, complaining of vague pains and of great weakness.
>
> Exactly eight days after having witnessed his sister's crisis, he himself was taken with a similar crisis. At the beginning he too complained of pains in the right side. And he indicated the hepatic region as the seat of those pains, but it was established on palpation that the liver was not at all sensitive. His acts and his complaints were absolutely identical to those of his sister: he emitted the same cries, he grasped at his right side with the same clasping fingers, as if to tear out what was hurting him. After a certain time, this same pain seemed to radiate towards the epigastric region, the chest and the lower abdomen. He writhed upon the bed eight days later in exactly the same manner as his sister. The scene could not be more perfectly imitated, and one might indeed have believed in a true hepatic colic, had the end of the attack not furnished evidence of a quite different origin.

The young man namely went into a Charcot-style attack of *grande hys-térie*.[55] For this patient the pain was probably real enough, but it was demonstrably psychogenic in origin.

Patients occasionally achieved insight into the psychological nature of their pain. In 1879 Weir Mitchell in Philadelphia received in his private clinic a woman of nineteen from a western state. She was brought in on a stretcher unable to walk, in constant pain, her eyes bandaged against the sunlight. She turned out to be a nervous case, and Mitchell cured her with the usual therapies. After returning home, she wrote him a letter.

Her headaches, she said, had begun in 1878 after some "mental and social strain. I had for two years before that time suffered from a weak back, had felt constantly tired, spent much of my time on the bed, and taken but little exercise." Then came the turn for the worse, she did less and less, staying in bed increasingly until her family sent her to the famous Doctor Mitchell. "I cannot now understand why. . . . I could not realize that the less I did the less I could do; but I was blind, and so was every one else. I thought it was some strange, mysterious disease that was taking away my strength. By summer, a few minutes' conversation or the walk of a block would make the pain in my head agonizing, and every sound become unendurable."

So bad did the pain become that she lay, she said,

in one position with closed eyes for eight weeks before going to Doctor Mitchell in a state of supposed helplessness. One thing I want to say in extenuation of myself, and that is that the pain was real, not fancied. Whatever its cause or however easily it might have been averted, it was genuine suffering at the time. . . .

In looking back over that year with the light of the present, I can only say that I believe there was nothing really the matter with me, only it seemed as if there was.[56]

What cannot be overemphasized in discussing the history of psychogenic pain is that it is not simulation. For patients, the pain is real. Many unsympathetic doctors have appeared in these pages, but sympathetic physicians since time out of mind have appreciated the reality of sensation for the patient. In 1889 Armand Hückel, on the staff of the university medical clinic in Tübingen, said: "The itching that someone can get who falls asleep in the woods and suddenly notices ants in his vicinity, can be quite painful for him, even though there is not a single insect on his body. For that person such sensations exist as reality, as though they were received from the periphery, and are perceived as reality in exactly the same manner as the psychotic patient perceives a hallucination."[57]

Medical awareness of hysterical pain as part of the central-nervous paradigm increased greatly during the nineteenth century. However, doctors' increasing sensitivity to hysterical pain does not constitute proof that the phenomenon itself increased in frequency. Yet in the typical interaction between a medical paradigm and the presentation of symptoms, medical acceptance of such pain (under the assumption that it was a functional nervous condition) gave patients "permission" to present it. As early as 1833, English psychiatrist John Conolly said: "Pains of variable severity, often very severe, are among the distresses of the hysterical." He described, among others, "*clavus hystericus,* the sensation of a nail driven into the forehead," and hysterical abdominal pain mimicking peritonitis, "which is most felt on slight pressure, and is often evinced on the gentlest touch, which is not commonly seen in instances of internal inflammation."[58] Hector Landouzy said in 1846:

One of the invariant characteristics of hysterical pain is its prodigious intensity, in the absence of local findings capable of explaining the violence of the distress. One gets a sense of this in the shrieks that the patients emit when the affected part is touched in the slightest. I remember two hysterics who, in hopes of disencumbering themselves of pain, asked in the one case for a knee amputation, in the other for an amputation of the thigh . . . ; she also wanted the resection of the sciatic nerve and the extraction of the head of the femur.

Landouzy had consulted in the cases of two other patients, aged twenty-three and thirty-five, whose breasts, despite the absence of any local findings, had been in danger of amputation by the Paris surgeons.[59]

The whole generation of London consultants of the 1860s and 1870s who were responsible for destroying the reflex paradigm also accepted the possibility of hysterical pain. In 1867 Frederic Skey and Dennis Hovell both provided descriptions of such pain. Skey said of hysteria in the form of local pain: "The most common seats are the female breast; the side of the trunk under the ribs" and seven other sites, including all the muscles, the joints and the entire spine.[60] Russell Reynolds maintained in 1872:

Hysteric patients constantly complain of "pain," more or less spontaneous in its development. Such pain, wherever it may be situated, usually requires several strong adjectives for its description, and the account given of it is sometimes tediously minute. I have heard one hysteric lady enumerate and detail nine different kinds of pain in her chest! Of these some were bearable, some "intolerable," others "agonizing"; and four or five of them usually appeared together, and were present at the moment of description,—and yet the face was calm, and simply conveyed the expression of interest in the description.[61]

Here Reynolds was describing what the Salpêtrière school later referred to as *"la belle indifférence,"* the patient's apparently unaffected composure while reciting bloodcurdling complaints.[62]

The psychoanalytic tradition has established its own conventions for diagnosing pain of psychological origin. In 1895 Sigmund Freud said, apropos the case of Fräulein Elisabeth von R.:

I was struck by the indefiniteness of all the descriptions of the character of her pains given me by the patient, who was nevertheless a highly intelligent person. A patient suffering from organic pains will . . . describe them definitely and calmly. He will say, for instance, that they are shooting pains, that they occur at certain intervals, that they extend from this place to that, and that they seem to him to be brought on by one thing or another. Again, when a neurasthenic describes his pains, he gives an impression of being engaged on a difficult intellectual task to which his strength is quite unequal. His features are strained and distorted as though under the influence of a distressing affect. His voice grows more shrill and he struggles to find a means of expression. . . . He is clearly of opinion that language is too poor to find words for his sensations and that those sensations are something unique and previously unknown, of which it would be quite impossible to give an exhaustive description. For this reason he never tires of constantly adding fresh details, and when he is obliged to break off he is sure to be left with the conviction that he has not succeeded in making himself understood by the physician.[63]

In the Vienna of the 1880s and early 90s, Freud had obviously seen a number of patients with psychogenic pain.

By the turn of the century the psychological paradigm had become a major competitor of the central-nervous paradigm, and pain of psychological origin had become a familiar concept to physicians. Charles Stimson of Eaton Rapids, Michigan, who had graduated from the University of Michigan in medicine in 1891 and was very up-to-date, told the members of the Montcalm County (Michigan) Medical Society in 1908 about "psycho-therapy," "psycho-neurosis," and pain which was "psychological in origin." "The pain in itself is none the less real on this account," he said.[64]

Walter Alvarez of the Mayo Clinic was one of the key figures in American internal medicine in the first half of the twentieth century. He began practice in Mexico as a rural doctor in 1906, then trained after 1910 in internal medicine in San Francisco. Over the years Alvarez had acquired great experience with psychogenic pain, and a not inconsiderable number of antifemale and anti-Semitic prejudices, by the time he discoursed on pain for his fellow physicians in 1943:

> I learned early in my career that pain can be of psychic origin by noting that in the case of a young woman with a mild cyclic insanity and pathologic and prostrating fatigue, the successive removal by optimistic surgeons of the appendix, right uterine adnexa, right half of the colon, and the gallbladder did not affect the pain in the right side of the abdomen.

How could one tell if the pain was psychogenic?

> Real pain, especially severe pain, points to the presence of organic rather than of functional disease. On the other hand a burning, or a quivering, or a picking, pricking, pulling, pumping, crawling, boiling, gurgling, thumping, throbbing, gassy or itching sensation, or a constant ache or soreness strongly suggests a neurosis. In my experience intra-abdominal quivering is always a sign of nervousness, and epigastric "burning," especially in the Jew, points almost as certainly to a neurosis.[65]

In 1904 Otto Binswanger, professor of psychiatry at the University of Jena (and member of the Binswanger psychiatric dynasty whose clinic was in Kreuzlingen, Switzerland), coined the term *psychogenic pain*.[66] This created a face-saving alternative to the stigmatizing adjective hysterical. A whole medical lore about dealing with such patients began to be elaborated, its guiding principle that of the psychological paradigm in general: Reassure the patient that you take his or her pain seriously. "There is no such thing as unreal pain," Victor Johnston, a Canadian country doctor, soothingly titled a chapter of his autobiography. Some of his patients, for example, still imagined that they could feel a fishbone in their throats after he removed it:

> How could I explain what was happening to them? I learned I must never use the words *imagine* or *imagination*. I must never tell them they imagined there was a fishbone in their throat; it would be insulting. Nor could I tell a patient with a headache or pain that he imagined it. *There is no such thing as an unreal pain or headache.* Patients are

nearly always correct about their symptoms, but may be very wrong as to the cause. . . . The alternative to using the word *imagination* is to tel! the patient that he is hypersensitive to pain, has a low threshold to pain, or that his subconscious mind is playing tricks on him. Most people will accept the last explanation and this was my favorite.[67]

Alfred Schofield on Harley Street addressed his colleagues more scathingly: "Let us remember that a disease of the imagination is not an imaginary disease. . . . To tell neurasthenics or hysterics that there is nothing the matter with them . . . is to confess oneself unfit to deal with functional nerve-diseases."[68] It is clear that in the real world of medical practice, the concept of psychogenic pain became firmly established in the first half of the twentieth century.

Does this increase in medical references to psychogenic pain mean that the incidence of such pain itself had increased? Or merely that, as pain acquired the reputation of being treatable, its frequency in the doctor's office rose? These are difficult questions, but an approach to answering them may lie in noting late-nineteenth-century medical opinion. A number of physicians became convinced that pain was the commonest hysterical symptom, as opposed to earlier doctors who knew fits as the mark of hysteria. In 1863 Graily Hewitt, who had a large gynecological and obstetrical practice in London, told the medical students of St. Mary's Hospital that, "The most distressing symptoms presented by hysterical patients, and for which relief is most urgently sought, are flatulence, headache, and pain in the side." He clearly thought these symptoms more salient in a middle-class, urban population than "hysterical convulsions," to which he came later in his lecture.[69] Mary Jacobi said in 1888 of her practice in New York: "Of all hysterical disorders, pain is the most frequent, the most distressing, and often the most perplexing, either for diagnosis or treatment."[70] Semi Meyer, sanatorium physician in Danzig, said in 1909 of his hysteria patients:

> Pain is the most usual symptom. Because hysteria seeks to reproduce a clinical picture of disease that will be more or less convincing, it quite naturally seizes upon pain. . . . Hysterical pain is exactly as real as an anesthesia or any other hysterical symptom, merely we cannot see it in the same manner as hysterical vomiting or paralysis. The patients do not imagine their paralyses, vomiting or anesthesias. Why therefore should they be imagining their pain. One can imagine that one's head is empty or that one's brain does not function anymore, but that one's head aches awfully: no one can imagine that.[71]

291

A fair amount of such testimony suggests that the urban middle classes represented the leading edge in seizing pain for the patients' new
paradigm.

With time, the fashionability of such a symptom would have trickled
down. There is some evidence that during the interwar years pain became the commonest presenting form of psychosomatic illness. In an
interesting juxtaposition of old- and new-style symptoms, many of the
working-class patients on the "nerve" ward of an insurance-company
hospital in Breslau were as late as 1925 still having fits and similar motor
attacks. Yet pain pervaded the unit. "Virtually every patient has the occasional headache," said director Felix Preissner, a disbeliever in organicity. "Migraine attacks are more often diagnosed than actually occur,
mostly on the basis of subjective complaints."[72] In 1925 fits were on their
way out and pain was on its way in. Such wards were therefore a sort of
crossroads for changing paradigms.

Further attempts to dig into the history of psychogenic pain smash
against the problem of headache. There is a scale of headaches, from
migraine, generally agreed on as organic, to conversion, generally believed to be psychological responses to stress.[73] Within this great range
it is difficult to disentangle the psychogenic from the somatogenic today,
let alone in past times, when the patients are dead and doctors cannot
assess them with technical aids that nineteenth-century headache specialists did not have at their disposal (not that such techniques definitively
separate the psychosomatic from the organic). With headache, unlike paralysis or chronic fatigue, it is impossible to decide whether given historical episodes are caused by stress and unhappiness, by physiological
changes in the brain, or whether (like irritable bowel syndrome) they represent an interaction of both. Neither the history of the illness nor the
response to treatment is conclusive, given the ease with which migraine
comes and goes. The tentative speculation remains that psychogenic head
pain, linked in tandem to chronic fatigue, may well have become more
common as the patients' paradigm of what constituted "true" illness
changed in sync with the doctors'.

Psychogenic pain, like chronic fatigue, seems to have afflicted women
more frequently than men in the first half of the twentieth century. In
the 1955–56 survey of the symptoms of English patients mentioned earlier, women's rates for "neuralgia and neuritis" (sciatica, trigeminal neuralgia, and brachical neuritis omitted) were 91 percent higher than men's;
for "pain in limb" 35 percent higher; and for "pain in back" 83 percent
higher.[74] Again, many somatogenic sources of pain may have been mixed
in (although such obvious somatic causes as infection, tumor, rheuma-

tism, and the like were reported elsewhere). But the core of these residual "pain" categories was undoubtedly psychogenic.

The pattern of symptoms in hysteria was in full transformation by the end of the nineteenth century. As Henri Schaeffer, a Paris physician and specialist in psychotherapy who had trained at Dejerine's Salpêtrière, said in 1929:

> The neuroses [les accidents névropathiques] never disappear. . . . Old as the world, they will vanish only with humanity itself. Hysteria is much the same: really just a manner of speaking. It symptoms have changed in form, although somewhat less than generally imagined, because the times and the culture have changed. The patients we see nowadays no longer present the stigmata of the old-style hysteria because they have not had the same conditioning [éducation]. What matters is to try and observe the new forms and determine their causes.[75]

What caused this paradigm shift among patients? Three different levels of explanation must be involved: First came improvements in medical ability to diagnose disease. The Babinski test of the upgoing toe must have canceled much motor hysteria. After 1900, not wanting to have their symptoms proved unreal, many patients who might formerly have selected paralyses, chose symptoms much more difficult to "disprove," such as headache and fatigue. Who, after all, could prove that someone was not tired or in pain?

Second, medical paradigms as such play a role in "shaping" symptoms. In the nineteenth century, patients presented those symptoms that reflex theory defined as evidence of "real" disease, such as paralysis, or that Charcot's grande hystérie predicted, such as fits in four stages, or that catalepsy called for, such as going stiff as a board. In the twentieth century those symptoms that the central-nervous paradigm called for or that the psychogenic paradigm was unable to rule out as invalid were brought to the doctor. After the revolution in molecular biology of the post-1960 era, those symptoms called for by immunology, such as "chronic immune dysfunction," would come to the fore.

Third, familial expectations of social roles help to shape the nature of symptoms. In the nineteenth century, when women were "weak," they produced fainting fits and paralyses. After the 1920s, when women became "strong," such evidence of physical incompetence started to seem anachronistic. My mind returns to a photograph of a young woman in Berlin in the 1920s: she is smoking and sitting astride a motorcycle.[76] It is a portrait of the new woman. Such a woman may have had headaches and, occasionally dismounted her motorcycle, weary, to rest. But she did not develop a hysterical paralysis.

In invoking the family, we are reminded that hysterical symptoms arise within a wider social context as well as within a medical dialogue between doctor and patient. Of the many dimensions of existence that formed that wider context, the family in particular was crucial, for symptoms often served as a means of communicating with others in intimate life. The family of the nineteenth century was hallmarked by a distinctive kind of intimacy, or "smother-love" if one will.[77] This intense intimacy neither characterized previous centuries, nor would it survive the generation of the flappers and the 1920s young women astride motorcycles. It is possible that hysterical paralysis, like anorexia nervosa, represented an emotional response to this overpowering, all-controlling familial intimacy. One did not walk, just as one did not eat, as a pathological, panic-stricken response to being fixed in the searing searchlight of parental attentiveness. If this analysis is correct, the weakening—though by no means the abandonment—of this system of intimacy early in the twentieth century would also permit the dismantling of the panicky symptoms to which this style of family life had originally given rise, namely paralysis.

11

Somatization at the End of the Twentieth Century

The psychosomatic symptoms of the 1990s are not very different from those of the 1920s. Now as then, pain and fatigue continue to be the commonest physical complaints. But there are two significant differences between the psychosomatic patients of the 1990s and those of the 1920s. Sufferers today are more sensitive generally to the signals their bodies give off, and they are more ready to assign these symptoms to a given "attribution"—a fixed diagnosis of organic disease. Many patients today have acquired the unshakable belief that their symptoms represent a particular disease, a belief that remains unjarred by further medical consultation.

This increase in illness attribution stems, at the level of the doctor-patient relationship, from the loss of medical authority and from the corresponding increase in the power of the media to suggest individuals into various fixed beliefs. At the cultural level, these new patterns come from a distinctively "postmodern" disaffiliation from family life. If the psychosomatic problems of the nineteenth century resulted from an excess of intimacy in the familial psychodrama, those of the late twentieth century have been the result of the opposite phenomenon: a splintering of close personal ties and the lack of intimacy. These changes of the late twentieth century have had the effect of making people more sensitive to bodily signals than ever before and more willing to shift the attribution of their plight from internal demons to external toxins.

A New Sensitivity to Pain

Our culture witnesses a kind of collective hypervigilance about the body, a sensitivity to variations in weight, for example, that has sufficed to make many fortunes in the industry devoted to dieting and slimming, or a bowel consciousness that keeps pharmacy shelves stocked high with medically unnecessary laxatives. This kind of extreme alertness to the body's normal functions is itself without historical precedent. But even more striking is a willingness to amplify bodily signals so that they become evidence of disease and justify seeking help or taking medication.

People today believe themselves to be highly symptomatic. After reviewing various studies, one scholar writes: "Only 5 to 14 percent of the general population do not experience symptoms in a given two-week period. The average adult has four symptoms of illness on one out of every four days." She concludes: "There are probably many people with vague symptoms in search of a diagnosis."[1]

Some of these symptoms are psychogenic; some come from organic disease. People today are more sensitive to both. Various household-interview surveys of a random sample of the American population asked how many episodes of "illness" respondents had had over the previous months. Whereas those polled in 1928–31 reported 82 episodes of illness from all causes per 100 population, those polled in 1981 had 212 illnesses per 100. This represented an increase of 158 percent, despite the enormous improvements in health care, antibiotic therapy, and nutrition over the preceding fifty years. If one interprets being sick as seeking care for an illness, the average person in our society today is "sick" more than twice a year, as opposed to less than once a year on average in the 1920s.[2] On the basis of surveys from the 1950s through the 1970s, Arthur Barsky, a psychiatrist at Harvard University, concludes: "The total numbers of days of restricted activity and days in bed for acute and chronic illness have risen sharply, and the proportion of people who report a permanent total disability has increased."[3] Clearly, there are more people who interpret internal sensations as illness today than ever before.

It is true that individuals in the eighteenth century experienced the full range of somatic woes as well. What has changed is that much more of this illness is now channeled to the doctor's office, as people redefine themselves as patients. They are, for example, more willing to bring headaches to the doctor. Among 3,062 patients seen in a private neurological practice in Pittsburgh before World War I, only 26 had headaches (0.8 percent of the total).[4] By contrast, a survey of the practices of 3,630 neurologists in the United States in the period 1976–78 showed that 6 percent of all "practice encounters" concerned headache and migraine.[5] In the clientele of a busy neurologist in the late 1980s—a man on the staff of a major tertiary-care hospital whose practice I observed for some months—around one-third of all patients complained headache.

People have probably become more sensitive to headache as well, whether the complaint is brought to the doctor or not, for headache today is ubiquitous. Of a sample of Britons in 1969, 38 percent complained of headaches.[6] In a telephone interview in the late 1980s of 10,200 residents aged 12 to 29 of Washington County, Maryland, 57 percent of the men and 77 percent of the women had had a headache within the previous four weeks.[7] Such figures illustrate how much a part of daily life headaches have become.

In the context of psychosomatic illness as a whole, there is no doubt that pain is the number-one complaint today. Among two hundred "undiagnosed" patients (meaning those without evident organic disease) seen in 1976 in general practice in Hampshire, England:

- 16 percent had abdominal pain
- 10 percent had sore throats
- 8 percent had pain in a limb
- 6 percent had headaches
- 5 percent had backaches

The only significant nonpain complaints among these patients were 14 percent with a cough and 4 percent with dizziness.[8]

In the chronic-care setting of a veterans' hospital in Minnesota, of the forty male patients reporting symptoms that were diagnosed as psychogenic, 58 percent had nonheadache pain or painlike strange sensations (hyperesthesias), 32 percent reported headache, and 25 percent had "heart attacks" and chest pain. In this population of veterans there were quite a few motor problems as well (42 percent with slight paralysis). Yet pain was clearly the commonest complaint.[9] After reviewing a number of studies of primary care, Wayne Katon and collaborators conclude: "The most common form of somatization in American society is the chronic pain syndrome."[10] Pain dominates primary care, where the patients have a mixture of psychogenic and somatogenic illness, and psychiatric care, where it often turns up as chronic neurosis ("somatization disorder" and the like).[11]

Chronic facial pain has taken on a salience unknown fifty years ago. This is not the acute pain of a toothache but rather a sensation often described as "a deep, dull severe ache which is unbearable at times." It flows easily into the feeling that one's mouth is burning up, and often is called "burning-mouth syndrome." This sort of persistent nonorganic pain in the face and mouth was quite unfamiliar to the Parkes Webers

297

and Hermann Oppenheims of the turn of the century. Perhaps it was merely owing to the increase in visits to the dentist after World War I that many patients began complaining of unendurable facial pain following minor dental procedures (also following trauma). After the 1950s these reports appeared in considerable number. Stanley Lesse, a New York neurologist, described eighteen such patients whom he had seen between 1951 and 1956. One patient, a single woman of thirty-seven, was obsessed with the idea that "her teeth were all dying." She finally found a dentist willing to pull them out. Another patient, a separated woman of forty-eight, had seen "no fewer than twenty-four different dentists over a two-year period" and had had every tooth ground down and recapped. All eighteen patients were obsessed with their pain, and went from dentist to dentist, or doctor to doctor, pitting one against the other.[12] An English dental surgeon described in 1969 a series of a hundred patients with "ill-defined facial pain for which no obvious organic cause could be found." About half of them, many women in their early forties, were finally decided to be somatizers ("atypical facial pain").[13]

Pain in the face and mouth is mentioned frequently in any setting where chronic pain is treated. In the 1980s in a psychosomatic medicine clinic, Mrs. A, a thirty-eight-year-old housewife whose father was a dentist, had suffered pain of spontaneous onset in her right jaw for the previous five years. The pain, so severe that she had been out of work for two years, had arisen just after her divorce, but a remarriage had not assuaged it. Mrs. A had had numerous unsuccessful procedures for the pain, and indeed it had become worse since the last surgery a year previously. A "tense, angry lady who wants a medical solution" to her problems, Mrs. A was not helped by a six-week stay at the clinic.

The problems of Mrs. B, forty-two, began six months previously, when a dental operation led to an abscess. Although the abscess was drained, she developed chronic pain in her upper-front gum, and now complained of "burning mouth." Three months before admission the severity of the pain caused her to resign from her middle-class job. After a two-month stay in the clinic the pain, though still present, was "a thousand percent better." Over a two-year period involving many admissions, there were five such patients with "burning mouth" and "atypical facial pain," a not-uncommon condition of late-twentieth-century life.[14]

A skilled tradesman came to the clinic, entirely well until six years ago. "I was a Rock of Gibraltar," he said. Then, out of the blue, began sudden feelings of fatigue and dizziness. The following year groin pain set in, spreading over the next twelve months down his entire left leg and into his left abdomen. Thereafter he experienced multiple hospitalizations for his pain, signing himself most recently out of a psychiatric hospital, furious that the doctors had not been able to find anything wrong. Currently he has pain in urinating, in defecating, a burning at the pit of his stomach, and pain in his perineum and left leg. The pain has made him impotent. His preoccupation with his symptoms has resulted in a marital separation. His children are angry at him because of his illness. Aside from his various appointments with physicians, he is socially isolated.

He wrote the clinic staff a note:

To whom it may concern:
I, ____, have extreme, uncontrolled, severe extkruchting [all
spelling unchanged], unbearable, shaking, radiating, cutting pains.
24 hrs. day, 7 days a week, progressively getting more severe and
intense and spreading in my abdomon, left and right, stomach,
hips, buttocks, lower back, kidney, groin, testicles, bones, muscles.
In legs, ankles feet and arms. Chest pains.
Symptoms. Sharp jarring pains when urinating in lower abdomin,
testicles, groin, lower extremities. Pain full powl movements,
diarrea, feeling nausseated, head pressed.
Facts. Diverticulitis, spastic colon, severe back problems, kidney
problems, stone, prostitis, mono! Nephritis.
The truth. I have being used and abused, misdiagnosed, drugged by
the medical field.

The case, which could be reproduced many times in any setting in which chronic pain is treated, represents forward- and backward-looking themes in the history of psychogenic pain. A familiar, or backward-looking, theme is the casting of symptoms in the form of pain, which could have been seized from the 1920s. Mistrust of physicians, however, is a relatively new theme, for until the 1960s near veneration of the doctor was the rule, the demigod in white whose patients would willingly sacrifice their ovaries to suit his theories. For this male patient in the 1980s there was no question of venerating doctors. He mistrusted them deeply. He had in fact "shopped" from doctor to doctor, never happy with the diagnosis he received from any. As an inpatient in the clinic he continued to express himself in the most disgruntled terms about the medical staff and what could be expected of them. Mistrust of the doctor and refusal to accept his or her reassurance gives somatization at the end of the twentieth century its particular stamp.

299

Fatigue

In addition to psychogenic pain, fatigue is the other great somatoform symptom of the end of the twentieth century. For many reasons one might expect people leading frenetic, compartmentalized lives in crowded cities to feel tired. But we are talking about fatigue as an illness rather than simply feeling tired at the end of the day. Many individuals who are chronically fatigued believe something is physically wrong with them and end up having more than just a symptom. From their physician or from some other source, they acquire the diagnosis of chronic fatigue syndrome. Accordingly, fatigue is both a symptom and a syndrome, or pattern of illness.

The symptom of fatigue is omnipresent. Two researchers, wishing to determine how common the symptoms often associated with drug reactions were in a healthy population taking no drugs, did a symptom survey of 385 members of the medical and hospital staff of Temple University in Philadelphia during the 1960s. They used another 285 persons in a nonmedical setting as a control group. Of those workers surveyed in the hospital setting, 41 percent complained of feeling fatigued within the last seventy-two hours. Was it just the stress of hospital work? No, 37 percent of those in the nonhospital setting were also fatigued. About one in seven of the hospital workers and of the community control group had headaches too, so again, the stress of the medical setting in and of itself caused neither the fatigue nor the headaches.[15] In a random survey of the U.S. population in 1974–75, 14 percent of the men and 20 percent of the women said they suffered from fatigue.[16]

Findings from Britain also show high levels of fatigue. In the mid-1970s, 23 percent of the thirteen hundred people registered with one medical practice in Glasgow said they felt "more tired than usual or generally run-down," a complaint second in frequency after runny noses.[17] In another survey of 7,400 adults at the end of the 1980s in a random sample of the population of England, Wales, and Scotland, 20 percent of the men and 31 percent of the women said they were "always tired."[18] Finally, a survey during the early 1980s of civil servants in their mid-twenties in the Home Office—presumably a healthy group in general—found that 37 percent of the women and 29 percent of the men were "fatigued."[19] It was not that they thought themselves ill with fatigue, merely that subjectively they were weary.

In the early 1960s Michael Shepherd and coworkers asked a number of general practitioners in the London area to survey patients who were consulting for nonpsychiatric reasons on the following points. Seventeen hundred patients were interviewed:

"Do you often get spells of complete exhaustion or fatigue?" Eleven percent of the men and 18 percent of the women said yes.

"Does working tire you out completely?" Men 11 percent; women 16 percent.

"Do you usually get up tired and exhausted in the morning?" Men 13 percent; women 21 percent.[20]

After a review of this and other literature, two researchers conclude: "There is no doubt that between 20 to 40 percent of people in the community . . . have significant fatigue lasting more than a few weeks."[21]

In medical practice today, fatigue is not common as a principal diagnosis, yet physicians often encounter it in primary care.[22] Researchers interviewed twelve hundred consecutive patients at an army hospital in San Antonio, Texas, seeing active-duty military plus dependents and retired soldiers. Twenty-eight percent of the women and 19 percent of the men said that fatigue was a "major problem." Of these twelve-hundred, 102 were selected for intensive investigation. Eighty-three percent of them were tired every day. Half were tired on awakening. Three-quarters had been tired for more than a year. Virtually none of the 102 had any biochemical abnormality.[23] Customarily a physical cause is discovered in a quarter to a third of patients complaining of fatigue.[24] Yet in the other two-thirds, the cause of the fatigue is likely to be psychogenic, a result of depression, perhaps, or life's stress.

Although tiredness is common in the doctor's office, it may not be so much more frequent than in the 1920s, when perhaps a fifth of all patients had come to the doctor because of "loss of pep."[25] What matters is not really whether small increases have occurred in the percentage of patients who perceive their fatigue as a medical problem, but that both in the 1920s and the 1990s patients, whatever difficulties they experience in life, unconsciously choose fatigue as an expression of their distress.

Fixed Illness Belief

Setting our own time off clearly from previous epochs is "fixed illness attribution": the readiness of a large number of people to cling tenaciously to a given diagnosis, refusing to abandon their belief despite medical reassurance to the contrary.

Let us contrast a patient with multiple bodily symptoms from 1900 and one from today. In 1904, at the age of fifty-two, Franz K. was admitted to the provincial Austrian asylum of Kierling-Gugging near Vienna. His first physical complaints had begun a year previously, and now he was showing signs of psychotic depression. A letter carrier in Vienna, he had earned extra income by playing in beer bands, in his words, "over-exerting himself, not getting proper rest." He had first started to experience a "pulling" sensation in his armpits and back. His hands seemed to go to sleep at work. He started having the feeling,

> as though hot water was climbing along his spine to his head and then shooting into his chest and through his arms, where it races back and forth in a flickering kind of fire [*zuckendes Feuer*], finally shooting into his middle finger and causing soreness. He says also there are knots in his arms and the rest of his body, for which he receives relief from massage and from sulfur baths. He has had therapeutic success with a laxative tea, which has given him some relief and even lets him blow his trumpet.[26]

Franz K., though highly symptomatic and filled with therapeutic beliefs about healing teas and the like, clung to no particular disease attribution. "Around Christmas [1903] he read a lot of medical textbooks and imagined that he has tuberculosis and tabes [*Rückenmarksleiden*, a euphemism for the tabetic form of neurosyphilis]. But he did not persistently believe in these diagnoses.

One contrasts Franz K. with Mrs. C., a patient from the psychosomatic medicine clinic of today. A woman of thirty-odd years with a history of marital and emotional tumult, she has been highly symptomatic for about six months. She has seventeen "chief complaints," which the admitting physician records:

1. Anorexia with a weight loss from 135 lbs. to 118 lbs.
2. Sweating, "rivers of sweat run down my pits"
3. Muscle spasms in her right leg, armpit and ribcage which increase when she walks
4. Shakes of her body and she spontaneously notes that she is not a drug taker or drinker
5. Waves of sickness which come over her and are accompanied by light-headedness, nausea, dizziness and high fever
6. Waves of energy and heat which radiate throughout her and are unpleasant
7. Problems with shaking inside her spinal column and in her eye sockets which produces a buzzing, shaking quality and produces "violent after images" when she closes her eyes

8. Stomach constantly upset, "it's cooking all the time"
9. Abnormal bowel movements fluctuating between "diarrhea, small little lumps, sawdust and only 1 or 2 normal stools"
10. Worry about her tongue which she thinks is coated with white yuck and has a lesion on the left side which she feels is cancerous
11. Unquenchable thirst
12. Skin on fire
13. Bruising easily, "I have little bruises all over my body," "Sometimes it looks like there has been an explosion of blood vessels under the skin but I know nothing has burst"
14. A pulsing sensation in her head like blood is trying to get through, which is accompanied by her ears ringing, a vice-like grip sensation around her head and a "weird pain" on top of her head
15. The experience of her intestines rising up in her abdomen and feeling like a "banana"
16. Abnormal sensory experiences such as colors jumping out of paintings at her and brown rice vibrating on a plate
17. Her period is now regular and she is upset about this as in the past it was always irregular

She attributes these symptoms to a number of diseases. At first she thought she had AIDS, and had this preoccupation for almost two years since reporting a marital infidelity to her husband. She also believed she had anal herpes following an earlier sexual encounter with a lesbian. More recently, she had a sexual encounter with a male who had "red dots" all over his body and who acknowledged to her that he had "a shaking sensation in his spinal cord and behind his eyes and that he feels as though a snake is moving about in his abdomen." Following this, she acuired the belief that she has rabies. Her physician noted: "She thinks that it is possible to have rabies for an extended period of time and that medical science just doesn't know this. As well, she has considered the possibility that she has Lassa fever or wonders if she might have acquired Swine flu after eating a small piece of pepperoni on a pizza several months ago."

Her husband informed clinic doctors that for three years she had been preoccupied with the fear that she had multiple sclerosis. More recently she has had "early Epstein-Barr-virus titres done. No early antigen was detected." (Many patients in the late 1980s attributed their symptoms to a possible infection with Epstein-Barr virus. Titres refers to a test for substances in the blood.)

If Franz K. was a typical patient of his time, symptomatic but essentially willing to accept the analysis of his physicians that he was depressed, Mrs. C. was a patient for our own time. She scored heavily on all three attributes of today's hypochondria: (1) amplification of bodily symptoms, so that innocuous movements of gas became "bananas" rising up inside her; (2) disease phobias, instructing her physicians to test her for Epstein-Barr virus; (3) the fixed, quasi-delusional conviction that she had a given disease, at one time multiple sclerosis, at another, rabies. Negative blood tests did not reassure her, and she believed that her physicians were quacks because they did not accept the possibility of hidden rabies.

Although the amplification of normal bodily symptoms and phobias about disease have existed in all times and places, it is really the third characteristic of hypochondriasis, this delusional clinging to the belief in a given illness, that marks the last decades of the twentieth century. At the university psychiatric clinic in Zurich, the percentage of patients afflicted with "hypochondriacal delusions" rose fourfold between World War I and the 1970s.[27] These patients with a major mental illness might well represent a sounding board for the receptivity of the culture as a whole to such quasi-delusional beliefs.

One can differentiate between two forms of fixed illness belief: the diagnoses that simmer in the background and those that spread epidemically. Among the constant but subdued illness themes in the background today are yeast infection, food allergies, temporomandibular joint (TMJ) syndrome (facial pain imputed to the joint which is the hinge of the jawbone), and "twentieth-century disease," also known as total allergy syndrome. Food allergies and TMJ disfunction of course exist, but most individuals who believe that they have these problems do not have them. Instead they belong to a kind of subculture of illness that spawns patient support groups, claques of sympathetic (and very pricey) physicians, and periodic media concern. This subculture embraces a broad range of more-or-less endemic fixed-illness beliefs.

Yet none of these beliefs has managed to achieve the notoriety of chronic fatigue, each lacking some of the preconditions required for an epidemic of illness attribution. In the 1990s it is above all chronic fatigue syndrome—consisting of a combination of severe fatigue, weakness, malaise and such mental changes as decreased memory—that has won out over its competitors, just as reflex hysteria triumphed over spinal irritation in the nineteenth century.

The saga of chronic fatigue syndrome represents a kind of cautionary tale for those doctors who lose sight of the scientific underpinning of medicine, and for those patients who lose their good sense in the media-spawned "disease-of-the-month" clamor that poisons the doctor-patient relationship. As a precondition, we have a pool of nonspecific symptoms in search of a diagnosis. These symptoms include, in the experience of Donna Stewart, a psychiatrist who has dealt extensively with fixed-diagnosis somatizers, "transient fatigue, headaches, muscle or joint aches, backaches, digestive upsets, respiratory complaints, vague pains, irritability, dizziness, poor concentration, and malaise." It is chronic somatizers, Stewart continues, who are "especially prone to elaborate on non-specific symptoms, and tend to embrace each newly described disease of fashion as the answer to long-standing, multiple, undiagnosed complaints."[28]

How does a given symptom become a disease of fashion? An epidemic of illness attribution, or epidemic hysteria, seems to involve two phases: (1) appropriating a genuine organic disease—whose cause is difficult to detect and substantiate—as a template; (2) broadcasting this template to individuals with often quite different symptoms, who then embrace this template as the explanation of their problems. This broadcasting is effected by sympathetic physicians, patient support groups, and the media.

A prototype for such epidemic spread, offering all of the characteristics of the above model save one, was brucellosis in the 1930s and after. Brucellosis, also known as undulant, or Mediterranean, fever, is a genuine bacterial infection spread from animals to humans, and constitutes an occupational-disease risk for farmers, meat-packers, and veterinarians. It is characterized by all the signs of an acute bacterial or viral infection: high fever, aches and pains, chills, malaise, and so forth. There are suggestive blood findings, and indeed the organism is often found in the blood, providing unmistakable physical evidence of infection. The notion of chronic brucellosis was first proposed in 1903 and became a prototype for the attribution of psychosomatic illness to "real" bacterial disease.[29] By "chronic brucellosis" was understood symptoms of fatigue, malaise, pain, and depression that persisted long after the causative organism itself had left the blood. Such symptoms cry out for attribution to a "real" organic disease because sufferers find them so bewildering and intolerable. And it is quite possible that many patients with chronic brucellosis were in fact suffering delayed sequelae of a previous acute infection, so that brucellosis offered a genuine organic template. But other victims of chronic brucellosis who once previously had experienced the real disease may well have been somatizers.

Chronic brucellosis accordingly illustrates a major dilemma. We have no way of knowing whether the persistence of symptoms was owed (a) to occult infection, (b) to a psychiatric illness such as depression (whose physical symptoms are similar to those of chronic brucellosis), or (c) to somatization in the absence of any other psychiatric pathology. As for this last possibility, some of the chronic brucellosis patients were undoubtedly somatizers who had fixed on this particular label. In this array of possibilities, many physicians in the 1930s might, in fact, have made an incorrect choice, labeling someone such as Alice Evans, a distinguished senior microbiologist at the United States Public Health Service, neurasthenic. Exposed to the disease throughout much of her professional life, she had every right to believe in the organicity of her own symptoms. (She believed, however, in the organicity of everyone else's as well, and thought that neurasthenia was simply misdiagnosed chronic brucellosis.)[30]

The point is that chronic brucellosis became available as a disease attribution for those who may never have been infected yet nonetheless had the symptoms, namely muscular aches and pains, fatigue, irritability, and depression. In this first phase of an epidemic, brucellosis had created an organic template onto which somatizing patients could project their symptoms. The diagnosis served as a ready-made attribution that individuals experiencing various nonspecific sensations could grasp.

Yet few seemed to have grasped it. Chronic brucellosis never spread as a chic diagnosis, perhaps because of its association with rural life, perhaps because medical authority in the 1930s and 1940s had not yet experienced the decline it later was to undergo. In 1959 several distinguished physicians pooh-poohed the diagnosis of chronic brucellosis in a major internal medicine journal. Although they did it in subdued tones, speaking of "psychologic factors [that] may be of importance in the pathogenesis of the illness," the message was clear: Medicine does not believe in your disease label.[31] In the 1960s chronic brucellosis disappeared as a disease attribution among somatizing patients. Although the conditions necessary for phase one of an epidemic of illness attribution had been met, those required for phase two were lacking. Instead the somatizing public encountered dubious media, unsympathetic doctors, and an absence of patients' rights groups and support groups, not only for chronic brucellosis but for any disease entity. Yet chronic brucellosis did serve as a prototype for linking nonspecific distress to a given organism, whether the organism was responsible for the symptoms or not.

Chronic fatigue syndrome is without a doubt the illness attribution that has dominated the last two decades of the twentieth century. One researcher estimated in 1990 that "at least one million Americans [are] currently carrying a diagnosis of CFIDS [chronic fatigue immune dysfunction syndrome], and possibly another five million are ill and yet to be diagnosed."[32] By 1990, some four hundred local support groups for the illness had arisen in the United States, and the Centers for Disease Control of the U.S. Government, in Atlanta, were receiving a thousand to two thousand calls a month about chronic fatigue syndrome.[33] Many similar stories of wildfirelike spread elsewhere could be told.

A whole subculture of chronic fatigue has arisen in which those patients too tired to walk give each other hints about how to handle a wheelchair and exchange notes about how to secure disability payments from the government or from insurance companies.[34] The whirl of activities within this subculture sounds so diverting that one can understand why the members would be reluctant to part with their symptoms. Among various local associations for chronic fatigue in England, for example, we encounter the following notices: "Berks and Bucks. On 21st May [1988] there will be a stall for M.E. [myalgic encephalomyelitis, the English version of chronic fatigue] at the Young Farmer's RALLY at the Child-Beale Wildlife Trust near Pangbourne. Please do look out for anything yellow that you can spare," wrote the local organizer, "and either post it to me or let me know so that I can arrange for its collection (Stall themes are colours)."

"Gloucestershire. Seventeen members, together with partners and friends, attended a coffee morning at Lapley Farm, Coaley on March 5th. This was an excellent turnout for such a large and scattered county. . . . Next: Family Ploughmans Lunch, also at Lapley Farm, on Saturday, June 4th. We are hoping to arrange a meeting for the autumn in Cheltenham."[35] Chronic fatigue thus can become a way of life.

The Epidemic of Chronic Fatigue

What are the origins of this illness attribution, which has gripped the imagination of all Western society the way colitis once riveted the upper classes of nineteenth-century Paris? The epidemic started out as four separate organic diagnoses, some of them true diseases, others illnesses of a more psychosomatic nature. These various diagnoses then were appropriated by individuals with psychosomatic illness who wished to confer the imputed organicity of the diagnosis on their own condition. These organic diagnoses represented templates on which patients suffering from a wide variety of nonspecific symptoms could model their complaints as they brought them to the doctor.

In the United States, chronic fatigue syndrome began as neuromyasthenia, or muscle weakness caused by supposed central-nervous disorder. The story of it goes back to 1934, to a presumed epidemic of atypical poliomyelitis among 198 employees of the Los Angeles County General Hospital. A large epidemic of polio was then in progress in Los Angeles; indeed, many cases had been admitted to that hospital. And it seemed quite plausible that health workers, too, might somehow have acquired the virus, except that none of them died of it; none displayed the characteristic changes in samples of their cerebrospinal fluid, and few presented with the classical flaccid localized paralyses of polio. Sixty percent of the cases had no fever. Sensory disturbances were much more pronounced than motor (polio affects the motor cells of the spinal cord). In fact, if polio had not been abroad at the time, it would probably not have occurred to many observers to call the crushing fatigue and muscle pain observed among these health workers polio, for the patients had no other evident signs of the disease. The physician of the U.S. Public Health Service who investigated the epidemic and who took it for true-bill organic disease, noted: "Certain observers were of the privately expressed opinion that hysteria played a large role in this outbreak."[36] In retrospect it is impossible to establish what actually occurred at this hospital. The employees may well have suffered a bout of undiagnosed viral illness—aching limbs and numbing fatigue being recognized consequences of some viral infections. (But one must bear in mind that the average person suffers about four viral infections a year, so these are by no means automatic sequelae of viral illness.)

The point is that this epidemic, and others like it, became templates for the new disease entity, neuromyasthenia. Patients who themselves had not been in epidemics but were experiencing the symptoms of weariness and muscle pain would start to hold the belief that they, too, had acquired neuromyasthenia.

Patients are most content if the imputed cause of the illness is some external factor, rather than something in themselves. In 1957 two articles in the *New England Journal of Medicine* on epidemic neuromyasthenia implied the spread of an "infectious agent." One article discussed an outbreak of a "polio-like" illness among student nurses in 1953 in a private psychiatric hospital near Washington, D.C. The other epidemic had occurred in 1956 in Punta Gorda, Florida.[37] In 1959, a widely cited article appeared in the same journal looking back on twenty-three separate epidemics of neuromyasthenia. Here we encounter the same phenomenon as in chronic brucellosis: Patients in some of these epidemics were undoubtedly suffering from an undiagnosed viral illness, displaying in five of the twenty-three epidemics such "hard" neurological signs of disease as stiff necks (a possible indication of meningeal inflammation); double vision was present in fourteen, and nystagmus (involuntary eye movements) in six. Featured in virtually all of the twenty-three epidemics were such subjective sensations as fatigue, muscle pain and muscle weakness, headaches, and emotional instability. Pain, fatigue, and "protracted debility" clearly dominated the picture in the twenty-three epidemics as a whole. The authors of the article attributed these outbreaks to a distinctive disease, epidemic neuromyasthenia, caused by an unknown organic agent.[38] The article became widely cited as evidence that external agents were responsible for chronic fatigue and pain.

With the realization that many sufferers had not been in epidemics, the first of a series of tactical relabelings occurred. Instead of epidemic neuromyasthenia, this collection of symptoms became known in 1985 as postinfectious neuromyasthenia. External toxins were still clung to, but anyone who exhibited the symptoms could now qualify for the diagnosis.[39]

Meanwhile, a second kind of organic template for chronic fatigue was being fitted into place: a genuine organic disease once called infectious mononucleosis and later Epstein-Barr virus infection. The virus had been discovered in 1964 by Michael Epstein and Y. M. Barr, and in 1968 it was established that this virus caused mononucleosis. Hence a quite legitimate renaming took place of an infectious disease: EBV.[40]

Infectious mononucleosis had been known as a disease entity since at least 1889 ("Pfeiffer's disease"). Familiar as well was the great sense of lassitude caused by it, a lassitude that could be called chronic in some cases: of 206 patients investigated in 1948 by Raphael Isaacs, a hematologist at Chicago's Michael Reese Hospital, 53 had symptoms that persisted from three months to four years or longer. All in the group were demonstrably ill from an organic disease, exhibiting in their blood the particular white cells characteristic of mononucleosis. Their symptoms were aching legs, fatigue, and depression (and some organic findings, such as a slightly enlarged spleen).[41] Thus mono became a second template on which to fashion the illness chronic fatigue, as the symptoms of both bore a certain resemblance.

Yet infectious mononucleosis never really achieved phase two—diffusion to large numbers of somatizers in an epidemic of symptom attribution—because doctors looked for the characteristic misshaping of cells before granting mono as a diagnosis. It was really after the discovery in 1968 of Epstein-Barr virus as the cause of mononucleosis that EBV became a disease of fashion, because the vast majority of the population bears EBV antibodies in the blood. Disproof was impossible. Finally "evidence" was at hand that sufferers were "really ill": Their blood tests (and everybody else's) showed the antibodies. This particular proof seemed to be dramatically delivered in 1984, when an epidemic of still-inscrutable character occurred at Lake Tahoe. EBV antibodies were detected in blood samples of some of the victims, and the case for organicity seemed to be clinched.[42] In the mid-1980s EBV was warmly embraced as the explanation of one's difficulties, a series of learned medical articles strengthening the supposition of organicity.[43] EBV was christened in the press "the Yuppie flu," an infection to which fast-tracking professionals were thought especially vulnerable.

Unfortunately, the very ubiquity of Epstein-Barr virus caused its downfall as an illness attribution. In 1988 Gary Holmes at the Centers for Disease Control, along with coworkers, realized that the correlation was poor between those patients who had hematological evidence of chronic EBV infection and those who had the symptoms of chronic fatigue. Holmes therefore rebaptized chronic Epstein-Barr virus infection as chronic fatigue syndrome, or CFS.[44] This renaming did not sit well with patient groups, who promptly renamed their condition CFIDS, chronic fatigue immune dysfunction syndrome, to better insist on its organicity.[45]

These two templates therefore, neuromyasthenia and mononucleosis-EBV, provided the presumption of organicity for self-labeled sufferers of chronic fatigue in the United States and Canada. Donna Greenberg, professor of psychiatry at Harvard, wrote of these diagnoses: "Chronic mononucleosis and chronic fatigue syndrome represent neurasthenia in the 1980s. . . . It is in the nature of chronic fatigue that [the diagnosis] will inevitably recruit subjects with depressive disorders, anxiety, personality disorders, and other common medical syndromes such as allergic rhinitis or upper respiratory infections."[46] Exactly as appendicitis had given way to colitis, and reflex neurosis to neurasthenia, so in the United States chronic EBV gave way to CFIDS as somatization attempted to keep one jump ahead of science.

In Britain the template was quite a different one. In 1955 an epidemic of apparently infectious origin affected 292 members of the medical staff of several different branches of the Royal Free Hospital in London. Known in the movement as the "Royal Free epidemic," this outbreak of possibly viral illness featured muscle pain and great fatigue in virtually all patients, and in some individuals enlarged lymph nodes in the neck and elsewhere, abdominal tenderness on palpation, and in 10 percent of those affected, stiffness of the neck.[47] First called encephalomyelitis, this collection of symptoms was rechristened in 1956 benign myalgic encephalomyelitis. It was "benign" because nobody died and there were no pathological findings, "myalgic" because of muscle pain, and "encephalomyelitis" because the brain (encephalo-) and spinal cord (myelo-) were presumably inflamed.[48] The "benign" was then dropped because patients experienced nothing benign about their sensations, and the condition came to be called simply myalgic encephalomyelitis, or ME. The disease label alone was a triumph of the longing for organicity over science.

Then the same symptom drift observed after the Los Angeles County Hospital polio epidemic occurred. As the disease label ME became generalized to patients who had not been in epidemics, the symptoms thought to accompany the condition underwent a subtle change from the relatively "hard" neurological and physical findings present in the Royal Free patients to the "soft" subjective findings of pain, fatigue, and emotional instability exhibited by most other sufferers. Simon Wessely, a psychiatrist at the Institute of Psychiatry in London, writes of this shift:

Gradually the emphasis changed to a sporadic disease which was neither epidemic nor contagious, but still paretic. Finally, interest in the conventional neurological features waned, and attention shifted to the importance of fatigue as the central symptom. At the same time etiological theories have also altered. From an acute infectious disease with one agent, albeit unknown, concepts changed to a post-infective illness following the same agent, and finally following a variety of agents. It is difficult to write a review of such an elusive and changing condition.[49]

What is quite astonishing is that the same syndrome flourished on both sides of the Atlantic under several different names. In Britain it was known as a kind of encephalitis, a major and often fatal inflammation of the brain, and muscle pain was stressed as the presenting symptom. But in fact it was not encephalitis. In the United States it was called neuromyasthenia, EBV, and the like, postulating a viral cause and focusing on fatigue. But in fact pain and fatigue occurred simultaneously in almost all patients. It was only these national diagnostic traditions that made them sound like different diseases.

The fourth template was fibrositis, or fibromyalgia. Whereas the above-mentioned disease labels stemmed from internal medicine and neurology, fibrositis was the rheumatologists' phrase for the condition of patients who exhibited the same kind of fatigue and pain. Why such a proliferation of terms? Like the blind men, each of whom described the elephant according to the various parts they touched, it was the rheumatologists who focused upon the connective tissue and skin and, finding pain at various points, announced that their pattern of findings represented a distinct rheumatological disease.

Patients who report diffuse aches and pains have long been known in medicine. In 1838, for example, Charles Despine, the spa physician at Aix-les-Bains, described eight female patients who had, in addition to "catalepsy" and hysterical paraplegia, "local pain or *points hystériques,* varying in seat, form and position, depending on the case but occurring commonly at the front and top part of the head [*sinciput*] or the left side of the chest [*la pointe du coeur*].[50] Then in 1904 the great English neurologist William Gowers proposed the term *fibrositis* for these diffuse aches and pains.[51]

Fibrositis came as though heaven-sent to doctors as a diagnostic label for pain patients who displayed an important neurotic component in their illness. In 1918, for example, Frederick Parkes Weber, the Harley Street internist, wondered if a longstanding female patient of his, now sixty-one, might not have "fibrositis." She had a lengthy history of insomnia, a possible morphine addiction, and "nervous irritability."

July 2, 1916: "X has lately had troublesome lumbago-like symptoms."

December 28, 1917: "Troublesome abdominal pains," thought linked to a dropped kidney.

December 7, 1918: Parkes Weber raised the question of "so-called fi brositis," to which he believed a family tendency was present. In the same note he commented on her constant headaches.[52] Although Parkes Weber accepted the diagnosis as truly organic, it is interesting that he did not apply it to any of his male patients.

In the 1920s and after, a good deal of work was done on "muscular rheumatism" or nonarthritic rheumatism. Researchers were stymied by the fact that, although the patients were highly symptomatic, they displayed no clear-cut organic pathology.[53]

Then, in the 1970s, the diagnosis fibrositis, simultaneously with ME and EBV, experienced a renaissance. The scientific starting bell for this resurgence was an article in 1968 by Eugene Traut, an internist at the University of Illinois College of Medicine in Chicago, in an influential clinical journal, drawing together the pattern of insomnia, muscle pain, and fatigue into a distinctive clinical entity.[54] Rheumatologists now possessed a clear disease label when they encountered such patients, who exhibited all the distinctive characteristics of somatization in the twentieth century. Medical enthusiasts blossomed on both sides of the Atlantic, giving media interviews, encouraging the formation of patient support groups and all the other mechanisms necessary for the diffusion of a psychic epidemic.[55] From a grab-bag of scattered bodily pains, fibrositis (or fibromyalgia as some preferred to call it after muscle inflammation had failed to materialize) passed to being a specific disease: "The features are now well recognized," wrote one of its advocates in 1989, "the most important and common being generalized pains, fatigue, and disturbances of sleep." There might also be headaches and bowel problems. Four-fifths of the patients were women.[56]

Fibrositis accordingly became the fourth template for "chronic fatigue syndrome." The penny began to drop as it was realized that the abovementioned symptoms also characterized EBV, myalgic encephalomyelitis, and all the other diseases of fashion. This awareness dawned in both the camp of the medical skeptics and that of the patient advocates. Among the skeptics, Thomas Bohr, a neurologist then at the school of medicine at Stanford University, questioned the existence of the whole fibrositis syndrome: "There simply has never been good evidence for it as a syndrome distinct from affective disorders." He scoffed at enthusiasts' use of the "dolorimeter"—a spring-loaded device that applies given pressures to predetermined "tender points"—to confirm the diagnosis, "as if this quasi-scientific device supports the existence of anything other than plain old aches and pains. Any medical student knows that using a stethoscope does not take the subjectivity out of auscultation [listening with a stethoscope]." Bohr considered fibrositis to be a form of depression.[57] Simon Wessely thought fibromyalgia a form of chronic fatigue: "The distinction between fibromyalgia and CFS is largely arbitrary, and both overlap with affective disorder."[58] After studying a group of forty patients with the diagnosis of fibrositis, a group of Israeli researchers concluded that the condition was a well-delineated psychiatric ailment in which childhood deprivation caused depression in later adult life, depression presenting primarily as pain.[59] Although many rheumatologists continued to cling to the organicity of fibrositis,[60] mainstream medicine had started to shy away from it, just as English neurologists had once shunned Charcot's hysteria.

Remarkably, the sufferers' organizations as well—normally so resistant to psychiatric guidance—began accepting the suggestion that fibrositis and chronic fatigue were the same disease. Except that the patients and their counsellors considered both to be viral in origin, not psychiatric. "In most cases, fibromyalgia is probably ME," said Byron Hyde, one of the main medical boosters of ME, in a patients' newsletter.[61] At a "national conference for persons with fibromyalgia" in April 1990 in Ohio, the gist of the discussion was that the two conditions were identical.[62]

It is clear that chronic fatigue, the illness attribution that in the late twentieth century has experienced a more rapid growth than all its competitors, has had four distinct "organic" roots from which to draw its conviction of organicity: in the United States, epidemics of "polio-like" neuromyasthenia and Epstein-Barr virus; in the United Kingdom, similar epidemics of myalgic encephalomyelitis; and within the specialty of rheumatology a misguided vogue for fibrositis and fibromyalgia. What these four had in common with their ancestor, chronic brucellosis, was a presumption of organicity and of an external causal factor. What chronic brucellosis lacked, however, was media acceptance, for it was diffusion by the media that has given these disease labels such enormous popularity.

The Media and the Loss of Medical Authority

An avidly read popular press existed before World War II, yet the paradigms that patients accepted were basically those the doctors proposed: reflex theory and central-nervous theory. What is different about the end of the twentieth century is that the authority of the mass media has started to take precedence over what was once called medical authority. The dominant medical paradigms of our own time fall unheeded in the babble of media interviews of physician-enthusiasts and wrenching accounts of patients' suffering. At the end of the twentieth century the psychological paradigm remains the dominant medical explanation of somatoform symptoms, but this paradigm excites little interest among a press eager for sensation.

To what extent has medicine itself complied in this trouncing of the psychological paradigm? Since the 1960s a major resurgence of the central-nervous paradigm has in fact occurred in the form of biological psychiatry, an orientation that treats mental illness as disease of the brain. But this group of researchers has concentrated on such major disorders as schizophrenia and manic-depressive illness and has come up with little in regard to an organic-brain basis for somatization. The very real progress in biological psychiatry has left the psychological paradigm intact in the area of psychosomatic illness.

Patients' groups and physician-enthusiasts of CFS have seized with glee a trickle of inchoate immunological findings. Since the 1960s immunology has become the queen bee of the medical sciences, in the way that pathology was in the nineteenth century the foundation of all further knowledge. Advanced greatly by the techniques of molecular biology, immunology offers the brightest prospect of plumbing the secrets of such illnesses as AIDS, cancer, and multiple sclerosis. In the public eye the discipline, in other words, has become a symbol of all that is new and worthwhile. Quite naturally, psychosomatic patients who want their symptoms to keep abreast of scientific progress wish to see the underlying source of their problems as immunological in nature.

Yet the standard-bearers of immunology themselves have displayed little interest in the diseases of fashion. They are more interested in the major organic illnesses of our own time. In a curious inversion of the normal diffusion of scientific findings, the media advocates of CFS seize immunological data as they become available in the lab and apply them willy-nilly to their pet illnesses. "Not just the blues," trumpeted *Newsweek,* as a cover story of November 12, 1990, on chronic fatigue syndrome alerted readers to new findings about "a newly discovered herpes virus called HHV-6." Research on patients' "interleukin-2" levels had also proved promising, the story said.[63] Although individual sufferers may display disparate immunological abnormalities, no pattern of findings has emerged common to CFS patients as a whole. Nor is it clear how widespread these abnormalities are in the general public, nor to what extent they are shared by individuals with other psychiatric illnesses. Driving forward the pseudoscience underlying CFS has not been the medical profession itself—it has been the media.

In the United States, a widely read story in *Rolling Stone* magazine in 1987 gave the signal for converting chronic fatigue into a media frenzy. Entitled "Journey into Fear: The Growing Nightmare of Epstein-Barr Virus," the journalist-sufferer, once "in control of my career and my life," explained how an "enigmatic disease" had rendered her "unable to lift my toothbrush or remember my phone number." Of course her physicians had been unhelpful. "After rendering their diagnoses, my doctors made it clear they had served me to the limit of their ability. One of them, the internist, tried to comfort me: 'At least it isn't terminal.'" The writer cried a good deal and felt "a sadness akin to the raw grief of mourning." Then one day she read about the Lake Tahoe "epidemic" and realized what she had.

The writer located a physician-enthusiast. Because she carried with her copies of all her blood reports "rolled up and stuffed in my bag," she pulled them out for him to look at. Sure enough, she had the Lake Tahoe disease. He explained to her that her reports displayed the "reactivation phenomenon," a phenomenon unknown to his medical colleagues generally.

"I understand there are doctors who leave the room after speaking to one of these patients and can't stop laughing," he told her.

The message to *Rolling Stone* readers was that a terrible epidemic was ravaging the country and that a mainline physician was the last person one would want to put one's trust in.[64]

In England a milestone was a "factsheet on ME" offered by the *Observer* newspaper in 1986: Fourteen thousand readers applied for a copy.[65] It was after reading such a newspaper story that sufferer Peter Vaughan (who later became an information officer for the ME Association) acquired his disease conviction. After a bout of pneumonia, he had developed "foul-smelling urine . . . accompanied by bladder and testicular pain, which was often almost sickening. There was also deep seated retro-orbital [behind the eyeballs] pain associated with a feeling of grittiness in the eyes. . . . Spontaneous minor bruising and depression and moodiness often prevailed as did almost uncontrollable itching particularly at night."

It was on his return from vacation that his wife said, "I know what your illness is."

"Preposterous, too ridiculous for words," he thought.

"Read this," she said as she handed him an article entitled "Gaining Credence: The Disease That Isn't All in the Mind," which had appeared in the *Daily Telegraph* a few days previously.

"The symptoms were indeed identical and I felt sure that this was the illness which I was suffering from."[66]

A sympathetic story on fibromyalgia in the *New York Times,* featuring a chart of where the painful spots were supposed to be, provided a virtual roadmap for the unconscious.[67] Thousands of readers must have been suggested into coalescing their inchoate bodily symptoms into fibromyalgia as a result of this story.

Television has spread this plague of illness attribution even more rapidly than the print media. A "chronic fatigue" story on "TV Ontario," for example, prompted more than fifty-one thousand viewers to try to phone the station during the forty-minute segment.[68] A short spot on chronic fatigue on Channel 3 in Philadelphia produced seven hundred calls to the station—a record for that particular program—and a further two thousand inquiries to the CFIDS Association.[69]

On September 23 and 30, 1989, NBC aired a two-part show in the "Golden Girls" series, featuring Dorothy's struggle with chronic fatigue. Her first doctors, mainline physicians, had been beastly. As Dorothy is about to leave for an appointment with "her virologist," her friend Rose tells her: "Good luck, I hope he finds something wrong with you. . . . Oh, I don't mean something *wrong* wrong, I just mean something wrong so you'll know you're right when you know there's something wrong and you haven't been wrong all along." (This is the exact functional equivalent of nineteenth-century young women hoping to be admitted to hospital for ovariotomies.)

In the program Doctor Chang, the virologist, reassures Dorothy that "she really is sick and not merely depressed. . . . There are new diseases arising all the time," he says.

"So," Dorothy says with relief, "I really have something real."[70]

Dorothy's encounter with chronic fatigue demonstrates the oppositional stance to mainline medicine of this subculture of invalidism, a refusal to accept medical reassurance. The chronic fatigue sufferers of today are far more skeptical of medical authority than were victims of ovarian hysteria in the 1860s or brucellosis patients of the 1930s. In 1990 *Woman's Day* bannered "The Illness You Can't Sleep Off." "Can you imagine," asked the author, "how it feels to know there is something terribly wrong with you and have one doctor after another tell you there can't be?"[71] This theme of medical incompetence and indifference runs throughout the movement, which elevates the patients' subjective knowledge of their bodies to the same status as the doctors' objective knowledge. This presumption of privileged self-knowledge of one's body dovetails perfectly with media marketing strategies.

The rejection of psychiatric diagnoses by chronic fatigue patients is much more violent than are the normal reactions of medical patients to psychiatric consultation, and is itself a characteristic of the illness. Anything smacking of psychiatry or psychology is completely taboo. The chronic fatigue subculture evaluates internists, for example, not on the basis of the quality of their clinical judgment but their friendliness to the diagnosis. The work of Stephen Straus, a distinguished internist at the National Institutes of Health in Bethesda, was initially greeted by hosannas because in 1985 he seemed to take the EBV explanation at face value. Three years later, however, Straus became an object of vilification when he said that psychopathology might help to explain the symptoms as well.[72] "Expecting Stephen Straus to talk about CFS for very long without inevitably mentioning psychiatric disorders is like expecting Blaze Starr to walk without jiggling," wrote one disappointed sufferer.[73]

The chronic fatigue subculture brims with folklore about choosing physicians thought to be sympathetic. How does one pick a doctor? A patients' organization advised selecting one who would share test results and let the patient keep a copy—a bizarre request in the context of normal medical practice.[74] Chronic fatigue patients, reluctant to disclose emotional symptoms, are often quite resistant to psychological probing of any kind from the doctor.[75] Needless to say, psychiatrists are unwelcome in the subculture of chronic fatigue. The several psychiatrists who appeared at a chronic fatigue symposium in 1988 in London were called, by one physician-enthusiast, "colourful and frankly strange remnants of prehistoric medicine" and "as mad as hatters."[76] Behind this fear of psychiatry is the horror that one's symptoms will be seen as "imaginary," which characterizes most patients with fixed illness attributions. Thus

317

patients welcome the occasional blood abnormalities that turn up in their testing.[77]

Another characteristic of the subculture of invalidism is its "pathoplasticity," the willingness to change symptoms and attributions as new fads appear. Chronic fatigue sufferers are quite willing to believe that they also have other illnesses that are stylish at the moment. Monilia infections, sometimes called candida or total body yeast infections, enjoyed a certain currency during the 1980s. "Could Yeast Be Your Problem?" headlined one American chronic fatigue newsletter.[78] An English sufferer suggested an "anti-candida diet," including "half an avocado pear sprinkled with lemon juice."[79] A number of English patients expressed their concerns about yeast in letters to Doctor Dawes: "I put myself on an anti-candida diet, and persuaded my doctor to give me Nystatin [a fungicide]," wrote one patient. "He is gradually reducing the amount of Nystatin I am taking but he was reluctant to allow me to have Nystatin in the first place. I am not sure that he is the best judge of how much I should be taking." (Doctor Dawes responded: "A number of people need to take it for a year or two.")[80]

Other patients believe they have chronic fatigue and multiple food allergies ("causing immediate sensations in my stomach and legs").[81] Pyramiding the syndromes one atop the other, one person wrote to a physician-enthusiast, "I have CFS and was recently told I have Candida and given a special diet that excluded food items to which Candida sufferers are allergic. I was about to start when I saw you on TV and now wonder, what happens if I am also allergic to foods on the Candida diet."[82]

Still other patients believe that they have chronic fatigue and hypoglycemia ("It took me two years to find a doctor who understood.")[83] Or that they have TMJ syndrome, polio, and Lyme disease. One sufferer believed she was being poisoned by the mercury fillings in her teeth. She failed, however, to get better after having all the fillings removed.[84] Indeed, the only current disease chronic fatigue patients are sure they do *not* have is highly stigmatized AIDS. The occasional suggestion that whatever organism ails them is similar to the one producing AIDS is greeted with dismay.[85]

One study has demonstrated how closely the diseases of fashion are interwoven with one another. Fifty patients with "environmental hypersensitivity," a disease attribution closely related to chronic fatigue, were asked what else they thought they had. Ninety percent were found to be "suffering from at least one other media-popularized condition," including EBV, food allergy, candidiasis hypersensitivity, and fibrositis. More than 10 percent of the patients reported eight or more diseases of fashion. In 1985, when the study began, all patients attributed their problems to environmental sensitivity, but by 1986 many had shifted to *Candida albicans* as the main cause, and by 1987 EBV had become particularly popular. Most of the patients were on disability; none expected to return to his or her former job (88 percent were women). The author concluded: "These patients are suggestible and at high risk for acquiring diagnoses that are popularized by the media."[86]

Such hypersuggestibility is conceivable only in a population that has quite lost its moorings in the folk culture of body knowledge. In the United States there was once a common set of assumptions, or folk culture, about health and illness that was handed down from generation to generation. These assumptions gave people a commonsensical understanding of their own sensations. Instead, individuals today are buffeted by every new "finding" on television or in the morning paper. Accompanying this loss of contact with a folkloric inheritance and its tranquil interpretation of bodily symptoms, has been a loss of willingness to believe in "what the doctor says." For example, the percentage of patients in the United States willing to use the family doctor as a source of "local health care information" declined from 46 percent in 1984 to 21 percent in 1989.[87] As for selecting which hospital to attend, more than 50 percent of patients polled in 1989 said that "they or their family have the most influence in selection of a hospital"—as opposed to listening to the doctor—up from 40 percent in previous years.[88] (Non-American readers will recall that private American hospitals compete for patients.) According to a Gallup poll in 1989, 26 percent of patients said they respected doctors less now than ten years ago (14 percent said more). And of those who respected doctors less, 26 percent said, "they [the doctors] are in it for the money." Seventeen percent claimed that doctors "lack rapport and concern."[89]

The late twentieth century is writing a new chapter in the history of psychosomatic illness: fixed belief in a given diagnosis. The diagnosis itself may be changeable, based on fashion, but the fixity of belief remains the same, a questing after certainty resulting from the rising influence of the media upon public opinion and the corresponding decline of medical authority.

Given that some cultural shaping of symptoms always occurs, are patients better off if physicians do the shaping, or if the media carries out the task? These are the only two real alternatives, for men and women are social animals, loathe to be thrown back on the resources of their own wild imaginations. There are costs to either approach. When medical authority prevails and doctors shape symptoms under the influence of various "paradigms," patients risk having their ovaries needlessly removed or their spines cauterized. When the media takes on the job, patients are whipped about by the disease-of-the-month syndrome, because the desire of the press for novelty is relentless. But there must be some cultural interpretation of what we hear from our bodies. We must somehow draw upon the cultural symptom pool for models of illness to help us amplify and make sense of our own dim physical perceptions. Otherwise the mind cannot understand what the body is saying.

Somatization and Postmodern Life

Loss of medical authority is not the only factor behind the distinctive patterns of somatization in our own time. In family and social life in particular, the postmodern period has increased people's vulnerability to fixed ideas about illness. The same kinds of cultural changes that patterned psychosomatic illness in the nineteenth century have washed upon the late twentieth century as well.

Although the term *postmodern* has been bandied about in a nonspecific way, it does have a specific meaning in the area of family life: the triumph of the desire for individual self-actualization over commitment to the family as an institution.[90] This kind of larger commitment, not a commitment to specific individuals but to the ideal of "family," characterized the modern family of the nineteenth- and early-twentieth century. In the postmodern family, the notion of "relationship" has taken priority over the concept of the family as a building block of society. Indeed since the 1960s the relationship has often supplanted the concept of marriage itself. Sexual relationships involving periods of living together are becoming the antechamber to marriage.[91] Adulterous relationships often exist on the side for both partners, and after divorce the partners are spun once again into the world of relationships. So the notion of "relationship" has deeply pervaded the institution of marriage.

The intrinsic logic of the relationship lies in achieving self-actualization, or personal growth, instead of pursuing communitarian objectives. It is this search for individual psychological fulfillment for the individual partners that gives the postmodern family its remarkable fragility, for once personal growth ceases within marriage, the marriage itself terminates. Thomas Glick, a senior demographer at Arizona State University, wrote in 1987: "The relatively fragile state of American family life at present is undeniable in view of the prospect that close to one-half of the first and second marriages of young adults will end in divorce."[92] Accordingly, instability is becoming the rule rather than the exception.

The keynote of postmodern life is the solitude and sense of precariousness arising from ruptures in intimate relationships. As the average age at marriage rises, the number of young people living alone increases. Divorce further accelerates singlehood. And the social isolation of the elderly has greatly increased. The proportion of one- and two-person households rose in the United States from 20 percent in 1900 to 54 in 1980. And even over the short term, changes have been considerable: households consisting of a single woman rose from 8 percent of the total in 1960 to 14 percent in 1983; those with a single man climbed from 5 to 9 percent. Most of this growth in aloneness occurred in the younger age groups.[93] The growth in singleness reflects an unintended result of the logic of postmodernity: that individuals seeking to maximize their self-actualization in relationships find themselves spending much time alone between relationships.

The increase in solitude has been especially dramatic with respect to the elderly. The custom of older people co-residing with their married children has virtually vanished. According to one study, around 1900 only one old person in four lived alone or with a spouse. Almost 60 percent lived with one of their children. Another 13 percent lived with relatives or friends. In 1975 by contrast, more than eight out of ten old people lived alone or with their spouse; only 12 percent lived with a child, and only 4 percent with kin.[94] The postmodern imperative of maximizing individual privacy in order to enlarge the space available for intimacy has thus been especially brutal for the elderly. Previously sheltered by an institutionally oriented modern family, they find themselves cast outside the perimeter of the postmodern relationship. But the logic of solitude and loneliness embedded in the core of postmodern life affects all age groups.

What are the consequences of postmodernity for psychosomatic illness? People who are socially isolated tend to have higher rates of somatization in general than those who are not. One scholar concluded, after a review of the literature on health and loneliness, that "loneliness is linked with reported feelings of ill health, somatic distress, and visits to physicians as well as physical disease."[95] A comparative study for the period 1975 to 1978 of 109 frequent attenders (with 86 controls) in a medical practice in Whitehaven, England, showed that 12 percent of the male frequent attenders were divorced (vs. virtually none of the male controls). Of the frequent female attenders, not so much divorce as widowhood loomed as a risk factor: 13 percent of the female frequent attenders were widows (vs. 7 percent of the controls). The frequent attenders were found high in neuroticism and to have histories of poor health.[96] In a study of 94 patients with "intrapersonal problems" in a general practice in Hamilton, Ontario, 60 percent turned out to be widowed, separated or divorced (vs. 46 percent of the controls). Patients with interpersonal problems "were found to have a significantly greater number of . . . hospital admissions, major surgical procedures, number of visits to the practice [and] gastrointestinal disorders . . . when compared to controls." They had a far greater rate of in-patient psychiatric admissions.[97] Lonely elderly people tend to become strongly symptomatic. After a review of the literature, one scholar concluded, "Both lonely [elderly] males and females complained of multiple psychosomatic illnesses. . . . Negative self-assessments of health, fatigue, physician visits, and medication consumption were also more prevalent among the lonely rather than non-lonely subjects."[98] A substantial body of evidence shows, in other words, that a willingness to define internal states as "disease" accompanies the splintering of social relationships that has marked postmodern life.

What is the mechanism? By removing "feedback loops," social isolation intensifies the tendency of individuals to give themselves fixed self-diagnoses. The advantage of living closely with others is that one can test one's ideas. I'm feeling poorly today. Do I have chronic fatigue syndrome? No, it's because you slept poorly last night. This is the kind of feedback that occurs routinely in living together with others. We profit from the collective wisdom about health and illness of our co-residents. These feedback loops cease to function when one lives alone, and function imperfectly in living solely with one other individual, for one is either cut off from the collective wisdom entirely or has substantially reduced access to it.

The unmarried, divorced, and widowed tend to be easy prey for chic media-spawned diseases because they have few "significant others" with whom they may discuss interpretations of their own internal states. Of fifty patients with chronic fatigue syndrome seen at Toronto Hospital, "most were unmarried women and at least 4 had been divorced." Their average age was thirty-three, and fully 50 percent had had a major depression before the onset of the fatigue.[99] Of eight patients in one study who were "allergic to everything," four were married, two divorced and two single.[100] As for "twentieth-century disease," psychiatrist Donna Stewart describes a population of young, middle-class female sufferers whose personal lives were in chaos. Of her original eighteen patients reported in 1985, seven were married, eight single, and three divorced.[101] Lacking feedback loops, such individuals have only the media against which to test readings of their internal sensations, and the media purvey the most alarmist view possible.

In the nineteenth century the "restricted" Victorian woman gave us an image of the motor hysteria common among women. In the late twentieth century somatization has become the lot of both sexes. Both men and women have been victims of the shattering of the family, and both experience the kinds of pain and fatigue distinctive to our century. It is the lonely and disaffiliated who give us the image of our own times, who are the latter-day equivalent of the hysterical nineteenth-century woman in her hoop skirts and fainting fits. The difference is that, whereas the nineteenth-century woman was virtually smothered by the stifling intimacy of family life, the disaffiliated of the late twentieth century expire in its absence.

The development of psychosomatic symptoms can be a response to too much intimacy or too little. And if our forebears of the "modern" family suffered the former problem, it is we of the postmodern era who endure the latter. The disaffiliated, having lost their faith in scientific medicine and unable to interpret body symptoms in social isolation, seek out alternative forms of cure. The therapies are largely placebos, if not directly harmful to the body as in the case of colonic irrigation—a revival of the outdated practice of curing reflex neurosis by "getting those poisons out of there." This alternative subculture represents a population that has lost its faith in medical reassurance, that in the absence of folkloric family wisdom seeks its knowledge of the body from the media, and that has taken the full blow of the "relationship" stresses of postmodern life. It is a generation that did not invent psychosomatic illness, but finds itself singularly vulnerable to pain and fatigue that have no physical cause.

Notes

ABBREVIATIONS USED IN NOTES

AJO	American Journal of Obstetrics
AJP	American Journal of Psychiatry
BJP	British Journal of Psychiatry
BKW	Berliner Klinische Wochenschrift
BMJ	British Medical Journal
BMSJ	Boston Medical and Surgical Journal
DMW	Deutsche Medizinische Wochenschrift
JAMA	Journal of the American Medical Association
JNMD	Journal of Nervous and Mental Disease
LMG	London Medical Gazette
MMW	Münchener Medizinische Wochenschrift
MTG	Medical Times and Gazette
NCB	Neurologisches Centralblatt
NEJM	New England Journal of Medicine
PNW	Psychiatrisch-Neurologische Wochenschrift
Prog. méd.	Progrès médical
WKW	Wiener Klinische Wochenschrift
WMP	Wiener Medizinische Presse
WMW	Wiener Medizinische Wochenschrift
ZBG	Zentralblatt für Gynäkologie

CHAPTER 1
Doctors and Patients at the Outset

1. See Ari Kiev, *Transcultural Psychiatry* (New York: Free Press, 1972), pp. 66–70. Some authors consider this an "anxiety state," yet the patients are symptomatic in that they believe they can feel the penis beginning to retreat.

2. Robert Musil, *Der Mann ohne Eigenschaften* (1930); reprint, Reinbek bei Hamburg: Rowohlt, 1978), vol. 1, p. 22.

3. In using *somatization* as a more up-to-date synonym for *psychosomatic*, I follow Z. J. Lipowski, "Somatization: The Concept and Its Clinical Application," *AJP*, 145 (1988), pp. 1358–1368.

4. For biblical examples see Julius Preuss, *Biblisch-talmudische Medizin: Beiträge zur Geschichte der Heilkunde und der Kultur überhaupt* (1911; reprint, New York: Ktav, 1971), pp. 341–355; examples, pp. 346–348; for an English translation and commentaries, see Fred Rosner, "Neurology in the Bible and Talmud," *Israel Journal of Medical Sciences*, 11 (1975), pp. 385–397.

5. E. M. Thornton argues that these fits had nothing psychogenic, or "hysteric," about them and constituted undiagnosed instances of temporal-lobe epilepsy (what now would be called complex partial seizures). *Hypnotism, Hysteria and Epilepsy: An Historical Synthesis* (London: Heinemann Medical Books, 1976). Yet a prominent component of "acting out" in many of these fits, such as trying to bite bystanders, makes a psychological origin more likely than a neurological.

6. Gregory Smith, ed., *The Spectator*, vol. 2 (London: Dent Everyman's Library; reprint, 1945), pp. 142–143.

7. Vanessa S. Doe, ed., *The Diary of James Clegg of Chapel en le Frith, 1708–1755*, 3 vols. (Matlock: Derbyshire Record Society, 1978–81), vol. I, p. 93.

8. Peter Templeman, ed., *Select Cases and Consultations in Physick by the late eminent John Woodward* (London, 1757), pp. 2–6.

9. Ibid., pp. 58–62.

10. John Purcell, *A Treatise of Vapours, or Hysterick Fits*, 2nd ed. (London, 1707; 1st ed., 1702), pp. 1, 7–8.

11. Robert Peirce (also Pierce), *The History and Memoirs of the Bath* (London, 1713), pp. 109–110.

12. C.-M. Rebord, *Gerbe de notes et documents* (Annecy, 1922), pp. 205–320, chronicles the various cures introduced in evidence at the hearings that began in 1656. Of the paralyses, thirteen affected men, twenty-one women. These paralyses represent a minuscule proportion of the great number of miracle cures from fevers and the like. Examples cited from pp. 199–200 and 223. See also *Pouvoir de Saint François de Sales ou miracles et guérisons opérés par le Saint Évêque . . .*, 2nd. ed. (Bourg, 1911). In a study of miraculous cures in eleventh- and twelfth-century France, Pierre-André Sigal found that a third of all cures concerned pseudoneurological symptoms, and

that 18 percent of these affected the lower limbs. Thus the "paralyzed" leg has long been in the symptom pool of Western society. *L'Homme et le miracle dans la France médiévale (XIe–XIIe siècle)* (Paris: Editions du Cerf, 1985), pp. 239–242. See also Ronald C. Finucane, *Miracles and Pilgrims: Popular Beliefs in Medieval England* (London: Dent, 1977), pp. 144–145, on miracles reported in England in the twelfth and thirteenth centuries. Among the lower classes, "cripples" were the commonest type of miraculous cure.

13. Quoted in Gerhard Schormann, *Hexenprozesse in Deutschland* (Göttingen: Vandenhoeck & Ruprecht, 1981), pp. 16–17. See also Armin Steyerthal, "Die Stigmata Diaboli," *PNW,* 13 (March 30, 1912), pp. 520–536.

14. Pierce, *Memoirs Bath,* pp. 12–14.

15. G. L. W. Hohnstock, *Über Hysterie und Hypochondrie und deren Heilart* (Sondershausen, 1816), pp. 26–27.

16. Evidence for this assertion is the success of psychotherapy in cases of irritable bowel syndrome, which this example constitutes. See Paul R. Latimer, *Gastrointestinal Disorders: A Behavioral Medicine Approach* (New York: Springer, 1983), pp. 113–135.

17. See Fraser N. Watts, "Attributional Aspects of Medicine," in Charles Antaki and Chris Brewin, eds., *Attributions and Psychological Change* (London: Academic Press, 1982), pp. 135–155, especially p. 141 on the "three main components" of hypochondriasis.

18. Modern medical thinking on this subject goes back to the professor of medicine in Halle, Johann Christian Reil (1759–1813). For an overview, see Jean Starobinski, "A Short History of Bodily Sensation," *Psychological Medicine,* 20 (1990), pp. 23–33, especially pp. 24–25 on Reil.

19. See, for example, Michael MacDonald, *Mystical Bedlam: Madness, Anxiety and Healing in Seventeenth-Century England* (Cambridge, England: Cambridge University Press, 1981), pp. 208–217. On medical adherence to this belief, see Oskar Diethelm, "The Medical Teaching of Demonology in the 17th and 18th Centuries," *Journal of the History of the Behavioral Sciences,* 6 (1970), pp. 3–15. For a bibliography of eighteenth-century writings linking witchcraft and demonic possession to fits and the like, see Glafira Abricossoff, *L'Hystérie aux XVIIe et XVIIIe siècles (étude historique)* (Paris: méd. diss., 1897), pp. 140–142.

20. The seven were (1) Dudley Ryder, in William Matthews, ed., *The Diary of Dudley Ryder, 1715–1716* (London, 1939), both years studied; (2) Mary Wollstonecraft, in Ralph M. Wardle, ed., *The Collected Letters of Mary Wollstonecraft* (Ithaca, N.Y.: Cornell University Press, 1979), years 1779–1797 studied; (3) Bridget Byng (née Forrest), whose illnesses were recorded in the diary of her husband John Byng, in C. Bruyn Andrews, ed., *The Torrington Diaries, Containing the Tours Through England and Wales of the Hon. John Byng (later Fifth Viscount Torrington) Between the Years 1781 and 1794,* 4 vols. (London, 1934), years 1781–1794 studied; (4) James Woodforde, in John Beresford, ed., *The Diary of a Country Parson; The Reverend James*

Woodforde, 5 vols. (London, 1924–31), years 1766–1792 studied; (5) Thomas Gray, in Paget Toynbee and Leonard Whibley, eds., with corrections and additions by H. W. Starr, *The Correspondence of Thomas Gray,* 3 vols. (Oxford, 1935; reprint, 1971), years 1742–1771 studied; (6) Elizabeth Smithson (née Percy), Duchess of Northumberland, in James Grieg, ed., *The Diaries of a Duchess. Extracts from the Diaries of the First Duchess of Northumberland (1716–1776)* (London, 1926), years 1760–1774 studied; and (7) Fanny Burney, in Joyce Hemlow, ed., *The Journals and Letters of Fanny Burney (Madame D'Arblay),* 12 vols. (Oxford: Clarendon Press, 1972), 1794 only studied. I am grateful to Jeffrey Coatsworth, who conducted the analysis of data. On the background of medical practice in this period, see Dorothy Porter and Roy Porter, *Patient's Progress: Doctors and Doctoring in Eighteenth-Century England* (Cambridge, England: Polity Press, 1989).

21. Her birthdate is unknown. Her husband was born in 1742.
22. Chart 1895/35 in the Austrian state asylum at Kierling-Gugging outside Vienna. Josef P. died of his disease on September 5, 1895.
23. It is beside the point that Dr. Andree thought he was dealing with an organic illness, a disorder of menstruation. John Andree, *Cases of the Epilepsy, Hysteric Fits, and St. Vitus Dance . . .* (London, 1746), pp. 170–174. Many of the patients described by Dr. Charles Perry in a similar work could have been suffering from any acute disease imaginable: Some of them turned "yellow as saffron," others died. See Perry's *A Mechanical Account and Explication of the Hysteric Passion* (London, 1755), for example, p. 191. For an instance of death from hysteria, see William Rowley, *A Treatise on Female, Nervous, Hysterical, Hypochondriacal, Bilious, Convulsive Diseases . . .* (London, 1788). The author, who in the course of more than thirty years of medical practice had performed many autopsies, said, "In nervous hysteric cases, I have found, more or less, the viscera diseased; and in convulsive cases the vessels of the brain extremely turgid or effusions of blood. This last shows the danger of giving emetics to nervous people" (p. 71).
24. Edward Baynard, *Health, A Poem,* 8th ed. (London, 1749; 1st ed., 1719), p. 37.
25. Johannes Baptist Friedreich, *Historisch-kritische Darstellung der Theorien über das Wesen und den Sitz der psychischen Krankheiten* (Leipzig, 1836), p. 185. In the context of German psychiatry, Friedreich was an influential "somatocist," a believer in physical illness as the cause of mental illness. On the role of the temperaments Friedreich cited Karl August Diez.
26. On Hippocratic doctrines of "suffocation of the mother" (uterus), or what the late eighteenth century would call hysteria, see James Palis et al., "The Hippocratic Concept of Hysteria: A Translation of the Original Texts," *Integrative Psychiatry,* 3 (1985), pp. 226–228.
27. John Sadler, *The Sick Womans Private Looking-Glasse* (London, 1636); quotes from pp. ii, 61, 68.

28. William Harvey, "Anatomical Exercises on the Generation of Animals . . ." (1651), reprinted in Robert Willis, trans. and ed., *The Works of William Harvey, M.D.* (London, 1847), p. 542. A useful overview of premodern doctrines of obstetrics and gynecology, in which issues of functional nervous illness appear, is Audrey Eccles, *Obstetrics and Gynecology in Tudor and Stuart England* (London: Croom Helm, 1982).

29. Jane Sharp, *The Midwives Book, or the Whole Art of Midwifery . . .* (London, 1671), quotes from pp. 129, 317. Among Mrs. Sharp's conclusions, "If one womb in a woman be the cause of so many strong and violent diseases, she may be thought a happy woman of our sex that was born without a womb" (p. 335).

30. William Sudlow Roots, "Hysterical Paralysis," *St. Thomas's Hospital Reports*, 1 (1836), pp. 248–260; quote p. 258.

31. Robert Sommer, *Diagnostik der Geisteskrankheiten* (Vienna, 1894), p. 126.

32. John Aitken, *Principles of Midwifery*, 2nd ed. (Edinburgh, 1785; 1st ed., 1784), p. 135.

33. James Sims, ed., *The Principles and Practice of Midwifery . . . by Edward Foster, M.D., Late Teacher of Midwifery in the City of Dublin* (London, 1781), pp. 57–58.

34. Edme-Pierre-Chauvot de Beauchêne, *De l'influence des affections de l'âme dans les maladies nerveuses des femmes*, rev. ed. (Amsterdam, 1783; 1st ed. 1781), pp. 102–103.

35. Jean-Baptiste Louyer-Villermay, *Recherches historiques et médicales sur l'hypochondrie, isolée . . . de l'hystérie et de la mélancholie* (Paris, 1802), p. 58.

36. For a review see Étienne-Jean Georget, *De la physiologie du système nerveux . . . recherches sur les maladies nerveuses*, 2 vols. (Paris, 1821), vol. 2, pp. 251–255.

37. Jacob Friedrich Isenflamm, *Versuch einiger praktischen Anmerkungen über die Nerven zur Erläuterung . . . hypochondrisch und hysterischer Zufälle* (Erlangen, 1774); see, for example, pp. 268–271.

38. Laurent-Alexis-Philibert Cerise, ed., *Rapports du physique et du moral de l'homme par P. J. G. Cabanis*, new ed., 2 vols. (Paris, 1867); quote from vol. 2, p. 14.

39. Xavier Bichat, *Anatomie générale appliquée à la physiologie et à la médecine*, 4 vols. (Paris, an X–1801); quotes from vol. I, pp. 227–228. In his *Recherches physiologiques sur la vie et la mort* (Paris, an VIII–1799), Bichat had already established the effects of "passions" on the various viscera, for example, pp. 62–80. On Bichat generally, see Elizabeth Haigh, *Xavier Bichat and the Medical Theory of the Eighteenth Century* (London: Wellcome Institute for the History of Medicine, 1984).

40. See Owsei Temkin, *The Falling Sickness: A History of Epilepsy from the Greeks to the Beginnings of Modern Neurology*, 2nd ed. (Baltimore: Johns Hopkins, 1971).

41. For an account of Hoffmann's life and work, see August Hirsch. ed., *Bio-*

graphisches Lexikon der hervorragenden Ärzte aller Zeiten und Völker, 2nd ed., vol. 3 (Berlin, 1931), pp. 256–259.

42. Richard Blackmore, *A Treatise of the Spleen and Vapours: or, Hypochondriacal and Hysterical Affections* . . . (London, 1725), p. 109. Blackmore allowed that the causation could flow in the opposite direction as well, from the abdomen to the head.

43. Giovanni Battista Morgagni's *De sedibus et causis morborum*, 2 vols. (Venice, 1761) was translated into English by Benjamin Alexander as *The Seats and Causes of Diseases Investigated by Anatomy*, 3 vols. (London, 1769), quotes from vol. 2, pp. 628–629. Morgagni conceded, however, a certain role to the pelvic organs (p. 632).

44. On Cullen's work see José M. López Piñero, *Historical Origins of the Concept of Neurosis*, trans. D. Berrios (Cambridge, England: Cambridge University Press, 1983), pp. 11–15. The term *neurosis* appears for the first time in Cullen's 1769 book.

45. See Erwin H. Ackerknecht, "The History of the Discovery of the Vegetative (Autonomic) Nervous System," *Medical History*, 18 (1974), pp. 1–8.

46. Edward Hody, ed., *Cases in Midwifery Written by the Late Mr. William Giffard* (London, 1734), pp. 327–328.

47. Examples from Thomas Denman, *An Introduction to the Practice of Midwifery*, 2 vols. (London, 1794–95), vol. I, pp. 336–337. Andrew Wilson, *Medical Researches: Being an Enquiry into the Nature and Origin of Hysterics in the Female Constitution* . . . (London, 1776), p. 90.

48. Charles Singer and E. Ashworth Underwood, *A Short History of Medicine* (Oxford: Clarendon, 1962), p. 153. On Haller's intellectual predecessors, see Owsei Temkin, "The Classical Roots of Glisson's Doctrine of Irritation," *Bulletin of the History of Medicine*, 38 (1964), pp. 297–328.

49. Brown's "Elementa medicinae" appeared in English as John Brown, *The Elements of Medicine, translated from the Latin with Comments and Illustrations by the Author*, rev. ed., 2 vols. (London, 1795). Brown died in 1788.

50. See, for example, Erna Lesky, *Die Wiener Medizinische Schule im 19. Jahrhundert* (Graz: Böhlau, 1978), pp. 23–28.

51. The founder of modern doctrines on inflammation was the surgeon John Hunter, *A Treatise on the Blood, Inflammation, and Gun-Shot Wounds* (London, 1794).

52. See, for example, Broussais's *Examen des doctrines médicales et des systèmes de nosologie*, 2 vols. (Paris, 1821), vol. 2, p. 531f. on irritation in the "névroses." See also Erwin H. Ackerknecht, "Broussais or a Forgotten Medical Revolution," *Bulletin of the History of Medicine*, 27 (1953), pp. 320–343. Broussais was also a supporter of the anatomical-clinical approach that was simultaneously flourishing in Paris, and not just a system builder.

53. John Burns, *Dissertations on Inflammation*, 2 vols. (Glasgow, 1800), vol. 1, p. 119.

54. In this exposition of the history of the reflex arc, I rely on Edwin Clarke

and L. S. Jacyna, *Nineteenth-Century Origins of Neuroscientific Concepts* (Berkeley: University of California Press, 1987), chap. 4, "The Reflex." See pp. 103–105 on Whytt.

55. Robert Whytt, *Observations on the Nature, Causes, and Cure of those Disorders Which Have Been Commonly Called Nervous, Hypochondriac, or Hysteric: To Which Are Prefixed Some Remarks on the Sympathy of the Nerves,* 2nd ed. (Edinburgh, 1765; 1st ed. also 1765); quotes from pp. 111, 173–177, 230–231. This edition spells the author's name Whyte. On Whytt see also R. K. French, *Robert Whytt, The Soul, and Medicine* (London: Wellcome Institute of the History of Medicine, 1969).

56. See Clarke and Jacyna, *Nineteenth-Century Origins* (1987), pp. 105–106; Lesky, *Wiener Schule* (1978), pp. 89–94.

57. For details see Clarke and Jacyna, *Nineteenth-Century Origins* (1987), p. 111.

58. Pierre Pomme, *Traité des affections vaporeuses des deux sexes,* 3d ed. (Lyon, 1767; 1st ed., 1763), pp. 20, 32–36. "Je dis que la cause prochaine et immédiate des affections vaporeuses doit être attribuée au racornissement du genre nerveux. Si le terme choque par sa nouveauté . . . je dirai que la sécheresse des membranes et des nerfs forme elle-même ce racornissement, qui seul produit tous les différens symptomes de la maladie que j'attaque" (pp. 20–21). Although Pomme does not use the phrase *nervous disease,* he refers to "vapours" involving the postulated nerves throughout the text.

59. Jan Petersen Michell, *Abhandlung von den Nervenkrankheiten* (Vienna, 1798; Latin original 1787), pp. 1, 51.

60. Isenflamm, *Versuch* (1774), pp. 196–199.

61. James Makittrick Adair, *Medical Cautions for the Consideration of Invalids: Those Especially Who Resort to Bath* (Bath, 1786), pp. 13–14.

CHAPTER 2
Spinal Irritation

1. For accounts by medical historians see José M. López Piñero, *Historical Origins of the Concept of Neurosis* (Cambridge, England: Cambridge University Press, 1983), pp. 64–68; Francis Schiller, *A Möbius Strip: Fin-de-siècle Neuropsychiatry and Paul Möbius* (Berkeley: University of California Press, 1982), pp. 70–71.

2. For an overview see the work of John Abercrombie, an early Edinburgh neurologist, *Pathological and Practical Researches on Diseases of the Brain and the Spinal Cord* (Edinburgh, 1828).

3. For example, Edward Sutleffe's diagnosis of "delicate spine" in a girl of twelve, presenting as an orthopedic defect. He treated her with rest and an issue of antimony tartrate ointment. "The child was, in less than a month, so improved that it appeared superfluous to urge the continuance of any further scientific interference." Sutleffe, *Medical and Surgical Cases, Selected During a Practice of Thirty-Eight Years* (London, 1824), p. 471. Frankfurt

physician Salomon Stiebel described a fourteen-year-old girl who came to him with abdominal pain, a tender spine, and trouble walking. He treated her with two *Fontanellen* (a kind of seton in which something like a pea is implanted under the skin with a knife to cause a sore) on her vertebrae, and her symptoms vanished. Neither author used such terms as *reflex* or *irritation*. Stiebel, *Kleine Beiträge zur Heilwissenschaft* (Frankfurt am Main, 1823), pp. viii–x.

4. Letter to the editor of the *Quarterly Journal of Science, Literature and the Arts,* 12 (1821). I was unable to consult this volume of the journal, and rely on its quotation in Thomas Pridgin Teale, *A Treatise on Neuralgic Diseases, Dependent Upon Irritation of the Spinal Marrow and Ganglia of the Sympathetic Nerve* (London, 1829; reprint, Concord, N.H., 1830?), pp. 5–6.

5. In a letter dated December 4, 1822. *Quarterly Journal of Science, Literature and the Arts,* 12 (1822), pp. 296–298. On the manifold vocabulary of "counterirritation," which includes vesicants, moxas, issues, and so forth, see Richard Quain, *Dictionary of Medicine,* vol. 2 (London, 1886), pp. 311–314. In cupping, the application of hot glasses or cups raised a blood boil that then could be lanced; bleeding was done with a lancet; blistering meant raising a vesicle with a strongly caustic substance such as sodium hydroxide.

6. Benjamin Travers, *An Inquiry Concerning that Disturbed State of the Vital Functions Usually Denominated Constitutional Irritation* (London, 1826). See pp. 40–45 on "local irritation."

7. Abercrombie, *Pathological and Practical Researches,* pp. 403–404. He avoided the term spinal irritation.

8. Thomas Brown, "On Irritation of the Spinal Nerves," *Glasgow Medical Journal,* 1 (1828), pp. 131–160. Few diseases of the spinal cord may be diagnosed by simply pressing on the spinous processes of the vertebrae, as opposed to palpating deeply the paravertebral muscles (which these irritationists did not do). So unrevealing are local findings from the back that it is usually omitted in the standard neurological examination.

9. Teale, *Treatise Neuralgic Diseases,* pp. 18–20.

10. Although the term irritation is still occasionally used in clinical neurology, in the sense of dysfunction or subclinical inflammation, it has lost its scientific status in neuropathology. There is no such thing as physical irritation of the nerves.

11. T. N. Smart, "Hysteria," *LMG,* 6 (1830), pp. 687–689. Italics in original.

12. William Griffin and Daniel Griffin, *Observations on Functional Affections of the Spinal Cord and Ganglionic System of Nerves, in Which Their Identity with Sympathetic, Nervous, and Imitative Diseases is Illustrated* (London, 1834); William Griffin, "Medical Problems," *Dublin Journal of Medical Science,* 11 (1837), pp. 1–17. Only after moving to Limerick in 1830 did William Griffin start to become well known as a medical writer.

13. Isaac Parrish, "Remarks on Spinal Irritation as Connected with Nervous Diseases," *American Journal of the Medical Sciences,* 10, (1832), pp. 293–

314; cases from pp. 302–303, 311–312. For other early American reports, see James Bradbury, "Some Cases of Spinal Irritation," *BMSJ*, 6 (1832), pp. 236–238; and Austin Flint, "Observations on the Pathological Relations of the Medulla Spinalis," *American Journal of the Medical Sciences*, 7, (1844), pp. 269–296.

14. Riadore's three substantial works on the subject constitute a kind of encyclopedia of hysteria, in the sense of conversion disorders, among middle-class urban female patients of this period. John Evans Riadore, *Introductory Lectures to a Course on Nervous Irritation, Spinal Affections* . . . (London, 1835); *A Treatise on Irritation of the Spinal Nerves as the Source of Nervousness, Indigestion* . . . (London, 1843); and *A Treatise on Irritation of the Spinal Nerves, as the Source of Nervousness, Indigestion, Functional and Organical Derangements of the Principal Organs of the Body* . . . (London, 1853). See also John Marshall, *Practical Observations on Diseases of the Heart* . . . *Occasioned by Spinal Irritation* . . . (London, 1835).

15. Robert Bentley Todd, *Clinical Lectures on Paralysis, Certain Diseases of the Brain, and Other Affections of the Nervous System*, 2nd ed. (London, 1856; 1st ed., 1854), pp. 455–459.

16. Carl Haffter and Hermann Lei, eds., *Dr. med. Elias Haffter: Bezirksarzt und Sängervater, 1803–1861: Tagebuch, 1844–1853*, 2 vols. (Frauenfeld, Switzerland: Historisches Verein des Kantons Thurgau, 1985), vol. 1, p. 88.

17. *The Journal of Dr. John Simpson of Bradford* . . . *1825* (Bradford, England: City Libraries Division, 1981), p. 12.

18. Walter Johnson, *An Essay on the Diseases of Young Women* (London, 1849), pp. 149–151.

19. Allan Walters, "Psychogenic Regional Pain Alias Hysterical Pain," *Brain*, 84 (1961), pp. 1–18.

20. Benjamin C. Brodie, *Lectures Illustrative of Certain Local Nervous Affections* (London, 1837), pp. 54–55; different printings of this work have different paginations; the copy I consulted began at p. 33.

21. Frederic C. Skey, "Clinical Lecture on Hysteric Diseases," *Lancet*, i (February 24, 1855), pp. 205–207; quotes from pp. 205–206.

22. Reprinted in Oliver Wendell Holmes, *Medical Essays, 1842–1882* (Boston, 1911); quote p. 389. "Congestion of the portal system" was also quite serviceable, Holmes said.

23. "Letters from Our Special Paris Correspondent," writing on a "Suggestive Health Resort at Lake Maggiore," *BMSJ*, 155 (October 11, 1906), pp. 423–425; quote p. 424.

24. Moritz Benedikt, *Aus meinem Leben: Erinnerungen und Erörterungen* (Vienna, 1906), p. 141.

25. William N. Macartney, *Fifty Years a Country Doctor* (New York, 1938), p. 175.

26. William Alexander Hammond, *Spinal Irritation (Posterior Spinal Anaemia)* (Detroit, 1886), p. 23.

27. Ap Morgan Vance, "Hysteria as the Surgeon Sees It," *AJO*, 58 (1908), pp. 757–767; quotes pp. 757–760. In France, this cauterizing of the spine was called *pointes de feu* and associated with a quite retrograde variety of medical (as opposed to surgical) gynecology. For example, see Jules Batuaud, *La Neurasthénie génitale féminine* (Paris, 1906), p. 116.

28. Benedict Stilling, *Physiologische, pathologische und medicinisch-practische Untersuchungen über die Spinal-Irritation* (Leipzig, 1840), pp. 78–79, on men and women. Other Central European writers had previously touched on the subject, yet Stilling's book was first to legitimate the diagnosis. On Stilling, see Gerhard Aumüller, "Benedict Stilling (1810–1879): Untersuchungen über das Rückenmark: ein Wendepunkt in der neuroanatomischen Forschung," *Medizin Historisches Journal*, 19 (1984), pp. 53–69. Also Bernd Ottermann, "Benedict Stilling (1810–1879): Landgerichtswundarzt zu Cassel, *Würzburg Medizinisch-Historische Mitteilungen*, 4 (1986), pp. 253–287.

29. Romberg noted with some reserve the existence of "neuralgia spinalis (*Spinal irritation* der neueren englischen Autoren)." *Lehrbuch der Nervenkrankheiten des Menschen* (Berlin, 1840), vol. 1 (i), p. 155. Several years after Stilling's and Romberg's books, the Viennese psychiatrist Ernst von Feuchtersleben endorsed spinal irritation as the cause of hysteria and melancholy. Sometimes it originated in the uterus, he said. *Principles of Medical Psychology*, (London, 1847; 1st German ed., 1845), p. 227. Feuchtersleben died in 1849 without further chance to amplify his views.

30. Charles-Prosper Ollivier (d'Angers), *De la moelle épinière et de ses maladies*, 3rd ed. (Paris, 1838), vol. II, p. 285. I have not seen this book; the citation is from Axenfeld, cited below.

31. August Axenfeld, *Traité des névroses*, 2nd ed., expanded by Henri Huchard (Paris, 1883; first ed., 1863); see pp. 291–292, 306. Spa treatment, especially at St. Moritz, would also suit.

32. Pierre Briquet, France's main authority on hysteria before Charcot, considered spinal irritation irrelevant in psychiatry. Briquet said, "La moelle épinière n'est nullement en rapport avec les affections morales qui produisent l'hystérie." The brain was the seat of hysteria, not the spine. Pierre Briquet, *Traité clinique et thérapeutique de l'hystérie* (Paris, 1859), p. 604.

33. I consulted the English translation, Wilhelm Heinrich Erb, *Diseases of the Spinal Cord and Medulla Oblongata*, trans. Edward G. Geoghegan et al. (London, 1878; vol. 13 of Hugo Wilhelm von Ziemssen's *Cyclopedia of Medical Practice*); see especially 358–371. On Krafft-Ebing's views of "spinal neurasthenia" see *Psychopathia Sexualis;* I used the English translation of the twelfth German edition (New York, 1933), pp. 51–55, 88, and passim. Julius Wagner-Jauregg confided in his manuscript autobiography (1939) that Krafft-Ebing was not loved in ministry circles or among other medical professors because his book was thought to appeal mainly to perverts (p. 70; preserved in the Institut für Geschichte der Medizin in Vienna).

34. On spas in Europe, see Alfred Martin, *Deutsches Badewesen in vergangenen*

Tagen (Jena, 1906); Rolf Bothe, ed., *Kurstädte in Deutschland: Zur Geschichte einer Baugattung* (Berlin: Frölich und Kaufmann, 1984). On France, Lise Grenier (Institut français d'Architecture), ed., *Villes d'eaux en France* (Paris: Fernand Hazan, 1985).

35. Louis Verhaeghe, *Du traitement des maladies nerveuses par les bains de mer* (Brussels, 1850), p. 78.

36. Sébastien-Didier Lhéritier, *Eaux de Plombières: clinique médicale des paralysies, "deuxième année"* (Paris, 1854), p. 134. See, for example, the case of Lucie Pilot, *"faible et languissante"* from the age of twelve onward, cured of her *"irritation spinale"* at twenty-three by the healing waters (p. 138; a succession of similar cases follows to p. 162).

37. Georg Thilenius, *Handbuch der Balneotherapie* [founded by Hermann Ludwig Helfft], 9th ed., 2 vols. (Berlin, 1882), vol. 2, pp. 210-211, 230.

38. See Edward Shorter, "Private Clinics in Central Europe, 1850-1933," *Social History of Medicine,* 3 (1990), pp. 159-195.

39. Rudolph Burkart, who until 1883 had been chief physician of a sanatorium (*Wasserheilanstalt*) in Boppard am Rhein, advised his colleagues specifically against the massage component of the Weir Mitchell rest cure in spinal irritation. "Zur Behandlung der Hysterie und Neurasthenie," *BKW,* 23 (April 19, 1886), pp. 249-255, especially p. 255.

40. Hermann Determann, "Über Wirkung und Anwendung der Hydrotherapie bei der Neurasthenie," *Zeitschrift für diätetische und physikalische Therapie,* 3 (1899-1900), pp. 306-320; quote from p. 315.

41. Moritz Heinrich Romberg, preface to the second edition of his neuropathology textbook of 1851, reprinted in Romberg, *Lehrbuch der Nervenkrankheiten des Menschen,* 3rd ed. (Berlin, 1857), vol. 1, p. viii. Note that at this point Romberg had not yet abandoned the doctrine of reflex neurosis.

CHAPTER 3
Reflex Theory and the History of Internal Sensation

1. See, for example, the surgeon George Tate, *Treatise on Hysteria* (London, 1830), who brought irregular menstruation, spinal irritation, and hysteria into the same broth; or Thomas J. Graham, a surgeon in Glasgow, who without using the term *reflex* represented the view that sympathy carried uterine disease everywhere around the body, including to the brain in the form of madness. *On the Diseases of Females . . .* , 8th ed. (London, 1855; 1st ed. 1834). "I believe that the marked influence of the womb on the brain may account for the greater number of instances of madness found in females than in males" (p. 3).

2. Marshall Hall, *Commentaries on Some of the More Important Diseases of Females* (London, 1827).

3. Marshall Hall, *Practical Observations and Suggestions in Medicine* (London, 1845), p. 354.

4. On Hall's life see J. H. S. Green, "Marshall Hall (1790-1857): A Biblio-

graphical Study," *Medical History*, 2 (1958), pp. 120–133; Edwin Clarke and L. S. Jacyna, *Nineteenth-Century Origins of Neuroscientific Concepts* (Berkeley: University of California Press, 1987), pp. 114–123.

5. John Evans Riadore, *A Treatise on Irritation of the Spinal Nerves as the Source of Nervousness, Indigestion* . . . (London, 1843), p. 118.

6. Unsigned review of Hall's book, *A New Memoir on the Nervous System* (London, 1843), in the *Lancet*, ii (1846), pp. 154–157, 186–189, 244–247; quote from p. 247.

7. On how quickly Hall's ideas spread, see Ruth Leys, "Background to the Reflex Controversy: William Alison and the Doctrine of Sympathy before Hall," *Studies in History of Biology*, 4 (1980), pp. 1–66, especially pp. 58–59 n. 77. Hall, to my knowledge, does not actually use the phrase *reflex neurosis*.

8. Benjamin Travers, *A Further Inquiry Concerning Constitutional Irritation and the Pathology of the Nervous System* (London, 1835), pp. 29–43, 246.

9. Benjamin C. Brodie, *Lectures Illustrative of Certain Local Nervous Affections* (London, 1837), p. 38; pagination in this copy begins at p. 33. Doctor Wollaston's stomach was incriminated in this case, but in Brodie's view of women, it was the menses that caused local "hysterical" pains. See Brodie, "Clinical Remarks," *Lancet*, i (November 30, 1839), pp. 355–358, especially p. 357: "Hysteria in women is generally caused by a sudden stoppage of the menstrual discharge." On the whole, however, Brodie leaned more toward the central-nervous than the reflex paradigm.

10. Johann Wilhelm Arnold, *Die Lehre von der Reflex-Function für Physiologen und Ärzte* (Heidelberg, 1842); the expression *Reflex-Theorie* appears on p. 16. In addition to Hall, Johannes Müller of Berlin figured prominently in Arnold's exposé.

11. In 1843 Vienna's famous neurologist Ludwig Türck announced the discovery of *Reflexstellen* on the side of the spinal column, by pressing on which he was able to reactivate vanished peripheral symptoms. *Abhandlung über Spinal-Irritation, nach eigenen, grösstentheils im Wiener allgemeinen Krankenhause angestellten Beobachtungen* (Vienna, 1843), p. 3, and passim. Türck saw irritated peripheral organs reflexly causing spinal irritation, and vice versa. Thus he was closer to total-body-reflex theories than to the narrower concepts of spinal irritation viewed in the previous chapter.

12. Romberg initially presented his views on hysteria as "eine von Genitalienreizung ausgehende Reflexneurose" in his *Lehrbuch der Nervenkrankheiten des Menschen*, I(ii) (Berlin, 1846; part i published in 1840), p. 456, 788–793. By the time of the publication of a second edition of this work in 1851 he had amplified some of the above points. I have consulted the English translation of this second edition in 1851 of his work, *A Manual of the Nervous Diseases of Man*, trans. Edward H. Sieveking, 2 vols. (London, 1853), especially vol. 2, pp. 81–99, on hysteria.

13. Romberg, *Lehrbuch der Nervenkrankheiten des Menschen*, 3rd ed. (Berlin,

1857), vol. 1, p. 552. Romberg thought that the ovaries, pushing against an ulcerated uterine cervix, reflexly caused "das ganze hysterische Cortège."

14. On Laycock's life see obituaries in the *BMJ*, ii (September 30, 1876), pp. 448–449, and *Lancet*, ii (September 30, 1876), pp. 483–484.

15. Thomas Laycock, *A Treatise on the Nervous Diseases of Women . . . Spinal and Hysterical Disorders* (London, 1840), especially pp. 115–120, 197–198, 222–227. See also his "On the Reflex Function of the Brain," *British and Foreign Medical Review*, 19 (1845), pp. 298–311.

16. Charles Schützenberger, "Études sur les causes organiques et le mode de production des affections dites hystériques," *Gazette médicale de Paris*, 1846, pp. 422–425, 442–444, 482–486 on the uterus; for the case of Élise Richert, which formed part of a later series of articles on hysteria, pp. 749–750. In the French incrimination of the ovaries as a cause of nervous disease, see also Pierre-Adolphe Piorry, *Traité du diagnostic et de séméiologie*, 3 vols. (Paris, 1836–37). Following Schützenberger see also Charles Negrier, *Recueil de faits pour servir à l'histoire des ovaires et des affections hystériques de la femme* (Angers, 1858). The author claimed that, around 1827, he had been the first to realize that the ovaries regulated menstruation.

17. Merriley Borell, "Organotherapy, British Physiology, and Discovery of the Internal Secretions," *Journal of the History of Biology*, 9 (1976), pp. 235–268, especially pp. 237–244.

18. Brown-Séquard was alluding here to a tradition of medical scholarship beginning with Edward Stanley in 1833 that made major organic diseases responsible for paralysis and paresis. Most of the patients in this literature were grievously ill, their motor symptoms in no way psychogenic. I have therefore not considered this body of writing. For an overview of the "reflex paralysis" literature, see Ernst von Leyden, "Über Reflexlähmung," (*Volkmann*) *Sammlung klinischer Vorträge*, no. 2 (*Innere Medicin*, no. 1 n.d. about 1870), pp. 1–22.

19. These quotes from Brown-Séquard, "Course of Lectures on the Physiology and Pathology of the Central Nervous System . . . Lecture X (continued)," *Lancet*, ii (November 20, 1858), pp. 519–520.

20. Edwin Walker, "Reflex Irritation as a Cause of Disease," *JAMA*, 24 (February 2, 1895), pp. 165–166; quote from p. 165.

21. Erwin Kehrer, *Die physiologischen und pathologischen Beziehungen der weiblichen Sexualorgane zum Tractus intestinalis und besonders zum Magen* (Berlin, 1905). On "splanchnoptosis" causing "reflex hysteria," for example, p. 189. Although Kehrer pooh-poohed older reflex views to some extent, the text makes clear that he was a firm adherent of the whole concept.

22. Alfred Adler, *Study of Organ Inferiority and Its Psychical Compensation: A Contribution to Clinical Medicine*, trans. Smith Ely Jelliffe (New York, 1917; German ed. 1907), pp. 47, 73. Adler was unaware of the phenomenon of diabetic neuropathy.

23. Hélan Jaworski, "La Réflexothérapie," *Gazette médicale de Paris*, November 1, 1911, pp. 345–346; quote from p. 346.

24. I used Leonard Williams, *Minor Maladies and Their Treatment*, 6th ed. (Baltimore, 1933; 1st ed., London, 1906), pp. 170–188.

25. J. M. Hooper, "A Case of Reflex Paralysis," *International Record of Medicine (New York Medical Journal)*, 40 (November 8, 1884), p. 520.

26. For a sampler: Georges Apostoli, "Du traitement électrique de la douleur ovarienne chez les hystériques," *Association française pour l'avancement des sciences*, 12ème session, Rouen, 1883 (Paris, 1884), pp. 740–741. The author believed the uterus the true culprit. Heinrich Fritsch, *Die Krankheiten der Frau* (Braunschweig, 1881), chap. on "Hysterie." Fritsch, however, was one of the early warning voices against the castration of women for mental illness. Valentin Holst, "Über das Verhältnis der Hysterie und einzelner nervöser Symptome zu der Gynäkologie," *Archiv für Psychiatrie*, 11 (1881), pp. 678–692; Holst observed that the only lesions in the pelvis capable of causing hysteria were ovarian, because uterine malposition, cervical erosion, and the like did not cause the necessary "Reizzustände," or irritation, in the pelvic nerves that reflexly produced vasomotor phenomena elsewhere in the body (p. 680).

27. Richard Förster, "Über die Beziehungen der Krankheiten der Geschlechtsorgane zum Sehorgan," in Alfred Graefe et al., eds., *Handbuch der gesamten Augenheilkunde*, 7 vols. (1874–80), vol. 7 (5) (Leipzig, 1877), pp. 88–103; quotes from pp. 89–92. See also Salo Cohn, *Uterus und Auge: Eine Darstellung der Funktionen und Krankheiten des weiblichen Geschlechtsapparates in ihrem pathogenen Einfluss auf das Sehorgan* (Wiesbaden, 1890).

28. Hermann Wolfgang Freund, "Die Beziehungen der weiblichen Geschlechtsorgane in ihren physiologischen und pathologischen Veränderungen zu anderen Organen," *Ergebnisse der allgemeinen Pathologie und pathologischen Anatomie*, 3 (2) (1896), p. 170f.

29. Pierre Berthier, *Des névroses menstruelles* (Paris, 1874), pp. 10–12.

30. Victor Cornelius Medvei, *A History of Endocrinology* (Lancaster, England: MTP Press, 1982), p. 222.

31. Fleetwood Churchill, "On Some of the Reflex Irritations Resulting from Uterine Disease," *Dublin Quarterly Journal of Medical Science*, 2nd ser., 33 (1862), pp. 193–199 (For example, after Doctor Churchill had treated the leukorrhea of a woman crippled with leg pain, she became able to dance again, pp. 195–196). Arthur W. Edis, *Diseases of Women* (Philadelphia, 1882; first ed. London, 1881), pp. 137–142. Alfred Lewis Galabin, *Diseases of Women*, 6th ed. (London, 1903; 1st ed. 1879), p. 26. Henry Macnaughton-Jones, "Uterine Reflexes, Distant Lesions, and Remote Symptoms due to Uterine Irritation," *British Gynecological Journal*, 9 (1893–94), pp. 133–167 (the discussion following this paper was of particular interest); see also his *Points of Practical Interest in Gynecology* (London, 1901), passim to p. 92.

32. For a sampling see Henry Turman Byford, *Manual of Gynecology* (Philadelphia, 1895), pp. 136–140; Gunning S. Bedford, *Clinical Lectures on the Diseases of Women and Children*, 8th ed. (New York, 1866; 1st ed. 1855),

pp. 363–372 and passim; Thomas Addis Emmet, *Principles and Practice of Gynecology*, 3rd ed. (London, 1885; 1st ed., Philadelphia, 1879), pp. 36–39 and passim; George J. Engelmann, "The Hystero-Neuroses, with Especial Reference to the Menstrual Hystero-Neurosis of the Stomach," *American Gynecological Society. Transactions*, 2 (1877), pp. 483–518; Alexander J. C. Skene, *Treatise on the Diseases of Women*, 2nd ed. (New York, 1892; 1st ed. 1888), pp. 930–937.

33. Jean Sarradon, "Hystérie et lésions génitales chez la femme," *L'Écho médical des Cévennes*, 8 (1907), pp. 293–300; case from pp. 293–295.

34. Mary Putnam Jacobi, *Essays on Hysteria, Brain-Tumor and Some Other Cases of Nervous Disease* (New York, 1888), pp. 13–14. Jacobi was, moreover, a believer in Battey's operation for the removal of normal ovaries as a cure for nervous disease, pp. 79–80.

35. See Gail Pat Parsons, "Equal Treatment for All: American Medical Remedies for Male Sexual Problems," *Journal of the History of Medicine*, 31 (1977), pp. 63–69.

36. Alexander Peyer, "Über Magenaffektionen bei männlichen Genitalleiden," *(Volkmann) Sammlung klinischer Vorträge*, no. 356 (Innere Medizin no. 117 [n.d., about 1890]), pp. 3169–3204; cases from pp. 3174, 3189–90.

37. C. H. Ohr, "Genito-Reflex Neurosis in the Female," *AJO*, 16 (1883), pp. 50–64, 168–180; case from p. 64.

38. Alexander Berg, *Der Krankheitskomplex der Kolik- und Gebärmutterleiden in Volksmedizin und Medizingeschichte unter besonderer Berücksichtigung der Volksmedizin in Ostpreussen* (Berlin, 1935), pp. 36–37, 41.

39. Hermann Klotz, "Gynäkologische Mittheilungen," *WMW*, 32 (September 23, 1882), pp. 1129–33; quote from p. 1129. On this see also Michael Macdonald, *Mystical Bedlam: Madness, Anxiety, and Healing in Seventeenth-Century England* (Cambridge, England: Cambridge University Press, 1981), p. 203.

40. Dietrich Wilhelm Heinrich Busch, *Das Geschlechtsleben des Weibes in physiologischer, pathologischer und therapeutischer Hinsicht*, 5 vols. 1839–44, vol. 2 (Leipzig, 1840), p. 309.

41. Laycock, *Treatise Nervous Diseases Women* (1840), p. 227.

42. Hector Landouzy, *Traité complet de l'hystérie* (Paris, 1846), p. 42.

43. Fulgence Raymond and Pierre Janet, *Les Obsessions et la psychasthénie*, 2 vols. (Paris, 1903), vol. 2, p. 334.

44. One of the few from the turn of the century is told in Louis Rimbaud, "Un cas de boulimie hystérique," *Montpellier médical*, 29 (October 3, 1909), pp. 313–321.

45. H. Bousquet, "Une grenouille dans l'intestin! Guérison par suggestion due à l'emploi d'images radiographiques," *Bulletin médical*, 21 (1907), pp. 47–49.

46. Felix Preissner, "Die Abteilung für Nervenkranke des Krankenhauses der Landesversicherungsanstalt Schlesien in Breslau," *PNW*, 27 (December 26,

1925), pp. 533–537; case from p. 537. The surgeon was unnamed. The author felt placebo operations in such cases to be generally unsuccessful.

47. Olive Schreiner's implicit acceptance of reflex theory is too delicious to pass by. She once told Havelock Ellis: "When a man puts his penis into a woman's vagina it is as if (assuming of course that she responds) he puts his finger into her brain, stirred it round & round." Cited in Phyllis Grosskurth, *Havelock Ellis: A Biography* (Toronto: McClelland and Stewart, 1980), p. 323.

48. Benjamin Brodie, *Lancet* (1839); quote from pp. 357–358.

49. Robert Brudenell Carter, *On the Pathology and Treatment of Hysteria* (London, 1853), p. 70.

50. Joseph Amann, *Über den Einfluss der weiblichen Geschlechtskrankheiten auf das Nervensystem mit besonderer Berücksichtigung . . . der Hysterie* (Erlangen, 1868), pp. 10–11. Amann was not a reflex theorist and attributed to gynecological disease a secondary role in hysteria.

51. Philip Coombs Knapp, "The Alleged Reflex Causes of Nervous Disease," *American Journal of the Medical Sciences,* 110 (1895), pp. 406–414; quote from p. 409. Knapp preferred explanations involving functional nervous disease.

52. Edward A. Weiss, "A Consideration of Neurasthenia in Its Relation to Pelvic Symptoms in Women," *AJO,* 57 (1908), pp. 230–235; quotes from pp. 231–232.

53. Chauncey D. Palmer, "The Relation and Co-relations of Gynecological and Nervous Affections," ibid., 47 (1903), pp. 755–763; quote from p. 760.

54. T[homas] Clifford Allbutt, *On Visceral Neuroses* (London, 1884), pp. 25–27. In 1892 Allbutt became Regius Professor of medicine in Cambridge.

55. Ap Morgan Vance, "Hysteria as the Surgeon Sees It," *AJO,* 58 (1908), pp. 757–767; case from pp. 764–765. To cure this patient Doctor Vance employed a sort of nurse-disciplinarian and prescribed some placebo treatments. "The nurse was directed to stand her on her feet several times every day and require her to take a few steps each time, gradually increasing the distance. At the end of three weeks she was walking around the infirmary, shortly thereafter she went out on the streets, and is now in Memphis, Tenn., on a mission trying to make up the twenty-five years she lost!"

56. Raymond Belbèze, *La Neurasthénie rurale . . . chez le paysan contemporain* (Paris, 1911), p. 172.

57. See John Percy Lockhart-Mummery, *Diseases of the Colon and Their Surgical Treatment* (Bristol, 1910).

58. Miss X greatly risked a colectomy at Lane's hands. See his, "Remarks on the Results of the Operative Treatment of Chronic Constipation," *BMJ,* i (January 18, 1908), pp. 126–130. Lane also believed that intestinal "stasis" caused neurosis. See his "Civilization in Relation to the Abdominal Viscera, with Remarks on the Corset," *Lancet,* ii (November 13, 1909), pp. 1416–1418.

59. From Frederick Parkes Weber's casebooks, Contemporary Medical Archives Centre, Wellcome Unit for the History of Medicine, London, casebook for 1907-9. Miss X's records begin on p. 5 of the volume, starting with a clipping, P. Lockhart Mummery, "A Case of So-Called Chronic Neurasthenia Due to Abdominal Adhesions," *Lancet,* ii (September 10, 1910), pp. 800-801.

60. Daniel Webster Cathell, *The Physician Himself and What He Should Add to the Strictly Scientific* (Baltimore, 1882), p. 103.

61. August Rheinstädter, "Über weibliche Nervosität, ihre Beziehungen zu den Krankheiten der Generationsorgane und ihre Allgemeinbehandlung," *(Volkmann) Sammlung klinischer Vorträge,* no. 188 (Gyn. no. 56), n.d. (1884 or before), pp. 1493-1510; quote from p. 1495.

62. The notion that the nose is connected to other organs and body systems is not inherently absurd. Branches of the olfactory nerve (cranial nerve I) connect to the hippocampus of the brain and help explain why odor is strongly implicated in emotional and sexual experiences. Powerful nasal reflexes do exist that can affect the heart and lungs (see, for example, D. J. Allison, letter "Reflexes from the Nose," *NEJM,* 299 [December 28, 1978], p. 1468), suggesting a possible mechanism in sudden death from glue-sniffing. The nasal mucosa do respond to topical applications of estrogen (Hector Mortimer et al., "Atrophic Rhinitis: The Constitutional Factor: and the Treatment with Oestrogenic Hormones," *Canadian Medical Association Journal,* 37 [1937], pp. 445-456). Yet, contrary to the beliefs of the nasal-reflex theorists, the nasal mucosa do not become engorged during the menses (H. Toppozada, et al., "The Human Nasal Mucosa in the Menstrual Cycle: A Histochemical and Electron Microscope Study," *Journal of Laryngology and Otology,* 95 [1981], pp. 1237-1247). It is the sympathetic nervous system (to a much lesser extent the parasympathetic), not the cranial nerves, that controls the diameter of the small arteries and veins in the nose; therewith the scientific basis of nasal-reflex theory collapses. See Richard T. Jackson, "Pharmacologic Responsiveness of the Nasal Mucosa," *Annals of Otology, Rhinology,* 79 (1970), pp. 461-467.

63. Friedrich E. R. Voltolini, *Über Nasenpolypen und deren Operation* (Vienna, 1880); he cites his 1871 publication on p. 7.

64. Arthur Hartmann, "Partielle Resection der Nasenscheidewand bei hochgradiger Verkrümmung derselben," *DMW,* 8 (December 16, 1882), pp. 691-692.

65. Moritz Rosenthal, *Zur Diagnose und Therapie der Magenkrankheiten* (Vienna, 1883), pp. 3-4.

66. See, for example, Louis Elsberg (of New York), "Reflex and Other Phenomena Due to Nasal Disease," *Archives of Laryngology,* 4 (1883), pp. 253-255.

67. John Noland Mackenzie, "On Nasal Cough and the Existence of a Sensitive Reflex Area in the Nose," *American Journal of the Medical Sciences,* 86 (1883), pp. 106-116. Damaging the delicate mucous membrane of the nose may easily result in ozena, a fetid crusting of the nose's normal discharge.

68. Mackenzie, "Irritation of the Sexual Apparatus as an Etiological Factor in the Production of Nasal Disease," ibid., 87 (1884), pp. 360–365. See also Mackenzie's "The Pathological Nasal Reflex: An Historical Study," *New York Medical Journal* (August 20, 1887), pp. 199–205, in which he argued, among other things, that sneezing was a prodrome of hysteria. For a general history of the rise of nasal-reflex-neurosis theories see Frank J. Sulloway, *Freud: Biologist of the Mind* (New York: Basic Books, 1979), pp. 147–150, including an extensive biographical note on Mackenzie, p. 148 n. 8.

69. Wilhelm Hack, *Über eine operative Radical-Behandlung bestimmter Formen von Migräne, Asthma, Heufieber . . . Erfahrungen auf dem Gebiete der Nasen-krankheiten* (Wiesbaden, 1884), especially, pp. 59–78. Hack's preferred treatment was nasal cautery.

70. See for a review Adolph Bronner, "A Few Words on Some Common Forms of Reflexes of Nasal Origin," *Lancet,* ii (July 27, 1895), pp. 204–205.

71. Joseph Joal, "De l'épistaxis génitale," *Revue mensuelle de laryngologie,* 8 (1888), pp. 74–138; cases from pp. 83–84.

72. Leopold Löwenfeld, *Pathologie und Therapie der Neurasthenie und Hysterie* (Wiesbaden, 1894), pp. 77–78.

73. Parkes Weber papers, casebooks of 1894–1900, 1906–07.

74. See for example, Sigmund Gottschalk, "Ein Fall von Anosmie nach opera-tiver Entfernung beider Eierstöcke," *DMW,* 17 (June 25, 1891), pp. 823–824; Alfred Koblanck, "Über nasale Reflexe," ibid., 34 (June 11, 1908), pp. 1046–1049. Koblanck went on to write extensively on this topic, includ-ing *Die Nase als Reflexorgan des autonomen Nervensystems* (Berlin, 1930).

75. Alexander Peyer, "Über nervösen Schnupfen und Speichelfluss und den ätiologischen Zusammenhang derselben mit Erkrankungen des Sexualappar-ates," *MMW,* 36 (January 15, 1889), pp. 38–41; case from p. 41.

76. For examples of Fliess's influence, see Arthur Schiff, "Über die Bezie-hungen zwischen Nase und weiblichen Sexualorganen," *WKW,* 14 (January 17, 1901), pp. 57–65; F. Linder, "Über 'nasale Dysmenorrhoe,'" *MMW,* 49 (June 3, 1902), pp. 922–925; Gottfried Trautmann, "Zur Frage der Be-ziehungen zwischen Nase und Genitalien," *Monatsschrift für Ohrenheil-kunde,* 37 (1903), pp. 129–144; and Erwin Kehrer, *Die physiologischen und pathologischen Beziehungen der weiblichen Sexualorgane zum Tractus intesti-nalis und besonders zum Magen* (Berlin, 1905), p. 191.

77. For a detailed discussion of Fliess's work and his relationship with Freud, see Sulloway, *Freud* (1979), pp. 147–152. Sulloway somewhat bizarrely finds "an important grain of scientific truth" in Fliess's nasogenital theories (p. 152).

78. Perry Meisel and Walter Kendrick, eds., *Bloomsbury/Freud: The Letters of James and Alix Strachey 1924-1925* (New York: Basic Books, 1985), pp. 241–242.

79. Jeffrey Moussaieff Masson, ed., *The Complete Letters of Sigmund Freud to Wilhelm Fliess 1887-1904* (Cambridge: Harvard University Press, 1985),

pp. 49, 61, 130, 285. In the last letter I have changed the translator's word "suppuration" to "discharge." Freud did, however, rebuke genital reflex theories, rejecting the work of "Preyer" in "Draft C" that Freud sent to Fliess. Of course Freud meant Alexander Peyer, not the psychologist and physiologist Wilhelm Thierry Preyer; the confusion is clarified in Masson, p. 46 n. 2.

80. Adler, *Organ Inferiority,* p. 54.
81. Quoted in Vincent Brome, *Ernest Jones: Freud's Alter Ego* (New York: Norton, 1983), p. 132.
82. On Stekel's treating his own patients see his *Äskulap als Harlekin: Humor, Satire und Phantasie aus der Praxis* (Wiesbaden, 1911), p. 105, published under the pseudonym "Med. Dr. Serenus." See also Stekel, *Nervöse Angstzustände und ihre Behandlung* (Berlin, 1908), p. 38. Carl Jung, who was somewhat dubious about these theories, mentioned Stekel's views in a letter to Freud. See William McGuire, ed., *The Freud/Jung Letters: The Correspondence between Sigmund Freud and C. G. Jung* (Princeton: Princeton University Press, 1974), p. 167 n. 2.
83. Albrecht Hirschmüller, "Briefe Josef Breuers and Wilhelm Fliess 1894–1898," *Jahrbuch der Psychoanalyse,* 18 (1986), pp. 239–261; evidence from pp. 242–244.
84. August Heisler, *Dennoch Landarzt! Erfahrungen und Betrachtungen aus der Praxis,* 5th ed. (Munich, 1950; 1st ed. a pamphlet, 1913; 2nd greatly expanded ed., 1933), pp. 227–229. The author, who operated a sanatorium in the Black Forest and edited a medical periodical (*Der Landarzt*), had updated this edition of his book and presumably still believed in the doctrine. A quite psychologically insightful practitioner, he had in 1926 attended the first meeting of the "Allgemeiner ärztlicher Kongress für Psychotherapie" in Baden-Baden. Wladimir Eliasberg, *Psychotherapie. Bericht über den I. Allgemeinen ärztlichen Kongress für Psychotherapie in Baden-Baden, 17–19. April 1926* (Halle, Germany, 1927), p. 322.
85. Thomas H. Holmes, et al., *The Nose: An Experimental Study of Relations Within the Nose in Human Subjects During Varying Life Experiences* (Springfield, Ill.: Charles C Thomas, 1950), p. 90; on views of nasal-gastric relations, pp. 102–110.

CHAPTER 4
Gynecological Surgery and the Desire for an Operation

1. François-Joseph-Victor Broussais, *Examen des doctrines médicales et des systèmes de nosologie,* 2 vols. (Paris, 1821), vol. 2, pp. 531–563 and passim.
2. On "die Kopro-Psychiatrie" see Wilhelm Griesinger, *Pathologie und Therapie der psychischen Krankheiten* (Stuttgart, 1867; reprint Amsterdam: Bonset, 1964), p. 202. See also Konrad Alt, "Über das Entstehen von Neurosen und Psychosen auf dem Boden von chronischen Magenkrankheiten," *Archiv für Psychiatrie,* 24 (1892), pp. 403–451, especially p. 404.

3. See Edwin Clarke and L. S. Jacyna, *Nineteenth-Century Origins of Neuro-scientific Concepts* (Berkeley: University of California Press, 1987), pp. 124–125, 133.

4. John Conolly, "Hysteria," in John Forbes et al., eds., *The Cyclopedia of Practical Medicine*, 5 vols. (1833–59), vol. 2 (London, 1833), pp. 557–586; quote from p. 568.

5. Thomas Laycock, *A Treatise on the Nervous Diseases of Women* (London, 1840), p. 105.

6. C. E. Louis Mayer, *Die Beziehungen der krankhaften Zustände und Vorgänge in den Sexual-Organen des Weibes zu Geistesstörungen* (Berlin, 1869), p. 59. Mayer thought that the link between pelvis and brain was either reflex or a circulatory or metabolic disturbance.

7. C. E. Louis Mayer, "Menstruation im Zusammenhange mit psychischen Störungen," *Beiträge zur Geburtshülfe und Gynäkologie*, 1 (1872), pp. 111–135; case from pp. 117–118.

8. R. Schroeter, "Über das Verhalten der Menstruation bei Psychosen," *Beiträge zur Geburtshülfe und Gynäkologie*, 3 (1874), pp. 293–310.

9. S. Danillo, "Recherches cliniques sur la fréquence des maladies sexuelles chez les aliénées," *Archives de neurologie*, 4 (1882), pp. 171–188.

10. Joseph Wiglesworth, "On Uterine Disease and Insanity," *Journal of Mental Science*, 30 (1885), 509–531, see p. 511.

11. Henry Macnaughton-Jones, *Points of Practical Interest in Gynaecology*, 2nd ed. (New York, 1901 [1st ed. London, 1901]), p. 92. Only thirteen of these patients, the author pointed out, had actual mental illness. Thus pelvic reflex mechanisms were more conducive of neurosis than psychosis.

12. Henry Maudsley, *The Pathology of Mind* (London, 1879), pp. 208–213, 498. Postpartum psychosis is a genuine phenomenon, but its mechanism (still unknown) is certainly not reflex action.

13. Sheila M. Ross, "Menstruation in Its Relationship to Insanity," *Journal of Mental Science*, 55 (1909), pp. 270–280. She had left the Holloway Sanatorium at the time she wrote the article.

14. Auguste Voisin, *Leçons cliniques sur les maladies mentales et sur les maladies nerveuses* (Paris, 1883), pp. 134, 138.

15. Richard von Krafft-Ebing, "Untersuchungen über Irresein zur Zeit der Menstruation," *Archiv für Psychiatrie*, 8 (1878), pp. 65–107; also his "Über pollutionsartige Vorgänge beim Weibe," *WMP*, 29 (April 1, 1888), pp. 465–470.

16. Erwin Kehrer, "Experimentelle Untersuchungen über nervöse Reflexe von verschiedenen Organen und peripheren Nerven auf den Uterus," *Archiv für Gynäkologie*, 90 (1910), pp. 169–212 (see p. 169 on reflexes from the uterus to the brain). Bernard Sigmund Schultze, "Gynäkologische Behandlung und Geistesstörung," *BKW*, 20 (June 4, 1883), pp. 341–343: "Kein Uteruskatarrh . . . keine Retroflexion, kein alter Dammriss dürfte unerkannt in einer Irren-Heilanstalt verweilen" (p. 341).

17. Henry Macnaughton-Jones, "Uterine Reflexes, Distant Lesions, and Remote Symptoms due to Uterine Irritation," *British Gynaecological Journal,* 9 (1893–94), pp. 133–148; the discussion following this paper (pp. 148–167) reads like a parade of the dinosaurs in British gynecology of those years.

18. See Shorter, *History of Women's Bodies* (New York: Basic Books, 1982), pp. 276–281.

19. Of previous work on the history of sexual surgery, the only monographic treatment is G. J. Barker-Benfield, *The Horrors of the Half-Known Life: Male Attitudes toward Women and Sexuality in Nineteenth-Century America* (New York: Harper & Row, 1976). The present account diverges sharply on some points of interpretation.

20. See the extensive mid-nineteenth-century debates on the use of the speculum, as for example at the London Obstetrical Society's trial of the clitoridectomist Isaac Baker-Brown, *MTG,* 33 (April 6, 1867), p. 371.

21. Robert Brudenell Carter, *On the Pathology and Treatment of Hysteria* (London, 1853), p. 67.

22. See Edward Shorter, *Bedside Manners: The Troubled History of Doctors and Patients* (New York: Simon & Schuster, 1985), pp. 110–113.

23. Benjamin Fordyce Barker, "On the Diseases and Functional Disorders of the Sexual Organs in Women, as an Exciting Cause of Insanity," *Journal of the Gynaecological Society of Boston,* 6 (1872), pp. 335–350; case from pp. 346–347.

24. Heinrich Laehr, "Irrthümer der Diagnose in Psychosen," *Allgemeine Zeitschrift für Psychiatrie,* 26 (1869), pp. 369–372; quote from p. 369.

25. See the noted ovariotomist Spencer Wells's review of the operation's remote history, "Castration in Mental and Nervous Diseases: A Symposium," *American Journal of the Medical Sciences,* n.s. 82 (1886), pp. 455–471. For secondary accounts see Herbert R. Spencer, "The History of Ovariotomy," *Proceedings of the Royal Society of Medicine,* 27 (1934), pp. 1437–1444, and Lawrence D. Longo, "The Rise and Fall of Battey's Operation: A Fashion in Surgery," *Bulletin of the History of Medicine,* 53 (1979), pp. 244–267.

26. Alfred Hegar, "Die Castration der Frauen," *(Volkmann) Sammlung klinischer Vorträge,* nos. 136–138 (Gyn. no. 42 [n.d., about 1878]), pp. 925–1068; case history from p. 1057. Although Hegar specifically condemned Battey's indication of castration for ovarian neurosis (p. 1018), in fact Hegar admitted such operations through a kind of escape clause. Castration, in his view, was "only exceptionally justified," the presence of an ovarian neurosis being "exceedingly difficult to demonstrate and only in a few cases" (p. 1012). Battey did not disagree with this.

27. For details see Dr. David Yandell's interview with Battey in the October 1875 issue of the *American Practitioner,* reprinted as David W. Yandell and Ely McClellan (interviewers), *Battey's Operation* (Louisville, 1875); Rob-

ert Battey, "Extirpation of the Functionally Active Ovaries for the Remedy of Otherwise Incurable Diseases," *American Gynaecological Society Transactions,* 1 (1876), pp. 101–120; case from pp. 102–103; in a talk before the International Medical Congress in London in 1881, Battey explained how he had conceived the idea for the procedure and gave the exact date of the first. Summarized in *ZBG,* 5 (1881), pp. 403–406.

28. See James Marion Sims, "Remarks on Battey's Operation," *BMJ,* ii (December 29, 1877), pp. 916–918. Sims proposed that both ovaries invariably be removed; Battey on occasion had spared one.

29. Robert Battey, "Is There a Proper Field for Battey's Operation?" *American Gynaecological Society Transactions,* 2 (1877), pp. 279–305.

30. Alfred Hegar, "Castration als Mittel gegen nervöse und psychische Leiden," *Archiv für Gynäkologie,* 24 (1884), pp. 318–320; quote from p. 320.

31. On Wells's one thousand ovariotomies see editorial, *BMJ,* i (June 19, 1980), pp. 931–932; the very term *ovariotomy* presupposed organicity. On Tait's twelve-month operating record see his "Note on Oophorectomy," ibid., ii (July 10, 1880), pp. 48–49.

32. Alexander Russell Simpson, "History of a Case of Double Oophorectomy, or Battey's Operation," ibid., i (May 24, 1879), pp. 763–766; case from p. 763. She survived.

33. Heywood Smith, "Successful Case of Battey's Operation, or Oophorectomy," ibid., ii (July 12, 1879), pp. 41–45.

34. Discussion summarized in "I. Bericht über die Verhandlungen der gynäkologischen Section der Naturforscherversammlung zu Baden-Baden," *ZBG,* 3 (1879), pp. 181 181.

35. George J. Engelmann, "Battey's Operation; Three Fatal Cases, with Some Remarks Upon the Indications for the Operation," *AJO,* 11 (1878), pp. 459–481 (in two of the fatal cases the indications had been "reflex," in a third there was evidence of preexisting pelvic infection). William Goodell, "A Case of Spaying for Fibroid Tumour of the Womb," *American Journal of the Medical Sciences,* n.s., 76 (1878), pp. 36–50; the case of a "maiden literary lady" of thirty-three who had become a "monomaniac" on the subject of her ovary. She was a patient of Silas Weir Mitchell's, who also assisted at the operation. Goodell had by this time done one other castration as well. For further details see his comments in a discussion, *American Gynaecological Society Transactions,* 2, (1877), p. 301.

36. Doctor Barss operated at the encouragement of Boston neurologist George Lincoln Walton; see Walton, "A Contribution to the Study of Hysteria, Bearing on the Question of Oophorectomy," *JNMD,* 11 (1884), pp. 424–434; case from pp. 431–434; she was cured of most of her symptoms.

37. J. Taber Johnson, "A Case of Removal of the Uterine Appendages for the Cure of Nymphomania and Uterine Myoma. Death on the Ninth Day from Septic Peritonitis Caused by the Rupture of an Abscess," *AJO,* 21 (1888), p. 940.

38. Robert T. Edes, "The New England Invalid," *BMSJ*, 133 (July 25, 1895), pp. 77–81; quote from p. 77. Edes opposed the operation.

39. Frank Billings, "Gynaecology from the Standpoint of the Medical Man," *AJO*, 50 (1904), pp. 534–537 for his general comments; case from p. 536.

40. William R. Houston, *The Art of Treatment* (New York, 1936), p. 50.

41. I owe these statistics to a graduate research paper by Karen J. Bottomley, "The History of Oophorectomies: A Critique of the Feminist 'Male Dominance' Explanatory Model," University of Toronto, May, 1978. These statistics exclude a much larger number of articles on ovariotomies done for organic disease of the ovaries themselves. The surgeon general's *Index-Catalogue* distinguished between ovariotomies for cysts, tumors, et cetera and "ovariotomy not for ovarian tumors," a category synonymous with oophorectomy and Battey's operation.

42. "VIII. Internationaler medicinischer Kongress zu Kopenhagen, August 1884," *ZBG*, 8 (September 20, 1884), pp. 593–595. "Aus der Berliner Medicinischen Gesellschaft 9 April 1884," *DMW*, 10 (May 1, 1884), pp. 276–277, which summarized Leopold Landau's presentation of patients with "ovarie." For perspective on these meetings see Carl König and Georg Linzenmeier, "Über die Bedeutung gynäkologischer Erkrankungen und den Wert ihrer Heilung bei Psychosen," *Archiv für Psychiatrie*, 51 (1913), pp. 1002–1054, especially p. 1028. On oophorectomy in Germany generally see also Günter Burger, *Nerven- und Geisteskrankheiten als Indikationen für eine bilaterale Oophorektomie im späten 19. Jahrhundert* (Erlangen-Nürnberg med. diss., 1984).

43. Hermann Klotz, "Gynäkologische Mittheilungen," *WMW*, 32 (September 23, September 30, October 7, October 14, 1882); the case is presented on pp. 1194–1195 and 1209–1210 of the last two issues.

44. Josef Peretti, "Gynäkologische Behandlung und Geistesstörung," *BKW*, 20 (March 5, 1883), pp. 141–145; quote from p. 141.

45. Summary of a talk by Max Eduard Hermann Schede at a medical society meeting, *DMW*, 13 (June 23, 1887), pp. 555–556, case 7.

46. Sigmund Gottschalk, "Ein Fall von Anosmie nach operativer Entfernung beider Eierstöcke," *DMW*, 17 (June 25, 1891), pp. 823–824.

47. Pierre-Constant Budin, "Opération de Battey—Extirpation des ovaires," *Prog. méd.*, 6 (February 23, 1878), pp. 137–139; the Parisian surgeon Simon Emmanuel Duplay evidently performed the first in 1880, according to Charles Maygrier, in a review in ibid., 14 (February 20, 1886), pp. 162–163, of Léon Tissier's work, *De la castration de la femme en chirurgie (opération d'Hegar ou de Battey)* (Paris: med. thesis, 1885). Maygrier found that the operation had taken off in France in the last few years after an initial period of reserve.

48. François Villar, "Ablation des ovaires—opération de Battey," *Prog. méd.*, 16 (March 24, 1888), pp. 225–228; quote from p. 227. The great Paris surgeon Jules Péan was said to have performed the operation in 1882. Henri Cesbron, *Histoire critique de l'hystérie* (Paris, 1909), p. 171.

49. Georges Gilles de la Tourette, *Traité clinique et thérapeutique de l'hystérie*, 3 vols. (Paris, 1891–95), vol. 1, pp. 99–100, p. 320, on the "compresseur ovarien." See also Salpêtrien Romain Vigouroux's hostile remarks, in "Notice thérapeutique," an addendum to Fernand Levillain, *La Neurasthénie: maladie de Beard* (Paris, 1891), pp. 265–266. One of his young patients was castrated a month before she was to be married and died one day following the operation.

50. George H. Rohé, "The Relation of Pelvic Disease and Physical Disturbances in Women," *AJO*, 26 (1892), pp. 694–726. For his first operation, done October 13, 1891, see p. 704.

51. S. E. D. Shortt, *Victorian Lunacy: Richard M. Bucke and the Practice of Late-Nineteenth-Century Psychiatry* (Cambridge, England: Cambridge University Press, 1986), pp. 143–159. See also Wendy Mitchinson, "A Medical Debate in Nineteenth-Century English Canada: Ovariotomies," *Histoire sociale—Social History*, 17, (1984), pp. 133–147.

52. Thomas G. Morton, "Removal of the Ovaries as a Cure for Insanity," *American Journal of Insanity*, 49 (1893), pp. 397–401. The author opposed such procedures. He observed of the Norristown asylum that "several insane patients have already had their ovaries extirpated"(p. 397).

53. George H. Rohé, "The Etiological Relation of Pelvic Disease in Women to Insanity," *BMJ*, ii (September 25, 1897), pp. 766–769; quotes from p. 767. In this issue A. T. Hobbs also gave an account of his operations, "Surgical Gynaecology in Insanity," pp. 769–770.

54. George Henry Noble, "Traumatisms and Malformations of the Female Genital Apparatus and Their Relation to Insanity," *JAMA*, 35 (September 1, 1900), pp. 531–534.

55. Margaret Abbie Cleaves, *The Medical and Moral Care of Female Patients in Hospitals for the Insane* (n.p., 1879; reprint of a paper she delivered in June 1879 at the annual meeting in Chicago of the National Conference of Charities. Cleaves herself was a chronic somatizer. See her absorbing account of her symptoms, *The Autobiography of a Neurasthene* (Boston, 1910).

56. Constance M. McGovern, "Doctors or Ladies? Women Physicians in Psychiatric Institutions, 1872–1900," *Bulletin of the History of Medicine*, 55 (1981), pp. 88–107; detail from p. 100.

57. On the female physician at the Adams Nervine Asylum see Robert T. Edes, "Ovariotomy for Nervous Disease," *BMSJ*, 130 (February 1, 1894), pp. 105–107; case 1 from p. 105. Also Edes, "The New England Invalid," ibid., 133 (July 25, 1895), pp. 77–81; detail from p. 77. She had urged it upon female patients, then underwent the operation herself. She had been having fits and a hysterical blindness, going on to "hopeless insanity" after attempting to commit suicide by jumping out of a window.

58. Mary Putnam Jacobi, *Essays on Hysteria, Brain-Tumor and Other Cases of Nervous Disease* (New York, 1883), p. 79. Karen Bottomley (1978 research

paper) further cites the following sources, which I have not seen: Mary A. D. Jones, "Oophorectomy in Diseases of the Nervous System," *Medical and Surgical Reporter,* 68 (1893), pp. 797–806; Elizabeth C. Keller, "A Case of Laparotomy," *Reports of the Proceedings of the Alumnae Association of Women's Medical College* (1887), pp. 61–65; Amelia M. Fendler, "Report of Laparotomy for Removal of Ovaries," *Maryland Medical Journal,* 27 (1892), p. 974; Anita E. Tyng, "A Case of Removal of Both Ovaries by Abdominal Section for the Relief of an Exhausting Menorrhagia and Uterine Fibroid," *Transactions of the Rhode Island Medical Society,* 2 (1881), pp. 265–275. Sarah Stage erroneously writes, "For the most part, criticism of sexual surgery came from women who saw in male medical practice misogyny translated into medical treatment" (*Female Complaints: Lydia Pinkham and the Business of Women's Medicine* [New York: Norton, 1979], p. 81). As the above demonstrates, women physicians often supported sexual surgery. The main critics were male proponents of the central nervous paradigm.

59. Paul Flechsig, "Zur gynäkologischen Behandlung der Hysterie," *NCB,* 3 (October 1, 1884), pp. 433–439. Further cases followed.

60. See Westphal's case notes, as published in Karl Schröder, "Über die Castration bei Neurosen," *Zeitschrift für Geburtshilfe,* 13 (1886), pp. 325–338; notes on this case from pp. 330–335.

61. Moritz Benedikt, "Das Hinüber und Herüber in der Gynäkologie," *WMW,* 53 (January 3, 1903), pp. 14–21. Benedikt was responding to Kroenig's book *Über die Bedeutung der funktionellen Nervenkrankheiten für die Diagnostik und Therapie in der Gynäkologie* (Leipzig, 1902). In 1903 Kroenig became professor of gynecology at the University of Jena.

62. See Melchior Fremont Kranz, *Clitoridectomie historisch-kritisch dargestellt* (Strasbourg: med. diss., 1891), pp. 50–52.

63. Anthelme Richerand, *Nosographie chirurgicale,* 2nd ed, 4 vols. (Paris, 1808; 1st ed. 1805), vol. 4, p. 327.

64. Robert Thomas, *The Modern Practice of Physic,* 4th ed. (New York, 1817; 5th London ed. 1816), p. 619. The 3rd edition of this work (New York, 1811) contains no reference to clitoridectomy.

65. The anonymous family doctor reported the case, mentioning Graefe as the surgeon. "Heilung eines vieljährigen Blödsinns durch Ausrottung der Clitoris," [in Carl Ferdinand von Graefe's and Ph. von Walther's] *Journal der Chirurgie und Augen-Heilkunde,* 7 (1825), pp. 7–37, details of operation p. 29. In 1838 Berlin physician H. S. Michaelis approvingly summarized in ibid., (vol. 27, pp. 679–681) a similar case of clitoridectomy reported by "Riberi" in *Repertorio delle scienze mediche del Piemonte,* 1837.

66. Dietrich Wilhelm Heinrich Busch, *Das Geschlechtsleben des Weibes,* 5 vols. (Leipzig, 1839–44), vol. 4 (1843), pp. 686–687, vol. 5 (1844), p. 222. For further "traditional" literature on clitoridectomy, see references in Étienne-Jean Georget, *De la physiologie du système nerveux,* 2 vols. (Paris, 1821),

vol. 2, p. 168. John Macfarlane, senior surgeon at the Royal Infirmary in Glasgow, described the surgical excision of morbidly enlarged clitorises. *Clinical Reports of the Surgical Practice of the Glasgow Infirmary* (Glasgow, 1832), pp. 155–157.

67. Claude-Marie-Stanislas Sandras, *Traité pratique des maladies nerveuses*, 2 vols. (Paris, 1851), vol. 2, p. 233.

68. Jean-Baptiste Louyer-Villermay, *Recherches historiques et médicales sur l'hypochondrie, isolée, par l'observation et l'analyse, de l'hystérie et de la mélancholie* (Paris, 1802), p. 54.

69. Raoul LeRoy d'Étiolles, *Des paralysies des membres inférieurs ou paraplégies*, 2 vols. (Paris, 1856–57), vol. 1, p. 220.

70. Jacques Lisfranc, *Clinique chirurgicale de l'hôpital de la Pitié*, 2 vols. (Paris, 1842), vol. 2, p. 594. After discussing icepacks, phlebotomy, and so on, he said, "Je m'abstiens d'exposer certaine pratique honteuse et absurde que je signale seulement pour la blâmer et la rejeter à tout jamais."

71. Isaac Baker Brown, *On Surgical Diseases of Women*, 2nd ed. (London, 1861; 1st ed. 1854), pp. 233–234. I have not seen the 1st edition and it is possible that there he recommends clitoridectomy as well, but if so it aroused no comment.

72. London, 1866.

73. The above facts are according to Lawson Tait, "Masturbation," *Medical News*, 53 (July 7, 1888), pp. 1–3. Tait referred to Brown's very "extensive cerebral softening," a phrase that usually indicated general paralysis of the insane, or neurosyphilis. Lawson Tait mentioned that he himself had once done a clitoridectomy to stop chronic masturbation, apparently before 1867.

74. On this story see J. B. Fleming, "Clitoridectomy—The Disastrous Downfall of Isaac Baker Brown, F.R.C.S. (1867)," *Journal of Obstetrics and Gynaecology of the British Empire*, 67 (1960), pp. 1017–1034.

75. From "Obstetrical Society of London, Wednesday, April 3, Special Meeting," *MTG*, 33 (April 6, 1867), pp. 366–378 for the trial as a whole; quote from p. 375.

76. "On the Restoration of the Clitoris," ibid., 32 (October 27, 1866), p. 465.

77. William Murray, *A Treatise on Emotional Disorders of the Sympathetic System of Nerves* (London, 1866), p. 78.

78. R. S. Sisson, letter, *Lancet*, ii (July 28, 1866), p. 114.

79. Thomas Hawkes Tanner, "On Excision of the Clitoris as a Cure for Hysteria etc.," *Obstetrical Transactions*, 8 (1867), pp. 360–375, especially pp. 369–370. After these experiences Tanner rejected clitoridectomy in favor of Battey's operation.

80. Robert D. Harling, "Clitoridectomy," *BMJ*, i (January 12, 1867), pp. 40–41.

81. Clitoridectomy had never been as popular in France and elsewhere in Europe as in the Anglo-Saxon world, possibly because Continentals were less

exercised about the horrors of masturbation. Among the few midcentury reports of clitoridectomy I have seen are Gustav Braun, "Die Amputation der Clitoris und Nymphen: ein Beitrag zur Behandlung des Vaginismus," *WMW*, 15 (September 13, 1865), pp. 1325–1328; and Braun, "Ein weiterer Beitrag zur Heilung der Masturbation durch Amputation der Clitoris und der kleinen Schamlippen," ibid., 16 (March 14, 1866), pp. 329–331. Vigouroux, in Levillain, *La Neurasthénie*, p. 265, alludes ironically to clitoridectomy and operations on the labia in France as having "fait merveille chez nombre de névropathes." I have seen no detailed French reports.

82. Mentioned in J. Arkwright, "Excision of the Clitoris and Nymphae," *BMJ*, i (January 28, 1871), p. 88. The patient, a thirty-nine-year-old womar., evidently had anorexia nervosa. The procedure "cured" her.

83. See the discussion following Robert Barnes's paper, "On the Correlations of the Sexual Functions and Mental Disorders of Women," *British Gynaecological Journal*, 6 (1890), pp. 390–407 for the paper; pp. 407–430 for the discussion. Heywood Smith strongly defended it (p. 421). Percy Smith observed that some nameless physician had clitoridectomized a patient before she entered Smith's asylum (p. 425); Barnes himself displayed open-mindedness on the subject (p. 430).

84. Harry Gage Moore, letter on "Clitoridectomy," *Lancet*, i (June 23, 1866), p. 699.

85. Moritz Rosenthal, *Zur Diagnose und Therapie der Magenkrankheiten insbesondere der Neurosen des Magens* (Vienna, 1883), p. 20. For other German cautery references see Kranz, *Clitoridektomie* (1891), p. 95.

86. Macnaughton-Jones, *Points of Interest in Gynaecology* (1901), pp. 88–89.

87. For example, Lewis A. Sayre, "Spinal Anaemia with Partial Paralysis and Want of Coordination, from Irritation of the Genital Organs," *American Medical Association Transactions*, 26 (1875), pp. 255–274g, especially pp. 262–266. Newton M. Shaffer, who opposed the practice, said he had seen a number of patients in whom other physicians had performed clitoridectomy "for the cure of supposed reflex symptoms." "On Indiscriminate Circumcision," *Annals of Anatomy and Surgery*, 3 (1881), pp. 243–247; quote from p. 247.

88. See for example H. E. Beebe, "The Clitoris," and E. H. Pratt, "Circumcision of Girls," *Journal of Orificial Surgery*, 6 (1897–98), pp. 8–12 and 385–392, on the value of "freeing up" the clitoris.

89. For example, in the *American Journal of Obstetrics* see, Horatio Robinson Storer, "Obstinate Erotomania," 1 (1869), pp. 423–426; Horatio R. Bigelow, "An Aggravated Instance of Masturbation in the Female," 15 (1882), pp. 436–441; W. Gill Wylie, "Amputation of the Clitoris," 43 (1901), pp. 720–723; see neurologist Archibald Church's scathing comments on the practice in a discussion, 50 (1904), pp. 537–542; Carlton C. Frederick, "Nymphomania as a Cause of Excessive Venery," 56 (1907), pp. 807–812.

90. Walter C. Alvarez, *Nervousness, Indigestion and Pain* (New York, 1943), pp. 76–77. Alvarez came to the Mayo Clinic in 1926.
91. Carl Backhaus, in discussion, *ZBG*, 25 (1901), p. 1330.
92. William O. Priestly, "On Over-Operating in Gynaecology," *BMJ*, ii (August 3, 1895), pp. 284–287. Cf. Thomas Clifford Allbutt's strictures about women "entangled in the net of the gynaecologist." *On Visceral Neuroses* (London, 1884), p. 17.
93. For example, Vigouroux, in Levillain, *La Neurasthénie*, p. 267. Jules Batuaud, *La Neurasthénie génitale féminine* (Paris, 1906), pp. 187–188. It is interesting that both Batuaud and Priestly were thought by their colleagues to be rather old-fashioned and conservative.
94. Carlton C. Frederick, "Neurasthenia Accompanying and Simulating Pelvic Disease," *AJO*, 32 (1895), pp. 829–834; quote from p. 833.
95. Joseph Taber Johnson, "Four Cases of Oophorectomy, with Remarks," *American Gynaecological Society Transactions*, 10 (1885), pp. 119–146; case from pp. 123–124.
96. Paul Mundé, summary of talk, "Removal of the Ovarian and Fallopian Tubes, Followed by the Disappearance of Symptoms of Spinal Atrophy," *AJO*, 17 (1884), pp. 1162–1163. For a similar case of Mundé's, see his article, "My Experience with Oophorectomy for the Cure of Hystero-Epilepsy," *AJO*, 25 (1892), pp. 454–460; case from pp. 455–456. The patient committed suicide three months after the much-desired operation.
97. Schröder, *Zeitschrift für Geburtshilfe*, pp. 337–338.
98. George Bernard Shaw, *The Doctor's Dilemma: A Tragedy* (first published 1911) (Harmondsworth, England: Penguin, 1946), pp. 18–19.
99. Albert Krecke, "Die weibliche Asthenie und die Mania operatoria activa und passiva," *MMW*, 72 (July 24, 1925), pp. 1231–1232; quote from p. 1232.
100. Rudolf Schindler, "Die Psychotherapie des Organspecialisten," ibid., 72 (September 4, 1925), pp. 1517–1518.
101. Paul Chevallier, "Le Diagnostic d'hystérie n'est il qu'un aveu d'ignorance?" *L'Hôpital*, 11 (1923), pp. 548–550; case from p. 549.
102. Karl A. Menninger, "Polysurgery and Polysurgical Addiction," *Psychoanalytic Quarterly*, 3 (1934), pp. 173–199; case from pp. 194–196.
103. Mandel E. Cohen, "Excessive Surgery in Hysteria," *JAMA*, 151 (March 21, 1953), pp. 977–986. Among later contributions see George Winokur and Charles Leonard, "Sexual Life in Patients with Hysteria," *Diseases of the Nervous System*, 24 (1963), pp. 337–343; Ronald L. Martin et al., "Psychiatric Illness and Non-Cancer Hysterectomy," ibid., 38 (1977), pp. 974–980.
104. See Jürgen Ludwig and Ruth J. Mann, "Münchhausen Versus Munchausen," *Mayo Clinic Proceedings*, 58 (1983), pp. 767–769.
105. Joseph D. Bryant, "Report of the Fourth Laparotomy on a Hysterical Patient," *Medical Record*, 42 (December 24, 1892), pp. 726–728.

106. Carsten Holthouse, "Epilepsy . . . Operation of Castration," *Lancet*, i (January 22, 1859), pp. 81–82.

107. For Kroemer's theoretical acceptance of castrating males, see his "Beitrag zur Castrationsfrage," *Allgemeine Zeitschrift für Psychiatrie*, 52 (1896), pp. 1–74, 69–70, on males. On his actual castrating of hebephrenic (schizophrenic) and epileptic male patients, see Theodor Kirchhoff, ed., *Deutsche Irrenärzte: Einzelbilder ihres Lebens und Wirkens*, 2 vols. (Berlin, 1921–24), vol. 2, p. 264.

108. Richard Dewey, "Nervous and Mental Diseases in General Practice," *Wisconsin Medical Journal*, no. 5 (February, 1907), pp. 453–461; quote from p. 458.

109. Archibald Church, in discussion, *AJO*, 50 (1904), p. 537.

110. For examples, see J. H. Hunt, "Partial Paralysis from Reflex Action Caused by Adherent Prepuce," *Medical Record*, 10 (October 9, 1875), pp. 692–693; and Charles Fayette Taylor, "Genital Irritation," *Annals of Anatomy and Surgery*, 4 (1881), pp. 1–7; case from pp. 4–5.

111. Lewis Albert Sayre, "Partial Paralysis from Reflex Irritation, Caused by Congenital Phimosis and Adherent Prepuce," *American Medical Association Transactions*, 21 (1870), pp. 205–211; quote from 211.

112. Moritz Wiederhold, "Varicocele und Neurasthenie und Verwandtes, nach Beobachtungen in meiner Anstalt," *DMW*, 17 (September 10, 1891), pp. 1069–1070. See also his *Nervenschwäche: Ihr Wesen und ihre Behandlung* (Wiesbaden, 1895), p. 7. I noted his conviction for assault as reported in *Lyon médical*, 2 (1892), p. 242.

CHAPTER 5

Motor Hysteria

1. Robert Brudenell Carter defined "simple hysteria" as fits ("This convulsive paroxysm is the essential characteristic of the disease."), and "complicated hysteria" as entailing (1) psychological changes and (2) the whole range of motor and sensory phenomena, not just fits. *On the Pathology and Treatment of Hysteria* (London, 1853), pp. 2–3. The substantial secondary literature on the history of "hysteria" as a diagnosis has been drawn together by Mark S. Micale, "Hysteria and Its Historiography: the Future Perspective," *History of Psychiatry*, 1 (1990), pp. 33–124.

2. A. Jean-Albert Pitres, *Leçons cliniques sur l'hystérie et l'hypnotisme*, 2 vols. (Paris, 1891), vol. 1, p. 52.

3. Frederick T. Simpson, "Hysteria: Its Nature and Treatment," *Psychotherapy*, 3 (1909), pp. 28–47, case p. 32.

4. The clinical literature differentiating hysteria from epilepsy is enormous. For current accounts see Robert J. Cohen and Cary Suter, "Hysterical Seizures: Suggestion as a Provocative EEG Test," *Annals of Neurology*, 11 (1982), pp. 391–395; Harold Merskey, *The Analysis of Hysteria* (London: Baillière Tindall, 1979), pp. 106–107; James Purves-Stewart, *The Diagnosis*

of Nervous Diseases, 9th ed. (London, 1945), pp. 159–160 (this being the most straightforward of accounts, yet Cohen's and Suter's findings diverge somewhat); Terence L. Riley and Alec Roy, eds., *Pseudoseizures* (Baltimore: Williams and Wilkins, 1982), especially pp. 23–26; and Rege S. Stewart et al., "Are Hysterical Seizures More than Hysteria . . . ," *AJP,* 139 (1982), pp. 926–929. Historians who have written on the problem of psychogenic versus neurogenic seizures include E. M. Thornton, *Hypnotism, Hysteria and Epilepsy* (London: Heinemann Medical Books, 1976), pp. 115–135, who believes that hysterical seizures did not exist, and Owsei Temkin, *The Falling Sickness: A History of Epilepsy from the Greeks to the Beginnings of Modern Neurology,* 2nd ed. (Baltimore: Johns Hopkins, 1971). Many nineteenth-century psychiatrists, neurologists, and gynecologists attempted to differentiate hysteria and epilepsy, yet by "epilepsy" they understood mainly "grand mal" seizures (omitting partial complex seizures and absence seizures), and doubtlessly were overinclusive with the notion of hysteria. On the coexistence of psychogenic and neurogenic seizures see Sumiya Komai, "A Study of Superimposition of Hysteria upon Epilepsy," *Folia Psychiatrica et Neurologica Japonica,* 37 (1983), pp. 267–270; Venkat Ramani, "Diagnosis of Hysterical Seizures in Epileptic Patients," *AJP,* 137 (1980), pp. 705–709; Alec Roy, "Hysterical Seizures," *Archives of Neurology,* 36 (1979), p. 36; and Daniel T. Williams et al., "Neurogenic and Hysterical Seizures in Children and Adolescents: Differential Diagnostic and Therapeutic Considerations," *AJP,* 135 (1978), pp. 82–86.

5. Pierre-Adolphe Piorry, *Traité de médecine pratique,* 9 vols. 1841–51, vol. 8 (Paris, 1850), pp. 379–381.

6. Joseph Amann, *Über den Einfluss der weiblichen Geschlechtskrankheiten auf das Nervensystem* . . . (Erlangen, 1868), p. 24.

7. One scholar has speculated that they might arise from a sense of "bodily depersonalization" (*dépossession corporelle*) on the patient's part: "Your body escapes you, it withdraws itself from your control. It demonstrates visibly that it has a life of its own." Thus a psychic state of the "extériorité du corps," an externalization of the body, might be considered responsible for these fits. Gladys Swain, "L'âme, la femme, le sexe et le corps," *Le Débat,* no. 24 (March 1983), pp. 107–127; quote from p. 113. Swain further observes that twentieth-century women are probably the first in history not to have this sense of "dépossession corporelle."

8. Pierre Briquet, *Traité clinique et thérapeutique de l'hystérie* (Paris, 1859), pp. 495–496. In this work he gives the sample size as "les 400 et quelques malades que j'ai étudiées." In an article in 1881 on the subject, he refers to 450 cases seen at the Charité. "De la prédisposition à l'hystérie," *Bulletin de l'Académie de médecine,* Paris, 2nd ser., 10 (1881), pp. 1135–1153.

9. Ibid., p. 184. I have not included some of these lesser causes.

10. Jean-Baptiste Louyer-Villermay, *Recherches historiques et médicales sur l'hypochondrie, isolée . . . de l'hystérie et de la mélancholie* (Paris, 1802), pp. 41–44.

11. Thomas Addis Emmet, *Principles and Practice of Gynaecology,* 3rd ed. (London, 1885; 1st ed. 1879), pp. 185–187. J. Russell Reynolds told of a "married lady," mother of four, who came into University College Hospital, London, paraplegic and with a history of fits, also some loss of bowel control. "The first night that she was taken to the hospital, the evacuations occurred in bed; but she was told by the nurse that 'such things were not allowed,' and they never occurred again." "Remarks on Paralysis, and other Disorders of Motion and Sensation, Dependent on Idea," *BMJ,* ii (November 6, 1869), pp. 483–485; case from p. 485.

12. Moritz Benedikt, *Aus meinem Leben: Erinnerungen und Erörterungen* (Vienna, 1906), pp. 139–140, 161–162.

13. Robert Wollenberg, "Hysterie oder Simulation," *PNW,* 28 (May 8, 1926), pp. 211–212.

14. Henry Manning, *A Treatise on Female Diseases* (London, 1771), p. 204.

15. Adrian Wegelin, "Beobachtung, einer Nervenkrankheit nebst Heilung von Entstehung der Selbstbefleckung, bei einem Mädchen von 23 Jahren," *Johann Christ. Starks Archiv für die Geburtshülfe,* 4 (1792), pp. 101–109; details from pp. 103–105.

16. Felix Preissner, "Die Abteilung für Nervenkranke des Krankenhauses der Landesversicherungsanstalt Schlesien in Breslau," *PNW,* 27 (December 19, 1925), pp. 523–527.

17. Gerhart Pisk, "Über Veränderungen der hysterischen Symptomatologie in den letzten Jahren," *WKW,* 49 (1936), pp. 938–939. Once the "hysterical psychopaths" have been deducted from the men's total (there were no female psychopaths), fits represented 34 percent of the remaining total of men.

18. Israel S. Wechsler, *The Neuroses* (Philadelphia, 1929), p. 198.

19. Contemporary Medical Archives Centre, Wellcome Institute for the History of Medicine, London, Frederick Parkes Weber casebooks.

20. Margaret A. Cleaves, *The Autobiography of a Neurasthene, As Told by One of Them and Recorded by . . .* [the author] (Boston, 1910), pp. 99, 107, 115, 119. The autobiographical nature of the work is evident.

21. See Shorter, "Paralysis: The Rise and Fall of a 'Hysterical' Symptom," *Journal of Social History,* 19 (1986), pp. 549–582.

22. Jean-Baptiste Chevalier, "Mémoire et observations sur les effets des Eaux de Bourbonne-les-Bains en Champagne, dans les maladies hystériques et chroniques," *Journal de médecine,* 33 (1770), pp. 17–39 and 122–145, case pp. 30–33. Unfortunately Chevalier's evidence may have been somewhat contaminated by his pecuniary interest in publicizing the spa, for later contributors to the journal challenged the facts in some of the cases and suggested indeed that he had made some up. See Brun, "Réponse . . . ," ibid., pp. 255–259 and other letters ff. Chevalier had attacked the views of Pierre Pomme, an authority on nervous diseases, in his article. The editors saw the hand of Pierre Pomme behind several of the responses and defended Chevalier.

355

23. Louis Verhaeghe, *Du traitement des maladies nerveuses par les bains de mer* (Brussels, 1850), pp. 88–90.

24. For a bibliography of these studies see Glafira Abricossoff, *L'Hystérie aux xviie et xviiie siècles* (Paris: med. diss., 1897), pp. 142–145.

25. Charles-Humbert-Antoine Despine, *Observations de médecine pratique faites aux bains d'Aix-en-Savoie*, "premier numéro" (Annecy, 1838 [vol. actually published in 1839]), pp. 136–137.

26. Maurice Macario, "De la paralysie hystérique," *Annales médico-psychologiques*, 3 (1844), pp. 62–82; case from pp. 71–72. On the development of his own interest see Piorry, *Traité de médecine pratique* (1850), vol. 8, p. 384; on his treatments see pp. 397–398.

27. John Abernethy, *Surgical and Physiological Works*, 6th ed., 2 vols. (London, 1825), vol. 1, pp. 61–62; from his essay "On the Constitutional Origin and Treatment of Local Diseases," first published 1809.

28. John Abercrombie, *Pathological and Practical Researches on Diseases of the Brain and the Spinal Cord*, 3rd ed. (Edinburgh, 1836; 1st ed. 1828), pp. 403–404.

29. Hysteria was vastly overdiagnosed in the past, as many young women with that diagnosis probably had multiple sclerosis. Only with Joseph Babinski's discovery of the "cutaneous plantar reflex" in 1896 (upward-turning toe indicating the presence of an upper-motor neuron lesion), did the separation of MS and hysteria become more reliable, and even then it was not completely straightforward. The historian may not therefore accept contemporary diagnoses of hysteria at face value. Since World War II, several distinguished English neuropsychiatrists have argued that most hysteria was the result of undiagnosed organic brain disease. For a rebuttal of this hypothesis see Alec Roy, "Hysterical Neurosis," in Roy, ed., *Hysteria* (New York: Wiley, 1982), pp. 89–100.

30. A quintessential and common form of nonanatomical deficit were paralyses that just seemed to drift about the body, or "la paralysie erratique," as Paul Richer put it in his *Paralysies et contractures hystériques* (Paris, 1892), p. 45; see pp. 91–99 for the case of Albertine G.

31. Edward Sutleffe, *Medical and Surgical Cases, Selected During a Practice of Thirty-Eight Years* (London, 1824), pp. 292–293. For other early cases, see Henry J. Bond, "Tetanus and Hysteria," *LMG*, 9 (March 24, 1832), pp. 929–933, case of Mary Dockley; John Wilson, "Nervous Affections Peculiar to Young Women, Causing Contraction of the Muscles of the Extremities," *Royal Medico-Chirurgical Transactions*, 21 (1838), pp. 107–124, for a series of cases.

32. Arnold von Franque, "Vier Fälle von hysterischer Lähmung," *Correspondez-Blatt der deutschen Gesellschaft für Psychiatrie und gerichtliche Psychologie*, 7 (1860), pp. 33–42; case from pp. 33–34.

33. Jacques Lisfranc, *Clinique chirurgicale de l'hôpital de la Pitié*, 2 vols. (Paris, 1842), vol. 2, pp. 581–582.

34. Hector Landouzy, *Traité complet de l'hystérie* (Paris, 1846), pp. 106–107.

35. See Raoul LeRoy d'Étiolles, *Des paralysies des membres inférieurs ou paraplégies*, 2 vols. (Paris, 1856–57), vol. 1, pp. 188–190; J. B. T. Séraphin Barnier, *Des paralysies sans lésions organiques appréciables* (Paris: thèse . . . agrégation en médecine, 1857), p. 71.

36. Robert T. Edes, "The New England Invalid," *BMSJ*, 133 (July 18, 1895), pp. 53–57; quote from p. 56.

37. Henri Liouville and Georges-Maurice Debove, "Note sur un cas de mutisme hystérique, suivi de guèrison" *Prog. méd.*, 4 (February 26, 1876), pp. 145–146. At the St.-André Hospital in Bordeaux, paralysis was the second commonest form of hysteria following fits. Pitres, *Hystérie* (1891), vol. 1, p. 52.

38. According to Sébastien-Didier Lhéritier, *Eaux de Plombières: clinique médicale des paralysies*, "deuxième année," (Paris, 1854), p. 45; and Silas Weir Mitchell, *Lectures on Diseases of the Nervous System, Especially in Women* (London, 1881), pp. 20–21. According to Leopold Löwenfeld, however, while hemiplegias might be commoner in France, paraplegias were found more often in Germany. *Pathologie und Therapie der Neurasthenie und Hysterie* (Wiesbaden, 1894), p. 368.

39. See Ernest Mesnet, *Étude des paralysies hystériques* (Paris: med. thèse, 1852), p. 31. Auguste Axenfeld, *Traité des névroses* (1861), rev. ed. by Henri Huchard (Paris, 1883), p. 1012; the observation stems from the first edition. Paul Richer, *Paralysies et contractures hystériques* (Paris, 1892), p. 162. Armand Hückel, a medical lecturer in Tübingen, offered however the observation that paralyses of upper limbs were commoner than of lower. "Über psychische Lähmungen und ihre Behandlung," *MMW*, 36 (March 19, 1869), pp. 213–217; datum from p. 215.

40. LeRoy d'Étiolles, *Paralysies* (1856), vol. 1, p. 185, and Richer, *Paralysies* (1892), pp. 155–157, said monoplegias were commoner. Hermann Determann, at the time an assistant of Wilhelm Erb's in Heidelberg, said that monoplegias were rare, especially in Germany, and when they occurred they affected the upper limb rather than the lower. "Hysterische Monoplegie," *NCB*, 9 (1890), pp. 424–430; datum from p. 425.

41. Ap Morgan Vance, "Hysteria as the Surgeon Sees It," *AJO*, 58 (1908), pp. 757–767; case from p. 763. Dr. Vance, with his model bedside manner, said, "If it does draw up, I will break your d——d little neck." The limb, he adds, did not draw up and the child was cured.

42. See James N. Brawner, *The Mind and its Disorders* (Atlanta, 1942), pp. 196–197. The author owned a sanatorium in Smyrna.

43. William Gull, "Hysteric Paraplegia for Twelve Months," *Lancet*, i (January 17, 1863), pp. 62–63. They gave her purgatives and "electricity," and she was cured about five months later.

44. See J. S. Lawrence, *Rheumatism in Populations* (London: Heinemann Medical Books, 1977), pp. 211–212.

45. John Conolly, "Hysteria," in John Forbes et al., eds., *Cyclopaedia of Practical Medicine*, 5 vols., 1833–59, vol. 2 (London, 1833), pp. 557–586; quotes from p. 561.

46. Benjamin Travers, *A Further Inquiry Concerning Constitutional Irritation and the Pathology of the Nervous System* (London, 1835), pp. 272–273.

47. Benjamin C. Brodie, *Lectures Illustrative of Certain Local Nervous Affections* (London, 1837), pp. 48–53 (different printings have different paginations).

48. Mesnet, *Étude* (1852), p. 31. See also early accounts in Barnier, *Paralysies* (1857), p. 24, and LeRoy d'Étiolles, *Paralysies* (1856), vol. 1, pp. 208–209.

49. Sigismond Jaccoud, *Les Paraplégies et l'ataxie du mouvement* (Paris, 1864), pp. 653–654. Later writer was A. Duprat, *Contribution à l'étude des troubles moteurs psychiques; syndrome de Jaccoud (Astasie-Abasie)* (Paris: med. thèse, 1892), p. 15. Both of the cases Duprat reports sound like organic disease of the nervous system.

50. Paul Blocq, "Sur une affection caractérisée par de l'astasie et de l'abasie," *Archives de neurologie*, 15 (1888), pp. 24–51. Bloch received his medical degree that year, and the article was evidently part of his thesis. The only further contribution to shaping it came two years later from Otto Binswanger, professor of psychiatry at Jena, who saw it as a form of agoraphobia, a panicky fear of leaving the house. "Über psychisch bedingte Störungen des Stehens und des Gehens," *BKW*, 27 (May 19 and May 26, 1890), pp. 441–445, 473–478. Binswanger ridiculed the French desire to subdivide every symptom into many distinct "diseases."

51. Mitchell, *Lectures Diseases Nervous System* (1881), p. 48.

52. Lennart Ljungberg, *Hysteria: A Clinical, Prognostic and Genetic Study* (Copenhagen: Munksgaard, 1957), p. 44.

53. Semi Meyer, "Hysterie-Typen," *PNW*, 13 (April 8, 1911), pp. 16–18, quote p. 18.

54. Ernst von Leyden, "Ein Fall von Schrecklähmung," *BKW*, 42 (February 20, 1905), pp. 193–196. Case p. 193; on p. 196 it was added that she recovered after "faradization" (electrotherapy).

55. Theodor Clemens, "Paraplegia hysterica (Eine von Genitalienreizung ausgehende Reflexneurose)," *Deutsche Klinik*, 2 (1850), pp. 545–546.

56. Paul Maigre, *Quelques considérations sur l'astasie-abasie* (Paris: med. thèse, 1892); case from pp. 23–27.

57. Henry Charlton Bastian, *Various Forms of Hysterical or Functional Paralysis* (London, 1893), pp. 94–96. The pain later escalated into a full-blown paralysis of the left leg (cured with static electricity and injections of pure water).

58. Albert Charpentier, "Démarche à petits pas (Phobie hystérique de la marche)," *Revue neurologique*, 15 (1907), pp. 83–84.

59. Albert Beni-Barde, *La Neurasthénie: les vrais et les faux neurasthéniques* (Paris, 1908), pp. 65–68. Beni-Barde restored her from this "irritabilité de son système nerveux" with cold showers.

60. Auguste Voisin, *Leçons cliniques sur les maladies mentales et sur les maladies nerveuses* (Paris, 1883), pp. 188–189.

61. Historians of this large subject include E. Fischer-Homberger, *Die traumatische Neurose vom somatischen zum sozialen Leiden* (Berne: Hans Huber, 1975); Michael R. Trimble, *Post-Traumatic Neurosis: From Railway Spine to the Whiplash* (New York: Wiley, 1981); and Harold Merskey, "Shellshock," *London [Ontario] Psychiatric Hospital Bulletin,* 4 (1989), pp. 1–43.

62. Dennis De Berdt Hovell, *On Pain and Other Symptoms Connected with the Disease Called Hysteria* (London, 1867), p. 34.

63. Esnault, *Paralysies* (1857), pp. 28–29. Her medical attendants commenced cupping and scarifying her abdomen (des ventouses scarifiées). "On July 20 she could move the leg very slowly; fifteen leeches were applied." After further leeching the leg was restored to full mobility, and she could bear further uterine cauterization without incident.

64. Fraser, "A Case of Recovery from Reflex Paralysis," *MTG,* 32 (May 19, 1866), p. 518.

65. Louis Stromeyer, *Erfahrungen über Local-Neurosen* (Hanover, 1873), pp. 25–26.

66. Briquet, *Hystérie* (1859), pp. 504–507, both cases.

67. Jacob Friedrich Isenflamm, *Versuch einiger praktischen Anmerkungen über die Nerven zur Erläuterung . . . hypochondrisch- und hysterischer Zufälle* (Erlangen, 1774), p. 192.

68. Chevalier, *Journal de médecine* (1770), p. 133. He said of men, "Quoiqu'on ne puisse point les désigner, chez eux, sous le titre d'hystériques, il ne s'ensuit pas de-là qu'ils ne soient susceptibles du désordre des nerfs et de l'ataxie des esprits."

69. Travers, *Further Inquiry* (1835), pp. 266–269.

70. Landouzy, *Hystérie* (1846), p. 223.

71. Moritz Heinrich Romberg, *Lehrbuch der Nervenkrankheiten des Menschen,* 3rd ed. (Berlin, 1857), pp. 563–564.

72. Briquet, *Hystérie* (1859), pp. 15–17. For the discussion of male hysteria generally, see pp. 11–35.

73. Stromeyer, *Local-Neurosen* (1873), p. 39.

74. Maurice Krishaber, *De la névropathie cérébro-cardiaque* (Paris, 1873), pp. 6–9.

75. John W. Ogle, "A Case of Hysteria," *BMJ,* ii (July 16, 1870), p. 57 n.

76. Montrose A. Pallen, "Some Suggestions with Regard to the Insanities of Females," *AJO,* 10 (1877), pp. 206–217; quote from p. 207.

77. For this argument in greater detail, see Edward Shorter, *The Making of the Modern Family* (New York: Basic Books, 1975).

78. Josef Breuer and Sigmund Freud, "Studien über Hysterie" (1895), in *Gesammelte Werke,* vol. 1 (Frankfurt am Main: Fischer, 1952), p. 157 n.

79. Ernst von Leyden, *Lebenserinnerungen* (Stuttgart, 1910), p. 168.

80. Valentin von Holst, *Erfahrungen aus einer vierzigjährigen neurologischen Praxis* (Stuttgart, 1903), pp. 53–54.

81. Philip L. Harriman, "A Case of Hysterical Paralysis," *Journal of Abnormal Psychology,* 29 (1934–35), pp. 455–456.

82. Harry L. Parker, "Hysterical Paralysis," *Medical Clinics of North America*, 10 (3) (November, 1926), pp. 703–714; case from pp. 706–707.
83. Maria Rivet, *Les Aliénés dans la famille et dans la maison de santé* (Paris, 1875), pp. 227–233.
84. H. Sutter, "Weiterer Beitrag zur Kasuistik der nervösen Erkrankungen im Wochenbett," *ZBG*, 30 (August 25, 1906), pp. 945–954.
85. Albert E. Davis, *Hypnotism and Treatment by Suggestion*, 4th ed. (London, 1923; 1st ed. 1918), pp. 193–194.
86. John Thomas Banks, discussion comment following J. Russell Reynolds's paper, "Certain Forms of Paralysis Depending on Idea," *BMJ*, ii (October 2, 1869), p. 378. Doctor Banks cured her with a rhubarb pill, "and now she is able to walk miles."
87. On the role of anorexia nervosa in new-style emotional rivalries within the nineteenth-century family, see Shorter, "The First Great Increase in Anorexia Nervosa," *Journal of Social History*, 21 (1987), pp. 69–96; Joan Jacobs Brumberg, *Fasting Girls: the Emergence of Anorexia Nervosa as a Modern Disease* (Cambridge, Mass.: Harvard University Press, 1988), pp. 126–140.
88. William Osler, *The Principles and Practice of Medicine* (New York, 1892), p. 974.
89. Parker, *Medical Clinics North America* (1926), p. 703.
90. Ibid., p. 703
91. Byrom Bramwell, "Functional Paraplegia," *Clinical Studies*, n.s., 1 (1902–3), pp. 332–344; quotes from pp. 343–344.
92. Mitchell, *Lectures Diseases Nervous System* (1881), p. 31.
93. Brodie, *Lectures Nervous Affections* (1837), pp. 70–71. Brodie said, "The stump healed readily enough, but she obtained no relief. I had the opportunity of seeing her some months after the operation, suffering more than ever" (p. 71).
94. Frederic C. Skey, "Clinical Lecture on Hysteric Diseases," *Lancet*, i (February 24, 1855), pp. 205–207; reference from p. 207. ("Amputation of such limbs formerly practiced, left the diseased cause behind.")
95. Georg Friedrich Louis Stromeyer, *Erinnerungen eines deutschen Arztes*, 2nd ed., 2 vols. (Hanover, n.d. [1875]), vol. 2, p. 26. She did not have an anatomical deformity, and Stromeyer believed the problem would correct itself.
96. Benedikt, *Aus meinem Leben* (1906), p. 141.
97. Anna Robeson Burr, *Weir Mitchell, His Life and Letters* (New York, 1929), p. 184.
98. Abraham Myerson, "Hysterical Paralysis and its Treatment," *JAMA*, 105 (November 16, 1935), pp. 1565–1567; quote from p. 1565.
99. Vance, *AJO*, (1908), p. 762.

CHAPTER 6

Dissociation

1. For a *mise au point* see Nicholas P. Spanos, "Hypnosis, Nonvolitional Re-

sponding, and Multiple Personality: A Social Psychological Perspective," *Progress in Experimental Personality Research*, 14 (1986), pp. 1–62. One skeptical researcher is Graham F. Wagstaff, "Is Hypnotherapy a Placebo?" *British Journal of Experimental and Clinical Hypnosis*, 4 (1987), pp. 135–140.

2. See the somewhat neglected Traugott Konstantin Oesterreich, *Possession, Demoniacal and Other among Primitive Races, in Antiquity, the Middle Ages, and Modern Times* (1921), Eng. trans. (New Hyde Park, N.Y.: University Books, 1966).

3. For a list of various phenomena associated with somnambulism, see Friedrich Hufeland, "Ausserordentliche Erhöhung der Sensibilität; ein Beitrag zu den Erfahrungen über Somnambulismus und thierischen Magnetismus," *Archiv für die Physiologie*, 6 (1805), pp. 225–264, especially p. 234. On somnambulism as sleepwalking see (Karl Bernhard?) Brühl, "Feuilleton: Aus Pest," *WMW*, 2 (July 3, 1852), pp. 435–438, the story of "die Mondsüchtige," a twenty-two-year-old female servant who walked the rooftops at night.

4. John Jacob, "Case of Hysteria," *LMG*, n.s., 1 (1838), pp. 976–978. Jacob attributed her symptoms to irritation from the uterus and a constipated colon. Although Jacob's diagnosis of his patient's behavior may well have been influenced by talk of "animal magnetism" going on about them, he made no reference to it.

5. On different traditions of defining catalepsy, see Claude-Étienne Bourdin, *Traité de la catalepsie* (Paris, 1841), p. vii.

6. Pierre Pomme, *Traité des affections vaporeuses des deux sexes*, 3rd ed. (Lyon, 1767; 1st ed. 1763), pp. 36–37.

7. John Maubray, *The Female Physician* (London, 1724), pp. 405–406.

8. John Conolly, "Hysteria," in John Forbes et al., eds., *Cyclopaedia of Practical Medicine*, 5 vols. (1833–56), vol. 2 (London, 1833), p. 560.

9. Franz Xaver Mezler, "Beobachtung einer Starrsucht (Catalepsis)," *Medicinisch-chirurgische Zeitung*, 1 (1794), pp. 139–141.

10. J. Munk, "Über wirkliche und simulirte Katalepsie," *WMP*, 21 (May 23, 1880), pp. 677–680. Some consciousness returned, but for three weeks Schwartz could not speak nor open his eyes. He was "cured" after being transferred to the Allgemeines Krankenhaus in Vienna, and several months later remembered virtually nothing of the entire episode.

11. Silas Weir Mitchell, *Lectures on Diseases of the Nervous System, Especially in Women* (London, 1881), pp. 179–180.

12. Thomas Hall Shastid, *My Second Life* (Ann Arbor, 1944), pp. 907–908.

13. Joachim Friedländer, "Sind die in der Catalepsie vorkommenden Erscheinungen, die wächserne Biegsamkeit nämlich und der Starrkrampf, ihrer Natur oder dem Grade nach verschieden?" *Medicinische Jahrbücher des k.k. österreichischen Staates*, NF, 17 (1838), pp. 206–220; cases from pp. 209–211.

14. For a history of animal magnetism and hypnotism, written from the viewpoint of the true believer, see Eric J. Dingwall, *Abnormal Hypnotic Phenomena: A Survey of Nineteenth-Century Cases,* 4 vols. (London: Churchill, 1967–68). Dingwall himself wrote the monograph on France, which takes up the entirety of volume one.

15. The point of departure for all writing on Mesmer is Henri Ellenberger's magisterial *The Discovery of the Unconscious* (New York: Basic Books, 1970), p. 57 f. On Mesmer in France, see also Robert Darnton, *Mesmerism and the End of the Enlightenment in France* (Cambridge, Mass.: Harvard University Press, 1968).

16. See Ellenberger, *Discovery* (1970), p. 70 f.

17. I have compiled these from the four different "series" of subject listings of medical titles, published as *Index-Catalogue of the Library of the Surgeon-General's Office, United States Army* between the 1880s and the 1940s, the most important medical bibliography in the world for the pre–World War II period. I enumerated all books and articles under the headings "animal magnetism," "somnambulism" and "hypnosis-hypnotism." The decade totals for these years were: 1800–9, 16; 1810–19, 71; 1820–29, 61; 1830–39, 94; 1840–49, 190; 1850–59, 138; 1860–69, 77.

18. Carl Alexander Ferdinand Kluge, *Versuch einer Darstellung des animalischen Magnetismus* (Berlin, 1811), pp. iii–v, xi.

19. Heinrich Löw, "Über Bio-Magnetismus mit Bezugnahme auf die Dynamide Reichenbachs," *WMW,* 1 (August 30, 1851), pp. 345–348.

20. Jacques-Étienne Belhomme, in discussion, *Annales médico-psychologiques,* 3 (1858), p. 261.

21. See Maurice Macario, "De la paralysie hystérique," *Annales médico-psychologiques,* 3 (1844), pp. 62–82, especially p. 82; Piorry, *Traité de médecine pratique,* 9 vols., 1841–51, vol. 8 (Paris, 1850), p. 398, on the zealous medical student on Piorry's service who cured a case of hysterical paralysis with "passes magnétiques." Piorry himself gave a paper in 1859 on hypnotism to the Academy of Sciences in Paris, which I have not seen ("L'hypnotisme," *Compt. rend. Acad. d. sc.,* 49 [1859], p. 987 f.).

22. In Charles-Humbert-Antoine Despine's classification of "maladies nerveuses," or "phénomènes nerveux" that could be reproduced under animal magnetism, catalepsy, "spasmes hystériques," and somnambulism are placed along the same spectrum; in fact somnambulism was treated as a subform of catalepsy. *Observations de médecine pratique faites aux bains d'Aix-en-Savoie,* "premier numéro" (Annecy, 1838), pp. 277–278.

23. Joseph Skoda, "Geschichte einer durch mehrere Monate anhaltenden Katalepsis," *Zeitschrift der kais. kön. Gesellschaft der Ärzte zu Wien,* 8 (2) (1852), pp. 404–419; details from pp. 404–407. It is probable though not certain that Schoder's first name was Johann.

24. *Mémoire sur la découverte des phénomènes que présent la catalepsie et le somnambulisme, symptômes de l'affection hystérique essentielle* . . . "Seconde par-

tie" (n.p, 1787); I have not seen this edition but rather a later and possibly revised edition published anonymously by his son Félix Petetin, *Électricité animale, prouvé par la découverte des phénomènes physiques et moraux de la catalepsie hystérique . . . par M. Petetin* (Paris, 1808). Petetin died in 1808. This volume contains, paginated separately, a "Notice historique sur la vie et les ouvrages de J.-H. Désiré Petetin."

25. See, for example, Bourdin, *Catalepsie* (1841), who scorned all this talk of vision being transported to the stomach and so forth (pp. 5–6).

26. Petetin, *Électricité animale* (1808), pp. xi–xiii, 14, 112; see also the interbound memoir of his life, pp. 39–40.

27. Ibid, pp. 1–110.

28. Despine, *Observations* (1838), p. 242. A "Dr. Pizzati" had encouraged him to try it.

29. Ibid., pp. 227–228.

30. "Ecstasy" has a deeper meaning in the context of Third World anthropology: the soul on a mission leaving the body of a shaman—during which the shaman goes into a cataleptic trance—then returning to his body. Yet this dimension of ecstasy is absent in the phenomena under discussion here. See for example Mircea Eliade, *Shamanism: Archaic Techniques of Ecstasy* (1951), Eng. trans. (New York: Bollingen, 1964).

31. Despine, *Observations* (1838), pp. 228–229.

32. Ibid., pp. 230–232.

33. Letter of September 4, 1844, to Doctor Despine. The correspondence between Despine and Mme. L. is in the departmental archives of the Haute-Savoie department at Annecy, shelf no. 45 J 117. I am grateful to Herr Mario von Moos of Fehraltorf, Switzerland, for helping ascertain Mme. L.'s date of birth and identifying the distinguished family from the Vaud canton into which she was born. Unlike the names of Doctor Despine's other patients, hers is not a matter of public record.

34. Alexandre Brierre de Boismont, "Hystérie, extase, crises convulsives, avec trouble momentané de la raison," *Annales médico-psychologiques,* 3 (1858), pp. 250–259; quote from p. 254.

35. Wilhelm Schlesinger (Sr.?), "Magnetische Soiréen in Paris," *WMW,* 7 (August 8, 1857), pp. 595–597, quote p. 597.

36. Reports on catalepsy by decade in the *Index-Catalogue* are: 1800–1809, 10; 1810–19, 10; 1820–29, 12; 1830–39, 25; 1840–49, 29; 1850–59, 28; 1860–69, 31; 1870–79, 44; 1880–89, 5.

37. Etienne-Eugène Azam, *Hypnotisme, double conscience et altérations de la personnalité* (Paris, 1887), pp. 39–40. This book is mainly a collection of his previous articles, the article from which this observation was taken having apparently first been published in 1860.

38. Bourdin, *Catalepsie* (1841), p. 51.

39. George H. Savage, "Some Cases of Catalepsy," *BMJ,* ii (December 9, 1876), pp. 748–749.

40. Henri Claude and Henri Baruk, "Les Crises de catalepsie: leur diagnostic avec le sommeil pathologique, leurs rapports avec l'hystérie et la catatonie," *L'Encéphale*, 23 (1928), pp. 373–402. After almost four decades of silence there were in 1920–29 fourteen articles on catalepsy, in 1930–39, twenty-two.

41. F. Fischer, "Einige Beobachtungen über thierischen Magnetismus und Somnambulismus," *Archiv für die Physiologie*, 6 (1805), pp. 264–281; details from pp. 264–274. In states of "lucidity," Puységur's patients were able to diagnose disease, predict the course of it and prescribe therapy. See Ellenberger, *Discovery* (1970), p. 71.

42. Justinus Kerner, *Die Seherin von Prevorst* (1829; Stuttgart: Steinkopf, 1973), pp. 60–61.

43. Ibid., p. 100. "Er ist nicht der Herr mehr/von Händen und Füssen/Sie zittern, sie wanken/Wie Hirn und Gedanken./Doch soll er nicht zagen/Ich muss ihm was sagen:/Muss sagen, dass er dies trinke aus!/Dann wird es ihm besser/Kann schlafen, kann essen/Und geht aus dem Haus!"

44. Salomon Stiebel, *Kleine Beiträge zur Heilwissenschaft* (Frankfurt am Main, 1823). The case of Marianne, pp. 149–212, is especially interesting because some portion of her symptoms later turned out to be due to simulation. For this episode, see pp. 161–162.

45. Despine, *Observations* (1838), pp. 177–178.

46. Maurice Macario, *Des paralysies dynamiques ou nerveuses* (Paris, 1859), pp. 37–38.

47. Jean-Roch Laurence and Campbell Perry refer to the years 1878–1905 as "the golden years of hypnosis." *Hypnosis, Will, and Memory: A Psycho-Legal History* (New York: Guilford Press, 1988), p. 177.

48. Although Charcot is often credited for the revival of hypnotism in France, above all after his public lecture on the subject in 1882, other French authorities aside from Azam had also previously expressed interest. See, for example, Charles Richet, "Du somnambulisme provoqué," *Journal de l'anatomie et de la physiologie*, no. 4 (1875), pp. 348–378; Richet thought it of interest for research, not for therapeutics.

49. For some details of Hansen's life see Friedrich Zöllner, *Die transcendentale Physik und die sogennante Philosophie*, 4 vols., 1878–81, vol. 3 (Leipzig, 1879), pp. 556–558. For Hansen's 1879 tour in Germany see pp. 417f. Paul Julius Möbius also makes reference to Hansen, "Über den Hypnotismus," *Schmidt's Jahrbücher der in- und ausländischen gesamten Medicin*, 190 (1881), pp. 73–93; facts from p. 78.

50. Reminiscences of Ewald Hecker, *Hypnose und Suggestion im Dienste der Heilkunde* (Wiesbaden, 1893), pp. 1–2.

51. See Adolf F. Weinhold, *Hypnotische Versuche: Experimentelle Beiträge zur Kenntniss des sogennanten thierischen Magnetismus* (Chemnitz, 1879). See also Christian Bäumler, *Der sogenannte animalische Magnetismus oder Hypnotismus* (Leipzig, 1881), p. 14.

52. Hecker, *Hypnose* (1893), p. 3.
53. For these details see P. Börner, "Thierischer Magnetismus und Hypnotismus," *DMW,* 6 (February 21, 1880), pp. 89–96, especially p. 89.
54. Hecker, *Hypnose* (1893), p. 4.
55. Oskar Berger, "Experimentelle Katalepsie (Hypnotismus)," *DMW,* 6 (March 6, 1880), pp. 116–118.
56. The lecture was later published as a pamphlet, Rudolf Heidenhain, *Der sogenannte thierische Magnetismus: Physiologische Betrachtungen* (Leipzig, 1880).
57. Editorial, "Der magnetische Rummel in Wien," *Wiener Medizinische Blätter,* 3 (February 5, 1880), p. 146. A trial arose from Hansen's appearance in Vienna; see Laurence, *Hypnosis* (1988), pp. 217–218.
58. Sigmund Freud, "Selbstdarstellung" (1925), *Gesammelte Werke,* vol. 14 (Frankfurt am Main, 1948); quote from p. 40.
59. See Moritz Rosenthal, "Der sogennante thierische Magnetismus im Lichte moderner Wissenschaft betrachtet," *Wiener Medizinische Blätter,* 3 (February 12, 1880), pp. 153–155.
60. Moritz Benedikt, "Über Katalepsie und Mesmerismus," ibid., March 4, pp. 250–252. See also Benedikt's "Über Katalepsie und Mesmerismus," *Wiener Klinik,* 6 (1880), pp. 73–92. He induced catalepsy in patients by pressing on their eyelids when he was on staff in Johann Oppolzer's clinic in the mid-1860s (p. 86). See also Benedikt, *Aus meinem Leben: Erinnerungen und Erörterungen* (Vienna, 1906), pp. 324–325; and Rudolf von Urban (Urbantschitsch), *Myself Not Least: A Confessional Autobiography of a Psychoanalyst* (London: Jarrolds, 1958), p. 11.
61. Ernest Jones, *The Life and Work of Sigmund Freud, vol. 1: The Formative Years* (New York: Basic Books, 1953), pp. 251–252.
62. Heinrich Obersteiner referred to a lecture on "Der Hypnotismus" that he gave in 1885 to the Wissenschaftlicher Klub in Vienna in this book, *Der Hypnotismus mit besonderer Berücksichtigung seiner klinischen und forensischen Bedeutung* (Vienna, 1887), p 67.
63. Heinrich Obersteiner, *Die Privatheilanstalt zu Ober-Döbling* (Leipzig, 1891), pp. 144–147.
64. Obersteiner, *Hypnose* (1887), p. 80.
65. Richard von Krafft-Ebing, "Zur Verwerthung der Suggestionstherapie (Hypnose) bei Psychosen und Neurosen," *WKW,* 4 (October 22, 1891), pp. 795–799.
66. Hugo Gugl and Anton Stichl, *Neuropathologische Studien* (Stuttgart, 1892), pp. 20–21, 34–35, 108, 137–138. They do not explicitly mention hypnotism, but that does not necessarily mean they did not perform it. On the history of hypnotism in Vienna, see also Gerhard Fichtner and Albrecht Hirschmüller, "Freud et l'hypnose: un compte rendu encore inconnu de l'écrit d'Obersteiner *L'hypnotisme* (1887)," *Revue internationale de l'histoire de la psychanalyse,* 1 (1988), pp. 405–417.

67. See Shorter, "Psychotherapy in Private Clinics in Central Europe, 1870–1913," First European Congress for the History of Psychiatry, the Netherlands, October 14–16, 1990.

68. See Otto Winkelmann, "Albert Moll (1862–1939) als Wegbereiter der Schule von Nancy in Deutschland," *Praxis der Psychotherapie,* 10 (1965), pp. 1–7.

69. See Hans H. Walser, ed., *August Forel, Briefe/Correspondance, 1864–1927* (Berne: Hans Huber, 1968), p. 266 on Kraepelin (who left Tartu in 1890), p. 262 on Möbius, p. 215 on Ewald.

70. August Forel, *Der Hypnotismus; oder, Die Suggestion und die Psychotherapie: ihre psychologische, psychophysiologische und medizinische Bedeutung* (Stuttgart, 1889).

71. For an overview, see Hannah S. Decker, "The Lure of Nonmaterialism in Materialist Europe: Investigations of Dissociative Phenomena, 1880–1915," in Jacques M. Quen, ed., *Split Minds/Split Brains: Historical and Current Perspectives* (New York: New York University Press, 1986), pp. 31–62.

72. See Carl Gerster, "Beiträge zur suggestiven Psychotherapie," *Zeitschrift für Hypnotismus,* 1 (1892–93), pp. 319–335, especially p. 321. The author disliked even this use of "Somnambulismus," and felt that the term should be restricted to sleepwalking alone. John Milne Bramwell defined a "somnambule" as someone "unable when hypnosis terminated to recall the events of hypnotic life." "Hypnotic and Post-Hypnotic Appreciation of Time," *Brain,* 23 (1900), pp. 161–238; quote from p. 161.

73. On the Nancy school, see Ellenberger, *Discovery* (1970), pp. 85–89.

74. Publications on "suggestion"—inevitably a mixture of hypnosis and other techniques—were mentioned as follows for the years in which the *Index-Catalogue* used that rubric: 1880–89, 116; 1890–99, 46; 1900–1909, 102; 1910–19, 58; 1920–29, 31.

75. Shorter, "Psychotherapy Private Clinics" (1990).

76. Schnell, "Remarques sur la suggestion hypnotique chez les hystériques," *Marseille médical,* 25 (1888), pp. 464–485. To the credit of her clinicians, it must be said they realized early on that these were phenomena of suggestion.

77. Wellcome Institute for the History of Medicine, London, ms. 5157, cases 393, 413, 465, 475.

78. Chart at Psychiatrisches Krankenhaus der Stadt Wien. I am grateful to Prof. Dr. Eberhard Gabriel for access to this collection. The meaning of "Parme" is unclear.

79. Paul Sollier, *Genèse et nature de l'hystérie: recherches cliniques et expérimentales de psychophysiologie,* 2 vols. (Paris, 1897), vol. 2, pp. 4–7, 13. Charcot understood by "vigilambulisme hystérique," the "dédoublement hystérique de la personnalité." See Georges Guinon, ed., *Clinique des maladies du système nerveux, M. le professeur Charcot,* 2 vols. (Paris, 1892–93), vol. 2 pp. 168–265, for Charcot's teachings on the subject.

366

80. See Harold Merskey, "The Manufacture of Personalities: the Production of Multiple Personality Disorder," forthcoming, *BJP.* See also Ian Hacking, "Making Up People," in Thomas C. Heller, et al., eds., *Reconstructing Individualism: Autonomy, Individuality, and the Self in Western Thought* (Stanford: Stanford U.P., 1986), pp. 226–240; Hacking, "The Invention of Split Personalities (An Illustration of Michel Foucault's Doctrine of the Constitution of the Subject)," in Alan Donagan, et al., eds., *Human Nature and Natural Knowledge* (Dordrecht, the Netherlands: Reidel, 1986), pp. 63–85. An important contribution to the experimental literature is Nicholas P. Spanos, et al., "Hypnotic Interview and Age Regression Procedures in the Elicitation of Multiple Personality Symptoms: A Simulation Study," *Psychiatry,* 49 (1986), pp. 298–311.

81. Ellenberger, *Discovery* (1970), pp. 129–131. It is not a denigration of Ellenberger's great work, which covering as it does a large range of ground would inevitably include some errors, to point out that he misunderstands Despine's approach to the case. Ellenberger has Despine playing a close psychological game with Estelle: "One realizes how much experience Despine needed to become aware of his patient's tricks and to utilize the rapport [magnetism] to lead her skillfully out of her illness"(p. 892). Ellenberger likens Despine favorably to Josef Breuer's management of Anna O. (p. 484). In fact, Despine had virtually no psychological insight and simply applied mechanically the procedures of animal magnetism, writing "Le Magnétisme est l'action du fluide nerveux d'une personne sur une autre, ou sur elle même" (Despine, *Observations* [1838], p. 164). Ellenberger gives her surname as "L'Hardy" (p. 484). Despine writes it as "Lardy" (p. 195). Despine saw Estelle for the last time in April 1838.

82. Despine, *Observations* (1838), pp. 239–240, for a brief summary of the case, pp. 2–227 for details.

83. Ibid., p. 240.

84. Ibid., p. 145. "Un état partiel de crise, qui donnait à la malade, le sentiment intérieur d'une double existence".

85. Eberhard Gmelin, *Untersuchungen über den thierischen Magnetismus und über die einfache Behandlungsart* (Heilbronn, 1793; this is vol. 2 of Gmelin's *Materialien für die Anthropologie,* 2 vols. [Heilbronn, 1791–93]), case on pp. 2–45, details from pp. 3, 11, 22–28. Eric T. Carlson considers this the first historical case "of what would be today called multiple personality disorder." See Carlson, "Multiple Personality and Hypnosis: The First One Hundred Years," *Journal of the History of the Behavioral Sciences,* 25 (1989), pp. 315–322.

86. Fischer, *Archiv* (1805), p. 281.

87. Azam, *Hypnotisme* (1887), pp. 12–16, 63 f.

88. Pierre Janet, "Les Actes inconscients et le dédoublement de la personnalité pendant le somnambulisme provoqué," *Revue philosophique,* 22 (1886), pp. 577–592; dialogue from p. 589. On double personalities emerging in

367

similar written form, see William James, "Notes on Automatic Writing," *American Society for Psychical Research,* 1 (1889), pp. 548–564.

89. Joseph Collins, "Astasia-Abasia: Report of a Case Eventuating in Recovery after Many Years' Duration," *Medical Record,* 87 (April 24, 1915), pp. 673–679.

90. See Merskey, forthcoming, *BJP,* on this point.

91. Privately printed, Augusta, Ga.

92. On the background of this, see Shorter, *Bedside Manners: The Troubled History of Doctors and Patients* (New York: Simon and Schuster, 1985), chaps. 4 and 5. This book was republished with a new introduction by the author as *Doctors and Their Patients: A Social History* (New Brunswick, N.J.: Transaction Publishers, 1991).

CHAPTER 7

Charcot's Hysteria

1. Léon Daudet, *Devant la douleur: souvenirs des milieux littéraires, politiques, artistiques et médicaux de 1880 à 1905* (Paris, 1915), pp. 98–99.

2. Joseph Babinski, "Éloge de J.-M. Charcot," *Revue neurologique,* 32 (1925), pp. 746–756; detail from p. 747.

3. On the professors of medicine selecting mediocre but well-connected candidates in the *concours,* Daudet wrote, "Répétés chaque année, pendant vingt ans, à une douzaine d'exemplaires, ces actes de favoritisme avaient fini par rendre enragées deux générations de médecins." *Les Oeuvres dans les hommes* (Paris, 1922), p. 205.

4. For the story of his second *agrégation,* see Fulgence Raymond, "Leçon d'ouverture," *Prog. méd.,* 22 (November 24, 1894), pp. 399–407; anecdote from p. 400. Also Pierre Marie, "Éloge de J.-M. Charcot," *Presse médicale* (May 27, 1925), pp. 689–692; detail from p. 689. The bare facts of Charcot's early career are available in Georges Gilles de la Tourette, "Jean-Martin Charcot," *Nouvelle iconographie de la Salpêtrière,* 6 (1893), pp. 241–250; Georges Guillain, *J.-M. Charcot, 1825–1893: His Life, His Work,* Eng. trans. (London, 1959), pp. 5–6.

5. Marie, *Presse méd.* (1925), p. 689.

6. Jean-Martin Charcot, "Hospice de la Salpêtrière: Réouverture des conférences cliniques de M. Charcot," *Prog. méd.,* 8 (November 27, 1880), pp. 969–971; quote from p. 970.

7. Sigmund Freud, "Charcot," *WMW,* 43 (September 9, 1893), pp. 1514–1520; quote from p. 1516.

8. The list of Charcot's major scientific accomplishments is much longer. For a good, brief account of his life, see Georges de Morsier, "Jean-Martin Charcot," in Kurt Kolle, ed., *Grosse Nervenärzte,* 2nd ed., vol. 3 (Stuttgart: Thieme Verlag, 1970), pp. 39–56. A compact review of his achievements in neuropathology is on pp. 41–43. Alix Joffroy reviewed Charcot's scientific work in an obituary in the *Archives de médecine expérimentale,* 5 (1893),

368

pp. 577–606. For a detailed list of Charcot's publications, see René Seme-laigne, *Les Pionniers de la psychiatrie française*, 2 vols. (Paris, 1930–32), vol. 2, pp. 122–125, at the end of a rather sketchy monograph on Charcot himself, which moreover expropriates Charcot for "psychiatry" (*la médecine mentale*) (p. 116).

9. Alexandre-Achille Souques and Henry Meige, *Charcot (Jean-Martin)* (Paris, 1939, in the series "Les Biographies médicales," 13 [1], p. 333.

10. Léon Daudet, *Quand vivait mon père* (Paris, 1940), p. 213.

11. George Guillain, "Discours," *Revue neurologique*, 32 (1925), pp. 1164–68; quote from p. 1165.

12. Moses Allen Starr, "Memorial of Professor Jean-Marie [*sic*] Charcot," *Medical News*, 63 (October 14, 1893), pp. 433–437; quote from p. 434. The author had attended Charcot's lectures in the spring of 1883.

13. Georges Didi-Huberman has culled some of its published photographs in *Invention de l'hystérie: Charcot et l'Iconographie photographique de la Salpêtrière* (Paris: Eds. Macula, 1982). The *Iconographie* was a journal. Of course Charcot did not invent hysteria. He invented *one* hysteria.

14. These facts have been gleaned from various issues of *Progrès médical* in the 1870s and 1880s.

15. This list from *Prog. méd.*, 5 (November 3, 1877), p. 809.

16. Ibid., (November 10, 1877), p. 846.

17. Henri Colin believes that Charcot was the first chief physician to receive the sobriquet *patron;* after him it became generalized. "Charcot," *Annales médico-psychologiques*, 83 (1925), pp. 385–392; quote from p. 389.

18. For accounts of these evenings, see Daudet, *Douleur* (1915), pp. 19–20, and Daudet, *Oeuvres dans les hommes* (1922), pp. 208–210.

19. See J.-M. Charcot and Paul Richer, *Les Démoniaques dans l'art* (Paris, 1887).

20. Axel Munthe, *The Story of San Michele* (London, 1929), p. 285.

21. Daudet, *Douleur* (1915), pp. 12–13.

22. Daudet, *Quand vivait mon père* (1940), pp. 140–141. Surrealists Louis Aragon and André Breton, attributing their views to "Freud," believed the Salpêtrière a hotbed of sexual intrigue between doctors and patients. "Le Cinquantenaire de l'hystérie (1878–1928)," *La Révolution surréaliste*, no. 11 (1928), pp. 20–22.

23. Jules Claretie, "Charcot, le consolateur," *Les Annales politiques et littéraires*, 21 (September 20, 1903), pp. 179–180; quote from p. 179.

24. Daudet, *Oeuvres dans les hommes* (1922), p. 236.

25. Alexandre-Achille Souques, "Charcot intime," *Presse médicale* (May 27, 1925), pp. 693–698; detail from p. 695. The observation about France's lag in neuroanatomy is my own.

26. Edmond de Goncourt, *Journal: mémoires de la vie littéraire*, vol. 17 (1890–91) (Monaco: Les Éditions de l'imprimerie nationale de Monaco, 1956), pp. 178–179. His brother Jules de Goncourt, who collaborated in earlier volumes of the diary, died of neurosyphilis in 1870.

27. Daudet, *Quand vivait mon père* (1940), p. 256.
28. Joseph Babinski, "Recherches servant à établir que certains phénomènes nerveux peuvent être transmis d'un sujet à un autre sujet sous l'influence de l'aimant," *Revue de l'hypnotisme*, 1 (1886), pp. 181–183.
29. For this story see Vincente J. Iragui, "The Charcot-Bouchard Controversy," *Archives of Neurology*, 43 (1986), pp. 290–295.
30. Letter of Nov. 3, 1893, in Hans H. Walser, ed., *August Forel, Briefe/Correspondance, 1864–1927* (Berne: Hans Huber, 1968), p. 293. Italics in original. It was said that Charcot had initially opposed Dejerine's candidacy for the *agrégation* and was won over only after a personal confrontation. See Richard Satran, "Fulgence Raymond, the Successor of Charcot," *Bulletin of the New York Academy of Medicine*, 50 (1974), pp. 931–942; detail from p. 934. Léon Daudet said, that Charcot "brisa la carrière de Dejerine" (*Quand vivait mon père* [1940], p. 115).
31. Clément Simon made the point that most of Charcot's stigmata were on the sensory side, the motor list limited to contracture and muscle weakness. "Comment faut-il comprendre l'hystérie à la suite des travaux de M. Babinski?" *Journal de médecine et de chirurgie pratiques*, 84 (1913), pp. 401–410; see pp. 402–403. According to a tabulation by Mark Micale, 79 percent of Charcot's patients at the Salpêtrière had anesthesia or hyperesthesia, 76 percent some kind of visual abnormality, and 34 percent a paralysis or contracture. As for fits, 47 percent of all patients experienced some kind of partial seizure. Only 16 percent had two or more stages of the classic "attack," and only 12 percent received a diagnosis of "hysteria major." "Hysteria and its Historiography: The Future Perspective," *History of Psychiatry*, 1 (1990), pp. 33–124; statistics from p. 84.
32. Marie, *Presse médicale* (1925), p. 691.
33. Gilles de la Tourette, *Nouvelle iconographie* (1893), p. 245. Tourette was vague about when exactly Charcot first began making distinctions.
34. See Jean-Martin Charcot, *Leçons du mardi à la Salpêtrière. Policliniques, 1887–1888, Notes de cours* (Paris, 1887 [*sic*]), June 26, 1888, pp. 483–484. See also Sigmund Freud's comments in Freud, *Poliklinische Vorträge von Prof. J. M. Charcot, vol. 1, Schuljahr 1887–1888* (Leipzig, 1894), p. 371 n.
35. For these details see "B" (Desiré-Magloire Bourneville), "Les Erreurs de la *France médicale*," *Prog. Méd.*, 5 (November 10, 1877), pp. 845–847; Bourneville, "J.-M. Charcot," *Prog. Méd.*, 21 (August 26, 1893), pp. 137–143, especially p. 138. Bourneville was the intern on the hysteroepilepsy service in 1866, and remained in charge of this service until leaving the Salpêtrière in 1879.
36. Jean-Martin Charcot, *Leçons sur les maladies du système nerveux faites à la Salpêtrière*, 4th ed., vol. 1 (Paris, 1880), pp. 285–286, part of the "ninth lesson."
37. Ibid., lesson 11, pp. 320–346.
38. Ibid., pp. 341–342.

39. Ibid.

40. Jean-Martin Charcot, "Description de la grande attaque hystérique." *Prog. méd.*, 7 (January 11, 1879), pp. 17–20. See also *Leçons maladies système nerveux* (1880), pp. 432–445.

41. For an example see Morsier, "Charcot" (1970), p. 47, case of Th. L.

42. P. Poirier, "Des moyens d'arrêter les attaques hystéro-épileptiques, et en particulier, du compresseur des ovaires," *Prog. méd.*, 6 (December 28, 1878), pp. 993–994.

43. Charles Féré, "Compresseur de l'ovaire," ibid., 9 (November 26, 1881), pp. 941–942.

44. Desiré-Magloire Bourneville, "De l'influence de la compression ovarienne sur divers accident hystérique," ibid., 9 (January 8, 1881), pp. 22–23.

45. Charcot, *Leçons du mardi (1887-88)*, June 26, 1888, pp. 481–482.

46. Of course many refinements occurred to Charcot as time went on, such as the discovery of the hysterogenic and -frenic zones. See "Des zones hystérogènes: Résumé d'une leçon de M. Charcot," *Prog. méd.*, 8 (December 18, 1880), pp. 1036–1038. Although Charcot never codified his views in a single textbook, the works of several of his disciples do encompass the entire doctrine. See in particular Georges Gilles de la Tourette, *Traité clinique et thérapeutique de l'hystérie*, 3 vols. (Paris, 1891–95), and Paul Richer, *Études cliniques sur la grande hystérie ou hystéro-épilepsie*, 2nd ed. (Paris, 1885; 1st ed. 1881).

47. Jean-Martin Charcot, "Leçon d'ouverture," *Prog. méd.*, 10 (May 6, 1882), pp. 335–338; quote from p. 336.

48. On Burq's life and the circumstances surrounding this invitation, see Anne Harrington, "Hysteria, Hypnosis, and the Lure of the Invisible: the Rise of Neo-Mesmerism in *fin-de-siècle* French psychiatry," in W. F. Bynum et al., eds., *Anatomy of Madness: Essays in the History of Psychiatry, vol. 3: The Asylum and its Psychiatry* (London: Routledge, 1988), pp. 226–246. See also Harrington, "Metals and Magnets in Medicine: Hysteria, Hypnosis and Medical Culture in *fin-de-siècle* Paris," *Psychological Medicine*, 18 (1988), pp. 21–38. Harrington makes Burq the "discoverer" of therapy with metals, whereas he was in fact just part of an enormous tradition of applying magnets and metal plates to patients.

49. Bourneville, *Prog. méd.* (1893), p. 139. The "transfert" in particular would become, like "ovarie," one of the Salpêtrière's stock doctrines. See for example Charcot, *Leçons du mardi (1887-88)*, March 27, 1888, pp. 300–301, in which a patient, awaiting treatment for a paralyzed right hand in the electrotherapy room of the Salpêtrière, inadvertently placed her left hand near a machine which suddenly started up. She now found the left hand paralyzed and the right hand fine.

50. "Hospice de la Salpêtrière: M. Charcot," *Prog. méd.*, 6 (November 16, 1878), p. 875.

51. See Charcot, "Catalepsie et somnambulisme hystériques provoqués,"

ibid., 6 (December 21, 1878), pp. 973–975. "Stupéfaction générale" from Gilles de la Tourette, *Nouvelle iconographie* (1893), p. 246.

52. For an account see Arthur Gamgee, ". . . The Phenomena of Hystero-Epilepsy: And on the Modification which They Undergo under the Influence of Magnets and Solenoids," *BMJ*, ii (October 12, 1878), pp. 545–548.

53. Marie, *Presse médicale* (1925), p. 691.

54. Charcot, *Leçons maladies système nerveux* (1882), lesson 21, pp. 336–339, on *le grand hypnotisme* and its phases of lethargy, catalepsy, and somnambulism. See also Charcot's "Note sur les divers états nerveux déterminés par l'hypnotisation chez les hystériques," *Prog. méd.*, 10 (February 18, 1882), pp. 124–126.

55. Joseph Delboeuf, "Une Visite à la Salpêtrière," *Revue de Belgique*, 18 (1886), pp. 121–147, especially pp. 125–126.

56. A choice document is George M. Robertson, "Hypnotism at Paris and Nancy: Notes of a Visit," *Journal of Mental Science*, 38 (1892), pp. 494–531; the author quoted Charles Féré to the effect that, "The hypnotized hysterical woman is to be regarded as 'the psychological frog,' and that what the frog has done for physiology, the hysterical woman is to do for psychology" (p. 506).

57. Daudet, *Douleur* (1915), pp. 87–88. On Luys, see also Ernest Hart, *Hypnotism, Mesmerism and the New Witchcraft* (London, 1893), pp. 72–182.

58. Gilles de la Tourette, *Nouvelle iconographie* (1893), p. 247.

59. Charcot, *Leçons du mardi à la Salpêtrière, Policlinique 1888–1889* (Paris, 1889), October 23, 1888, pp. 2–9.

60. Charcot, *Leçons du mardi (1887–1888)*, March 27, 1888, pp. 305–309; May 1, 1888, pp. 388–391.

61. Charcot, ibid., May 1, 1888, pp. 391–395.

62. When Hack Tuke visited Charcot in Paris, mindful of Tuke's book Charcot said he had ruled out "expectant attention" (meaning suggestion) as an explanation of such phenomena as *le transfert*. See Daniel Hack Tuke, "Metalloscopy and Expectant Attention," *Journal of Mental Science*, 24 (1879), pp. 598–609; detail from p. 601. The book in question was Tuke's *Illustrations of the Influence of the Mind Upon the Body in Health and Disease* (London, 1872). Charcot considered such apparently objective phenomena as neuromuscular hyperexcitability produced under hypnotism to be evidence of the objective existence of hysteria as an organic condition, evidence that could not be simulated. See Charcot, "De l'électricité statique, particulièrement dans ses applications au traitement de l'hystérie," *Prog. méd.*, 9 (April 23, 1881), pp. 315–316.

63. Munthe, *San Michele* (1929), pp. 302–303.

64. Paul Dubois, *The Psychic Treatment of Nervous Disorders*, Eng. trans., 6th ed. (New York, 1909; 1st published in Paris in 1904 as *Les Psychonévroses et leur traitement moral*), pp. 15–16.

65. Jules-Joseph Dejerine, *Sémiologie des affections du système nerveux,* 2 vols. (Paris, 1914), vol. 1, p. 561.
66. G. Hahn, "Charcot et son influence sur l'opinion publique," *Revue des questions scientifiques,* 2nd ser., 6 (1894), pp. 353–379. "Vers 1878, le nom de la Salpêtrière envahit les revues de vulgarisation et les journaux quotidiens eux-mêmes"(p. 369).
67. Quoted in Robert G. Hillman, "A Scientific Study of Mystery: The Role of the Medical and Popular Press in the Nancy-Salpêtrière Controversy on Hypnotism," *Bulletin of the History of Medicine,* 39 (1965), pp. 163–182; quote from p. 166.
68. Ibid., p. 167.
69. Guy de Maupassant, "Le Tic" (1884), reprinted in Maupassant, *Qui Sait? et autres histoires étranges* (Paris: Union générale d'éditions, 1981), pp. 196–201; quote from p. 198. In this collection "Le Horla" and "Magnétisme" also reflect the climate of nervous illness surrounding the Salpêtrière and Charcot. On Parisian nervosity generally see also Octave Mirbeau, *Les Vingt et un jours d'un neurasthénique* (Paris, 1901). For a partial list of novels drawing somehow upon Charcot's hysteria see A. de Monzie, "Discours," *Revue neurologique,* 32 (1925), pp. 1159–1162.
70. Jules Claretie, *Les Amours d'un interne* (Paris, 1881), pp. 208–209.
71. Goncourt, *Journal,* vol. 16, p. 62. "La femme Lippmann, avec toutes sortes de gamineries et de gestes de toquée . . ."
72. Henri Huchard, "Caractère, moeurs, état mental des hystériques," *Archives de neurologie,* 3 (1882), pp. 187–211; quote from p. 190.
73. Léonce Bonamaison, "Un cas remarquable d'hypnose spontanée, grande hystérie et grand hypnotisme," *Revue de l'hypnotisme,* 4 (1890), pp. 234–243, especially 238–239, 242.
74. Jean-Albert Pitres, *Leçons cliniques sur l'hystérie et l'hypnotisme,* 2 vols. (Paris, 1891), vol. 2, p. 103.
75. Ibid., vol. 1, pp. viii–ix.
76. The local doctor reported this case to Paul Richer, "Notes et observations pour servir à l'histoire de l'hystéro-épilepsie ou grande hystérie," *Archives de neurologie,* 5 (1883), pp. 222–231. The attacks could be stopped by ovarian compression.
77. See Theodor Leber, "Die Anaesthesia retinae und hysterische Amaurose," in Alfred Graefe et al., eds., *Handbuch der gesammten Augenheilkunde,* vol. 5 (Leipzig, 1877), pp. 980–988. Johannes Kyri, "Beziehungen des cerebrospinalen Nervensystems zu den Funktionen und Erkrankungen der Geschlechtsorgane und insbesondere die Beziehungen des Sympathicus zu dem Gesammtnervensystem," *Verhandlungen der deutschen Gesellschaft für Gynäkologie,* 1893, pp. 385–390.
78. See Shorter, "Mania, Hysteria and Gender in Lower Austria, 1891–1905," *History of Psychiatry,* 1 (1990), pp. 3–31, especially p. 11.
79. Valentin von Holst, *Erfahrungen aus einer vierzigjährigen neurologischen Praxis* (Stuttgart, 1903), p. 50.

80. Josef Breuer and Sigmund Freud, "On the Psychical Mechanism of Hysterical Phenomena: Preliminary Communication," reprinted in Breuer and Freud, *Studies on Hysteria,* Eng. trans. James and Alix Strachey, *Standard Edition of the Complete Psychological Works of Sigmund Freud,* vol. 2 (London, 1955), pp. 67–68.
81. Ibid., p. 204.
82. Jeffrey Moussaieff Masson, ed., *The Complete Letters of Sigmund Freud to Wilhelm Fliess, 1887–1904* (Cambridge, Mass.: Harvard University Press, 1985), p. 120.
83. Ibid., p. 218.
84. See Freud's obituary of Charcot, *WMW,* (1893), p. 1520. On Freud's concerns about Jews and psychoanalysis, see his letter to Karl Abraham of May 3, 1908, in Hilda C. Abraham et al., eds., *Sigmund Freud/Karl Abraham: Briefe, 1907–1926,* 2nd ed. (Frankfurt am Main: Fischer, 1980), p. 47. For the grenadier, see Andrée and Knoblauch, "Über einen Fall von Hystero-Epilepsie bei einem Manne," *BKW,* 26 (March 11, 1889), pp. 204–207.
85. For a characteristic example of this process, see Karl Friedrich Westphal, "Über Metalloscopie," *BKW,* 15 (July 29, 1878), pp. 441–446. In view of the large German case literature on hysteria, which may be located through the *Index-Catalogue* of the U.S. surgeon general, Gilles de la Tourette's bitter judgment that the Germans had not absorbed the wise teachings of Charcot seems more a result of personal pique than a reflection of reality. *Traité hystérie* (1891), pp. 119–120.
86. Thomas Dixon Savill, *Lectures on Hysteria and Allied Vaso-Motor Conditions* (London, 1909), pp. 11–12. The young female with a hysterical paralysis, whose outraged father was responsible for Ernest Jones's exile from London to Toronto, had been a patient of Savill's. See Vincent Brome, *Ernest Jones: Freud's Alter Ego* (New York: Norton, 1983), pp. 49–50.
87. Savill, *Lectures* (1909), pp. 24, 30–31.
88. Cornelius William Suckling, "Cases . . . ," *MTG,* i (June 13, 1885), pp. 782–783.
89. Henry Charlton Bastian, *Various Forms of Hysterical or Functional Paralysis* (London, 1893), p. 119 n. 4.
90. I cannot accept Mark Micale's view that British lack of interest in Charcot's ideas stemmed from an exaggerated British definition of sex roles in which it became impossible to contemplate the notion of "male hysteria." This strikes me as an example of the perfervid theorizing that has deformed much of the social history of medicine. See Micale, "Hysteria Male/Hysteria Female: Reflections on Comparative Gender Construction in Nineteenth-Century France and Britain," in Marina Benjamin, ed., *Science and Sensibility: Gender and Scientific Inquiry,1780–1945* (Oxford: Basil Blackwell, 1991), pp. 200–239.
91. Samuel Wilks, "On Hemianaesthesia," *Guy's Hospital Reports,* ser. 3, 26 (1883), pp. 147–175, especially p. 175.

92. Bastian, *Various Forms* (1893), p. 120.
93. Samuel Alexander Kinnier Wilson, "Some Modern French Conceptions of Hysteria," *Brain*, 33 (1910), pp. 293–338; quotes from pp. 298, 300.
94. Sigmund Freud, "Selbstdarstellung" (1925), reprinted in *Gesammelte Werke*, vol. 14 (Frankfurt am Main: Fischer, 1948), p. 38.
95. Charcot, *Leçons maladies système nerveux* (1887), lesson 21, p. 335. See John Russell Reynolds, "Remarks on Paralysis and other Disorders of Motion and Sensation, Dependent on Idea," *BMJ*, ii (November 6, 1869), pp. 483–485.
96. Charcot described his use of "isolation" in "De l'isolement dans le traitement de l'hystérie," *Prog. méd.*, 13 (February 28, 1885), pp. 161–164. The interpretation that Charcot's experiences with isolation first brought him to the realization of hysteria as "une maladie psychique" is that of former intern Gilbert Ballet, "Le Domaine de la psychiatrie," *Presse médicale* (May 10, 1911), pp. 377–380, especially p. 378.
97. On the significance for Charcot of "l'hystérie de 1886," see Philippe Chaslin, *Éléments de sémiologie et clinique mentales* (Paris, 1912). In 1886 Charcot "commençait déjà à mêler à ce système somatique l'action discordante de l'idée, car il avait fini par s'apercevoir (pas assez!) de la puissance de la suggestion et de l'auto-suggestion et il commençait à parler de la puissance de l'idée." (p. 605).
98. Charcot, *Leçons du mardi (1887-1888)*, lecture of January 17, 1888, pp. 111–118; and lecture of May 1, 1888, pp. 373–387.
99. Ibid., lecture of January 17, 1888, p. 115.
100. On Janet's life and theories see Henri Ellenberger, *The Discovery of the Unconscious* (New York: Basic Books, 1970), p. 331 f.
101. Pierre Janet, "Quelques définitions récentes de l'hystérie," *Archives de neurologie*, 25 (June 1893), pp. 417–438, and in the July issue, vol. 26, pp. 1–29. The heading on p. 11 of this second installment reads "L'hystérie: maladie mentale."
102. Pierre Janet, *L'État mental des hystériques: les stigmates mentaux* (Paris, 1893). I have not seen this work.
103. Charcot, "La Foi qui guérit," *Archives de neurologie*, 25 (1893), pp. 72–87; quote from p. 87.
104. Chaslin, *Clinique mentale* (1912), p. 605; Souques, *Charcot* (1939), p. 345.
105. Edouard Brissaud, review, *Revue neurologique*, 1 (1893), p. 36. "Les symptômes hystériques reconnaissent toujours pour cause accidentelle une influence comparable à celle du traumatisme."
106. Chaslin, *Clinique mentale* (1912), p. 606. Paul Blocq attributed to Janet this new concept of hysteria as "une maladie mentale," but added that Charcot had given "sa haute autorité" to the doctrine. Blocq, "L'état mental dans l'hystérie," *Gazette des hôpitaux*, 66 (November 26, 1893), pp. 1273–1280; quote from p. 1273.
107. Ernest Jones gushed of Charcot's work, "Whatever the unknown neurolog-

ical basis of hysteria might be, the symptoms themselves could be both treated and abolished by ideas alone. They had a psychogenic origin. This opened the door to a medical motive for investigating the psychology of patients. . . . It put psychology itself on a totally different footing from its previous academic one and made possible discoveries concerning the deeper layers of the mind that could not have been made in any other way." *The Life and Work of Sigmund Freud,* vol. 1 (New York: Basic Books, 1953), p. 227. Thus Charcot as master psychologist! According to Esther Fischer-Homberger, the doctrine of "psychogenesis" is all that remained from Charcot's teachings. "So ist im Grunde Charcot's traumatische Hysterie zum Ausgangspunkt der psychologischen Neurosenlehre geworden." *Die traumatische Neurose: Vom somatischen zum sozialen Leiden* (Berne: Hans Huber, 1975), p. 112. Elisabeth Roudinesco demonstrates incomprehension of Charcot's basic doctrine of the "laws of hysteria." She writes: "[Charcot] donne un status précis à l'hystérie en créant un nouveau concept de névrose qui va être à l'origine de la decouverte de l'inconscient. En ce sens l'introduction de la psychanalyse en France commence en 1885, avec la rencontre entre Freud et Charcot, qui rend patente l'idée que l'hystérique invente des symptômes et qu'elle conduit le savant sur la voie de leur compréhension. Par cet évenement, le malade fabrique, montre, exprime et le médecin découvre." Elisabeth Roudinesco, *La Bataille de cents ans, Histoire de la psychanalyse en France,* 2 vols. (Paris: Seuil, 1982–86), vol. 1, p. 39. In fact, this is not a bad description of what happens in somatization, where the patient's unconscious mind does indeed invent symptoms. But it is not what Charcot believed. The laws of hysteria predetermined the fits, the hemianesthesias, the ovarie, and so forth. The patient had no unconscious lattitude in producing them. For Léon Chertok there are no figures in the literature on hysteria between the eighteenth century and Charcot, and it is Charcot who overturns the ancient uterine paradigms, introducing psychology to the understanding of the psychoneuroses ("a truly epistemological turning point"). "On the Centenary of Charcot: Hysteria, Suggestibility and Hypnosis," *British Journal of Medical Psychology,* 57 (1984), pp. 111–120; quote from p. 112. For what are, in my view, more reliable appreciations of Charcot's work, the reader may turn to the chapter in Ellenberger, *Unconscious* (1970), pp. 89–101; and Mark Micale, "Charcot and the Idea of Hysteria in the Male: Gender, Mental Science, and Medical Diagnostics in Late Nineteenth-Century France," *Medical History,* 34 (1990), pp. 363–411, which offers as well a good overview of the large secondary literature.

108. Fulgence Raymond, *Leçons sur les maladies du système nerveux (année 1894–1895)* (Paris, 1896), pp. 64–77 on hysteria, 78–86 on hypnotism. It is true that in 1902 Raymond wrote briefly on hysteria, yet without reference to the Charcot doctrines. "Clinique des maladies nerveuses," *Journal de médecine interne,* 61 (1902), pp. 194–199.

109. Those whom Joseph Babinski had followed over the years were cured of their symptoms. "Hystérie-pithiatisme," *Bulletins et mémoires de la société médicale des hôpitaux de Paris,* 52 (1928), pp. 1507–1521, see p. 1513. On those who stayed behind but "forgot" their symptoms, see Henri Schaeffer, "Conceptions nouvelles sur l'hystérie," *Presse médicale* (February 20, 1929), pp. 237–239. "[Around 1909] il existait encore dans le vieil hospice quelques anciennes des plus célèbres hystériques de l'époque de Charcot, mais elles ne présentaient plus aucune des manifestations de la névrose; elles n'y songeaient plus, elles les avaient oubliés" (pp. 237–238). For an anecdote about the supposedly telepathic powers of one of the patients who stayed on, see Edouard de Morsier, *Silhouettes d'hommes célèbres* (Geneva: Mont-Blanc, 1947), pp. 82–83. According to Dubois (*Psychic Treatment* [1909]), some of the "old horses" could still be persuaded to put on a show for foreign visitors (p. 16).

110. Babinski, *Bulletins* (1928), p. 1513.

111. Simon, *Journal de médecine* (1913), p. 402.

112. Paul Castin, in discussion of Martin-Sisteron, "Troubles nerveux fonctionnels. Leur rééducation," *Dauphiné médical,* 36 (1912), pp. 124–129; quote from p. 128.

113. J. Dejerine, "Le Traitement des psycho-névroses à l'hôpital par la méthode de l'isolement," *Revue neurologique,* 10 (1902), pp. 1145–1148; quotes from pp. 1147, 1148.

114. Wilhelm Stekel, "Gibt es noch eine Hysterie?" *Psychoanalytische Praxis,* 2 (1932), p. 208.

115. Joseph Babinski, "Sur le réflexe cutané plantaire dans certains affections organiques du système nerveux central," *Comptes rendus de la société de biologie* (Paris), 48 (1896), pp. 207–208.

116. Joseph Babinski, "Définition de l'hystérie," *Revue neurologique,* 9 (1901), pp. 1074–1080.

117. For contemporary reviews of these developments, see Henry Meige, "La Révision de l'hystérie à la société de neurologie de Paris: les prétendus stigmates hystériques, les troubles 'pithiatiques,' et les troubles trophiques soi-disant hystériques," *Presse médicale* (July 4, 1908), pp. 425–427; Henri Verger, "Le Bilan de l'hystérie d'après les discussions récentes," *Journal de médecine de Bordeaux* (June 19, 1910), pp. 401–404. This is not to say that Babinski's definition was universally accepted, for by this time he had the psychoanalysts to fight against, as well as such confirmed organicists ("un sommeil des centres cérébraux") as Paul Sollier. Babinski had also somewhat problematically excluded all symptoms referable to the autonomic nervous system from his definition. See Babinski, "Quelques remarques sur l'article de M. Sollier, intitulé: 'La Définition et la nature de l'hystérie,'" *Archives générales de médecine,* 84 (1907), pp. 271–283.

118. See for example Semi Meyer, "Die Diagnose der Hysterie," *Medizinische Klinik,* 6 (February 13, 1910), pp. 259–261.

119. Oswald Bumke, *Lehrbuch der Geisteskrankheiten*, 2nd ed. (Munich, 1924; 1st ed. 1919), p. 455.
120. Babinski, *Bulletins* (1928), pp. 1511–1512; for Alexandre-Achille Souques's comments in the discussion, especially on male hysteria, p. 1516. During his internship at Broussais Hospital in 1889 Souques had seen numerous cases of male hysteria.
121. Armin Steyerthal, "Neuere Anschauungen über Hysterie," *Deutsche medizinische Presse*, 15 (August 7, 1911), pp. 117–120; quote from p. 117. On the symptoms for which Steyerthal considered hydro- and electrotherapy appropriate, see his *Die Wasserheilanstalt Kleinen in Mecklenburg* (Wismar, Germany, 1900), for example, p. 47 on fatigue (*Neurasthenie*).
122. On this, see Claudia Huerkamp, *Der Aufstieg der Ärzte im 19. Jahrhundert (Göttingen: Vandenhoeck & Ruprecht, 1985).*

CHAPTER 8
The Doctors Change Paradigms:
Central Nervous Disease

1. Étienne-Jean Georget, *De la physiologie du système nerveux*, 2 vols. (Paris, 1821), vol. 2, p. 279.
2. Robert Brudenell Carter, *On the Pathology and Treatment of Hysteria* (London, 1853), p. 68.
3. Clara T. Dercum, "The Nervous Disorders in Women Simulating Pelvic Disease: An Analysis of Five Hundred and Ninety-One Cases," *JAMA*, 52 (March 13, 1909), pp. 848–851. Of 347 female patients with hysteria and neurasthenia, "the pelvic organs were entirely normal" in 181. She also found 209 patients with real pelvic disease in whom hysteria and neurasthenia were absent.
4. James Israel, "Ein Beitrag zur Würdigung des Werthes der Castration bei hysterischen Frauen," *BKW*, 17 (April 26, 1880), pp. 242–245. The story had an interesting sequel. The patient identified herself in press accounts of Israel's "Scheinoperation" and, realizing that she had been duped, became symptomatic again. She sought out Hegar in Freiburg, who performed the real operation on her. Alfred Hegar, "Zur Israel'schen Scheincastration," ibid., 17 (November 29, 1880), pp. 681–683.
5. Quotation from Victor Cornelius Medvei, *A History of Endocrinology* (Lancaster, England: MTP Press, 1982), p. 222.
6. For a brief review see Shorter, "The History of the Doctor-Patient Relationship," in William F. Bynum and Roy Porter, eds., *Encyclopedia of Medical History*, forthcoming.
7. Charles Bell Keetley, *The Student's and Junior Practitioner's Guide to the Medical Profession*, 2nd ed. (London, 1885; 1st ed. 1878), p. 19.
8. An anonymous acquaintance of Frederick Parkes Weber, quoted in Weber's obituary in the *Lancet*, i (June 16, 1962), pp. 1308–1309; quote from p. 1309.

9. This case in notebook for 1894–1900. Preserved at the Centre for Contemporary Medical Archives at the Wellcome Institute for the History of Medicine in London.

10. John Russell Reynolds, *A System of Medicine*, 2nd ed., 5 vols., 1866–1879, vol. 2 (London, 1872), p. 95.

11. Thomas Clifford Allbutt, *On Visceral Neuroses* (London, 1884), p. 28.

12. William Smoult Playfair, "Notes on the Systematic Treatment of Nerve Prostration and Hysteria Connected with Uterine Disease," *Lancet*, i (May 28 and June 11, 1881), pp. 857–859, 949–950.

13. William S. Playfair, "The Nervous System in Relation to Gynaecology," in Thomas Clifford Allbutt and W. S. Playfair, eds., *A System of Gynaecology by Many Writers* (London, 1896), p. 226.

14. Rudolf Kaltenbach, "Nochmals zur Frage der Hyperemesis gravidarum," *ZBG*, 15 (1891), pp. 537–540. He saw it as a form of hysteria, which was a systemic disease.

15. Each of the three published widely. For their antireflex views in 1901, see the report of the "Gesellschaft für Geburtshilfe zu Leipzig," meeting of July 15, 1901, ibid., 25 (1901), Windscheid, pp. 1316–19; Krönig, pp. 1320–27 (in which he took a swipe at Fliess's nasal-reflex theories); and Theilhaber, pp. 1330–1331. Franz Windscheid, *Neuropathologie und Gynäkologie: eine kritische Zusammenstellung ihrer physiologischen und pathologischen Beziehungen* (Berlin, 1897).

16. Luigi Maria Bossi, "Die gynäkologischen Läsionen bei der Manie des Selbstmordes und die gynäkologische Prophylaxe gegen den Selbstmord beim Weibe," *ZBG*, 35 (1911), pp. 1265–1272. Bossi, *A Proposito di malattie utero-ovariche e psicopatie: urgenza di riforme nel sistema manicomiale* (Varese, 1912), translated as *Die gynäkologische Prophylaxe bei Wahnsinn* (Berlin, 1912).

17. Gustav Ortenau, "Sieben Fälle von psychischer Erkrankung nach gynäkologischer Behandlung geheilt," *MMW*, 59 (October 29, 1912), pp. 2388–2391; see also a mildly favorable review of Bossi's 1911 article by Paul Michaelis, *PNW*, 13 (January 6, 1912), pp. 424–425.

18. Bernhard Sigmund Schultze, "Gynäkologie und Irrenhaus," *ZBG*, 35 (1911), pp. 1572–1575. Schultze's ideas around this time were still being received with favor in the United States. See a translation of a paper of his, "Diagnosis and Operative Treatment of the Diseases of the Genitalia in the Female Insane," *AJO*, 67 (1913), pp. 114–120.

19. Mayer, *ZBG*, 43 (1919), p. 451.

20. Josef Peretti, "Gynäkologie und Psychiatrie," *Medizinische Klinik*, 8 (November 17, 1912), pp. 1857–1862; quote from p. 1861.

21. Ernst Siemerling, "Bemerkungen zu dem Aufsatz von Prof. Dr. L. M. Bossi in Genua: 'Die gynäkologischen Läsionen . . . ,'" *ZBG*, 36 (January 13, 1912), pp. 33–39. See also the longer attack on Bossi by Carl König (a student of Siemerling's) and Georg Linzenmeier (on the gynecological

teaching staff at Kiel), "Über die Bedeutung gynäkologischer Erkrankungen und den Wert ihrer Heilung bei Psychosen," *Archiv für Psychiatrie*, 51 (1913), pp. 1002-1054.

22. See William F. Bynum, "Rationales for Therapy in British Psychiatry: 1780-1835," *Medical History*, 18 (1974), pp. 317-334; Roger J. Cooter, "Phrenology and British Alienists, c. 1825-1845," ibid., 20 (1976), pp. 135-151. For debates among various schools within German psychiatry in this period see Henri Ellenberger, *The Discovery of the Unconscious* (New York: Basic Books, 1970), pp. 210-228.

23. Johannes Baptist Friedreich, *Historisch-kritische Darstellung der Theorien über das Wesen und den Sitz der psychischen Krankheiten* (Leipzig, 1836), pp. 21, 115-116.

24. Wilhelm Griesinger, *Pathologie und Therapie der psychischen Krankheiten* (Stuttgart, 1845; 2nd [rev.] ed. Stuttgart, 1861. I consulted an unchanged reprint of this 1861 edition published in 1867. See pp. 203-210 for the role of the genital organs in insanity; "Hirnanämie" or "Hyperanämie" on p. 205. Griesinger first articulated his earlier-held reflex views in "Über psychische Reflexactionen, mit einem Blick auf das Wesen der psychischen Krankheiten," *Archiv für physiologische Heilkunde*, 2 (1843), pp. 76-113. The scholarly literature on Griesinger has gone little beyond the bare account offered by Theodor Kirchhoff, in Kirchhoff, ed., *Deutsche Irrenärzte: Einzelbilder ihres Lebens und Wirkens*, 2 vols. (Berlin, 1921-24), vol. 2, pp. 1-14.

25. ". . . Die Aetiologie der Geisteskrankheiten im Allgemeinen keine andere ist, als die Aetiologie aller übrigen Gehirn- und Nervenkrankheiten" (p. 135).

26. "G." (Griesinger), "Vorwort," *Archiv für Psychiatrie und Nervenkrankheiten*, 1 (1868), pp. iii, iv. I have translated "Nervenkrankheiten" here as "neurological illness" because of Griesinger's convictions of organicity. Later, as the term becomes a weasel word, "nervous disease" is a more appropriate translation. I have been unable to find in his work the phrase, often attributed to Griesinger, "Geisteskrankheiten sind Gehirnkrankheiten" (mental diseases are brain diseases). It captures, however, the essence of his thought.

27. Griesinger, *Pathologie* (1861), pp. 55, 162-163.

28. Heinrich Quincke, "Über ärztliche Spezialitäten und Spezialärzte," *MMW*, 53 (June 19, 1906), pp. 1260-1264, quote p. 1263. ("Aus der 'Irrenklinik' wird im Sprachgebrauch eine 'Nervenklinik.'")

29. Oswald Bumke, "50 Jahre Psychiatrie," ibid., 72 (July 10, 1925), pp. 1141-1143; the phrase comes, according to Bumke, from Franz Nissl.

30. Freud, "Selbstdarstellung" (1925), in *Gesammelte Werke*, vol. 14 (Frankfurt am Main: Fischer, 1948), p. 37.

31. Theodor Meynert, *Klinische Vorlesungen über Psychiatrie* (Vienna, 1890), p. III.

32. Oswald Bumke, *Erinnerungen und Betrachtungen: Der Weg eines deutschen Psychiaters* (Munich, 1953), p. 90 ("ganz aussichtslose Wissenschaft").

33. Letter of Dec. 29, 1878, in Hans H. Walser, ed., *August Forel, Briefe/ Correspondance, 1864–1927* (Berne: Hans Huber, 1968), p. 146.

34. Hermann Hesse, "Kurgast" (1924), in *Gesammelte Dichtungen*, vol. 4 (Berlin: Suhrkamp, 1957), pp. 24–25.

35. Caspar Max Brosius, *Aus meiner psychiatrischen Wirksamkeit: Eine Adresse an die practischen Ärzte* (Berlin, 1878), p. 33.

36. Brosius, *Aus meiner psychiatrischen Wirksamkeit: Eine zweite Adresse . . .* (Wiesbaden, 1881), pp. 3, 13. ("Das Irresein ist eine *Gehirn*krankheit.")

37. Ewald Hecker, *Über das Verhältnis zwischen Nerven- und Geisteskrankheiten* (Cassel, 1881), pp. 6–7.

38. Karl Kahlbaum, *Programm zur Betheiligung der Heilanstalt für Nervenkranke zu Görlitz an der diesjährigen Hygiene-Ausstellung (Allgemeine deutsche Ausstellung auf dem Gebiete der Hygiene und des Rettungswesens, Berlin, 1882/83)* (Görlitz, 1883), p. 8.

39. Andrew Wilson, *Medical Researches; Being an Enquiry into the Nature and Origin of Hysterics in the Female Constitution* (London, 1776). Wilson was physician at the Medical Asylum in London.

40. Benjamin Brodie, *Lectures Illustrative of Certain Local Nervous Affections* (London, 1837), pp. 65–66 (in the edition whose pagination begins at p. 33).

41. David D. Davis, *Principles and Practice of Obstetric Medicine*, vol. 1 (London, 1836), pp. 397–398.

42. Robert B. Todd, *Cyclopedia of Anatomy and Physiology*, 5 vols. (1835–59), vol. 3 (London, 1847), p. 722Q.

43. Pierre Briquet, *Traité clinique et thérapeutique de l'hystérie* (Paris, 1859), p. 100.

44. G. L. W. Hohnstock, *Über Hysterie und Hypochondrie und deren Heilart* (Sondershausen, Germany, 1816), p. 7.

45. See Dietrich Wilhelm Heinrich Busch, *Das Geschlechtsleben des Weibes*, 5 vols. (1839–44), vol. 2 (Leipzig, 1840), pp. 293–294, 307–309, 332–343; Anton Theobald Brück, *Bad Driburg in seinen Heilwirkungen* (Osnabrück, Germany, 1844), pp. 64–94; Joseph Amann, *Über den Einfluss der weiblichen Geschlechtskrankheiten auf das Nervensystem . . .* (Erlangen, 1868), pp. 58–69.

46. John Purcell, *A Treatise of Vapours or Hysterick Fits*, 2nd ed. (London, 1707; 1st ed. 1702), p. 164.

47. Busch, *Geschlechtsleben* (1840), vol. 2, p. 325.

48. Heinrich Laehr, *Über Irrsein und Irrenanstalten* (Halle, Germany, 1852), pp. 50–54.

49. Morel's *Traité des dégénérescences physiques* was published in 1857. For a good summary of the views of Morel see Werner Leibbrand and Annemarie Wettley, *Der Wahnsinn: Geschichte der abendländischen Psychopathologie* (Freiburg: Karl Alber, 1961), pp. 524–528; Magnan, pp. 528–533.

50. Joachim Heinrich Campe, *Allgemeine Revision des gesammten Schul und Erziehungswesens* . . . , vol. 8 (Vienna, 1787), p. 153, note. The author opposed fairy tales and other supernatural lore on the grounds that, "Es ist dies besonders in unsern phantasiereichen und nervenkranken Zeiten höchstgefährlich, weil der Mittel, phantastische Vorstellungen zu erwecken, leider schon zu viel in Bewegung gesetzt sind und weil nichts stärker auf die Nerven wirkt, als eine erhitzte Phantasie."

51. James H. Cassedy, *American Medicine and Statistical Thinking, 1800–1860* (Cambridge, Mass.: Harvard University Press, 1984), p. 158.

52. Paul Berger, *Führer durch die Privat-Heilanstalten* . . . (Berlin, 1889/90), pp. 5–6.

53. For a use of this term see S. W. Agar, "Some Social Questions in Connection with Nervous Disease," *Birmingham Medical Review,* 20 (1886), pp. 1–21. "There exists a steady increase of physical diseases of a certain nature, which have apparently developed side by side with our increased luxury and civilization. Broadly speaking, they may be designated modern diseases" (p. 3). On the phenomenon, see Andreas Steiner, *"Das nervöse Zeitalter": Der Begriff der Nervosität bei Laien und Ärzten in Deutschland und Österreich um 1900* (Zurich: Juris-Verlag, 1964).

54. Robert Musil, *Der Mann ohne Eigenschaften,* 2 vols. (1930–32) (Reinbek bei Hamburg: Rowohlt, 1978), vol. I, p. 458. "Es war Leben in ihr [die neue Zeit], Wandelbarkeit, Ruhelosigkeit, Standpunktwechsel. Aber sie spürten wohl selbst [die Menschen dieses neuen Zeitalters], wie das war. Es rüttelte an ihnen, es blies durch ihren Kopf, sie gehörten einem nervösen Zeitalter an, und es stimmte etwas nicht."

55. Leopold Löwenfeld, *Pathologie und Therapie der Neurasthenie und Hysterie* (Wiesbaden, 1894), p. 45. See also E. K. H. Bilfinger, who maintained that, "The signature of our epoch is an anemic, nervous race." "Unsere Zeitkrankheit und ihre Bekämpfung" (1892), reprinted in his, *Natürliche Heil- und Lebensweise* (Leipzig, 1901), p. 140. See also Wilhelm Erb, *Über die wachsende Nervosität unserer Zeit* (Heidelberg, 1893) as typical of the many writings on this theme.

56. Jules Chéron, *Introduction à l'étude des lois générales de l'hypodermie* (Paris, 1893), p. 267.

57. For example, see Henry Stedman, "Some of the Mental Aspects of Nervous Disease," *BMSJ,* 113 (August 6, 1885), pp. 123–127.

58. According to Michael Trimble, the Edinburgh psychiatrist Andrew Combe in 1831 was the first to use the term *functional* in relation to nervous disease, but meant by it disruption of function rather than the absence of a demonstrable organic lesion. Trimble, "Functional Diseases," *BMJ,* ii85 (December 18, 1982), pp. 1768–1770.

59. See for example August Axenfeld, the most distinguished of the pre-Charcotian French neurologists, *Traité des névroses* (1863), 2nd. rev. ed. Henri Huchard, ed. (Paris, 1883), p. 4; see pp. 29–31 for Axenfeld's classification of the "névroses," an anticipation of Charcot's mania for classification.

60. Richard von Krafft-Ebing, *Die Melancholie: eine klinische Studie* (Erlangen, 1874), p. 64. He said apropos autopsy findings in melancholic patients, "so lehrt die Erfahrung im Allgemeinen das Fehlen makroskopischer Veränderungen im Gehirn und dessen Hüllen. Wir sprechen deshalb von einer Psychoneurose, wohl bewusst jedoch, dass alle klinischen Symptome nur die Folge von Ernährungsstörungen der Rindenschicht des Grosshirns sein können, die sich aber beim gegenwärtigen Zustand unseres Wissens einer näheren Deutung und Bezeichnung entziehen." Krafft-Ebing developed his ideas about "psychoneurosis" as a nonhereditary form of insanity more fully in his textbook, *Lehrbuch der Psychiatrie* (1879), 3rd ed. (Stuttgart, 1888), pp. 319–325. For a major nonpsychoanalytic discussion of the "psychoneuroses" in the sense of psychogenic neuroses see Jules-Joseph Dejerine and Ernest Gauckler, *Les Manifestations fonctionnelles des psychonévroses, leur traitement par la psychothérapie* (Paris, 1911).

61. Forel, *Briefe* (1968), pp. 122–123; J. J. Honegger was acting chief of psychiatry in Zurich while Forel was away.

62. See Harold Neumann, "Die Entwicklung der deutschen Facharztordnung," *Nervenarzt*, 28 (1957), pp. 278–279. Of 18,600 physicians in 1906 in Prussia, 20 percent indicated themselves as "specialists." Two-thirds of these had received some kind of postgraduate training (of two or more years). Although the state of Saxony regulated use of the title "specialist" as early as 1902, not until 1924 did the official organization of German physicians begin systematically to define specialties and determine their certification.

63. Emil A. Gutheil, ed., *The Autobiography of Wilhelm Stekel* (New York: Liveright, 1950), p. 87.

64. For a convenient compilation of dates see Hans Laehr, *Die Anstalten für Psychisch-Kranke in Deutschland, Deutsch-Österreich, der Schweiz und den baltischen Ländern*, 6th ed. (Berlin, 1907), entries under various cities.

65. Leube was an internist, which reinforces the point that much "nerve doctoring" took place under the rubric of internal medicine. Such boasting occurred on the advertisement pages of spa and sanatorium guides. See for example Erwin Jaeger, *Illustrierter Führer durch Bäder, Heilanstalten und Sommerfrischen*, 6th rev. ed. (Leipzig, 1913), p. 603, for the advertisement of Abend's sanatorium in Wiesbaden.

66. See, for example, Ernst Beyer, "Mehr Nervenheilstätten!" *PNW*, 10 (April 18, 1908), pp. 29–33, especially p. 30.

67. For an example of attempts to wrest the neurologists and *Nervenärzte* to psychiatry, see the battle Emil Kraepelin had to wage in the late 1880s at the University of Dorpat (Tartu, Estonia), in Kraepelin, *Lebenserinnerungen* (written about 1922–26) (Berlin: Springer, 1983), pp. 48–49; see also Sidney I. Schwab, "The Neurologic Dilemma," *Archives of Neurology and Psychiatry*, 6 (1921), pp. 255–262. For the opposed attempt to maintain neurology as a separate field closely allied to internal medicine, Paul

Näcke, "Die Trennung der Neurologie von der Psychiatrie und die Schaffung eigener neurologischer Kliniken," *NCB*, 31 (1912), pp. 82–89.

68. For details see Shorter, "Private Clinics in Central Europe, 1850–1933," *Social History of Medicine*, 3 (1990), pp. 159–195.

69. Hermann Oppenheim, *Psychotherapeutische Briefe* (Berlin, 1906), p. 21.

70. Freud, "Selbstdarstellung" (1925), pp. 40–41.

71. Ernest Jones, *The Life and Work of Sigmund Freud*, vol. 1 (New York: Basic Books, 1953), pp. 228–229.

72. On Mendel's early days in Pankow see Hermann Kron's obituary of him, "E. Mendel," *DKW*, 33 (July 18, 1907), pp. 1182–1184. See also M. Stürzbecher, "Emanuel Mendel (1839–1907)," *Nervenarzt*, 60 (1989), pp. 764–765.

73. These details of Mendel's life stem from a variety of sources. See the account in Kirchhoff, *Deutsche Irrenärzte*, vol. 2, pp. 161–165. Arthur Stern offers a brief portrait in, *In bewegter Zeit: Erinnerungen und Gedanken eines jüdischen Nervenarztes, Berlin-Jerusalem* (Jerusalem: Verlag Mass, 1968), p. 42.

74. Kirchhoff, *Irrenärzte*, vol. 2 (1924), p. 164.

75. In fact the asylum psychiatrists took on more the air of gentleman farmers than physicians. Describing the life of the medical superintendent of the English asylum in the 1930s, Eliot Slater said: "Life could be quite leisured, and at that time it was still possible for the 'super' to live the life of a gentleman farmer, invited to tennis parties at the Rectory, fishing and even riding to hounds." "Psychiatry in the Thirties," *Contemporary Review*, 226 (1975), pp. 70–75; quote from p. 71.

76. Emanuel Mendel, *Die Manie: eine Monographie* (Vienna, 1881).

77. For an overview see Werner Janzarik, "Die klinische Psychopathologie zwischen Griesinger und Kraepelin im Querschnitt des Jahres 1878," in Janzarik, ed., *Die Psychopathologie als Grundlagenwissenschaft* (Stuttgart: Enke, 1979), pp. 54–57.

78. On the contrast see Friedrich Jolly, "Über Hysterie bei Kindern," *BKW*, 29 (August 22, 1892), pp. 841–845. Among Oppenheim's own writings, see especially his article. "Thatsächliches und Hypothetisches über das Wesen der Hysterie," ibid., 27 (June 23, 1890), pp. 553–556; whereas Charcot and Paul Julius Möbius considered hysteria the result of "ideas" (*Vorstellungen*), Oppenheim implicated "reizbare Schwäche." In his textbook he said that the mechanism of hysteria was "enorme Reizbarkeit," that of neurasthenia "die reizbare Schwäche." Oppenheim, *Lehrbuch der Nervenkrankheiten* (1894), 5th ed., 2 vols. (Berlin, 1908), vol. 2 pp. 1206, 1270.

79. Whereas at the end of the nineteenth century, only 5 percent of Berlin's population as a whole was Jewish, a third of the physicians were. See Rolf Winau, *Medizin in Berlin* (Berlin: de Gruyter, 1987), p. 325. On Vienna see Shorter, "The Two Medical Worlds of Sigmund Freud," paper for a

conference on "Sigmund Freud and the History of Psychoanalysis," Toronto, 1990. For a nominal list of physicians practicing in Berlin, see Verband der Ärzte Deutschlands, *Verzeichnis der Ärzte im Deutschen Reiche,* 2nd ed., 1908 (Leipzig, 1908), pp. 1–40, for the Landespolizeibezirk Berlin. On Juliusburger's altercation with Johannes Bresler, editor of the *Psychiatrisch-Neurologische Wochenschrift,* see Johannes Bresler, "Ist Religion Privatsache?" *PNW,* 31 (May 11, 1929), pp. 236–239; Otto Juliusburger, "Psychiater und Religion, ibid., (June 1), pp. 270–274. Juliusburger, a founding member of the Berlin Psychoanalytic Society, later moved to a private clinic in Berlin-Lankwitz.

80. See for example, Stern, *Bewegte Zeit* (1968), p. 57.

81. Claude-Marie-Stanislas Sandras, *Traité pratique des maladies nerveuses,* 2 vols. (Paris, 1851), "L'état nerveux constitue à peu près ce que M. [Laurent] Cerise a désigné sous le nom de névropathie-protéiforme." (vol. 1, p. 19).

82. Löwenfeld, *Hysterie* (1894), p. 15, made this point.

83. José M. López Piñero, *Historical Origins of the Concept of Neurosis* (Cambridge, England: Cambridge University Press, 1983), p. 73. According to information in F. G. Gosling, *Before Freud: Neurasthenia and the American Medical Community, 1870–1910* (Urbana: University of Illinois Press, 1987), the term was first used by an Italian physician in 1808 (p. 26 n. 2). For an example of the use of "neurasthenia" around the time of Beard, see Edwin Holmes Van Deusen, "Observations on a Form of Nervous Prostration (Neurasthenia) Culminating in Insanity," *American Journal of Insanity,* 25 (1868–69), pp. 445–461.

84. George Beard, "Neurasthenia, or Nervous Exhaustion," *BMSJ,* 80 (April 29, 1869), pp. 217–221.

85. On Beard's life see Charles E. Rosenberg, "The Place of George M. Beard in Nineteenth-Century Psychiatry," *Bulletin of the History of Medicine,* 36 (1962), pp. 245–259; Peter Gay, *The Bourgeois Experience, Victoria to Freud,* vol. 2: *The Tender Passion* (New York: Oxford University Press, 1986), pp. 341–348. On the history of the diagnosis of neurasthenia in the United States, see also Barbara Sicherman, "The Uses of Diagnosis: Doctors, Patients, and Neurasthenia," *Journal of the History of Medicine,* 32 (1977), pp. 33–54.

86. Beard, *Die Nervenschwäche (Neurasthenia). Ihre Symptome, Natur . . . nach der zweiten Auflage ins Deutsch übertragen* (Leipzig, 1881). This "second edition" of Beard's book also appeared in 1880. Oswald Bumke gave a scathing analysis of the triumphal march in Germany of Beard's neurasthenia in "Die Revision der Neurosenfrage," *MMW,* 72 (October 23, 1925), pp. 1815–1819.

87. Jean-Martin Charcot, *Leçons du mardi à la Salpêtrière, Policliniques, 1887–1888,* lecture of November 22, 1887, pp. 30–36. See also lecture of February 5, 1889, where Charcot says "our knowledge of these questions is

scarcely three or four years old." (Charcot, *Leçons du mardi* [1889], lesson of February 5, 1889, p. 284.) Not until 1895—two years after Charcot's death—did one of Beard's books appear in French. *Sexual Neurasthenia (Nervous Exhaustion). Its Hygiene, Causes* . . . (New York, 1884), was translated as *La Neurasthénie sexuelle; hygiène, causes* (based on 3rd U.S. ed. of 1891) (Paris, 1895). On Charcot's godfathering of neurasthenia see Fernand Levillain, *La Neurasthénie: maladie de Beard (Méthodes de Weir Mitchell et Playfair. Traitement de Vigouroux* (Paris, 1891), pp. 13–14. Charcot wrote the preface to this book. See also Joseph-Marie-Alfred Beni-Barde, *La Neurasthénie* (Paris, 1908), p. 361.

88. Paul Dubois, *The Psychic Treatment of Nervous Disorders (The Psychoneuroses and their Treatment)* (1904), Eng. trans. 6th ed. (New York, 1909), p. 18.

89. Alfred T. Schofield, *The Management of a Nerve Patient* (London, 1906). "You will probably meet at least six cases of neurasthenia for every one of hysteria," he advised fellow physicians (p. 105).

90. August Kühner, *Kranke, schwache und gesunde Nerven* (Mainz, Germany, 1901), pp. 10–11, 19.

91. Jeffrey Moussaieff Masson, ed., *The Complete Letters of Sigmund Freud to Wilhelm Fliess, 1887–1904* (Cambridge, Mass.: Harvard University Press, 1985), p. 51, letter of July 10, 1893. On Freud's own neurasthenia see Jones, *Freud*, vol. 1 (1953), p. 170.

92. Alfred W. Gruber and Erwin H. Ackerknecht, eds., *Constantin von Monakow, Vita Mea/Mein Leben* (about 1927), (Berne: Hans Huber, 1970), p. 237.

93. See Charles L. Dana, "The Partial Passing of Neurasthenia," *BMSJ*, 150 (March 31, 1904), pp. 339–344; Beni-Barde, *Neurasthenie* (1908), pp. 349–357.

94. See for example Edward E. Mayer, "The Present Status of the Psychoneuroses and of Psychotherapy," *New York Medical Journal*, 92 (December 10, 1910), pp. 1168–76, especially p. 1172.

95. Conrad Rieger, "Über die Behandlung 'Nervenkranker,'" *Schmidts Jahrbücher der in- und ausländischen gesamten Medicin*, 251 (1896), pp. 193–198; quote from p. 195.

96. Andrew Clark, "Some Observations Concerning What is Called Neurasthenia," *Lancet*, i (January 2, 1886), pp. 1–2; quote from p. 2.

97. David Drummond, "The Mental Origin of Neurasthenia and its Bearing on Treatment," *BMJ*, ii (December 28, 1907), pp. 1813–1816; quote from p. 1814.

98. George H. Savage, "A Lecture on Neurasthenia and Mental Disorders," *Medical Magazine*, 20 (1911), pp. 620–630; quote from p. 620.

99. Mary Putnam Jacobi, *Essays on Hysteria, Brain-Tumor and Some Other Cases of Nervous Disease* (New York, 1888), pp. 63–64.

100. William Osler, *The Principles and Practice of Medicine* (New York, 1892), pp. 979–980.

101. Rudolph von Hösslin, "Aetiologie," in Franz Carl Müller, ed. *Handbuch der Neurasthenie* (Leipzig, 1893), p. 66.

102. Thomas Dixon Savill, *Lectures on Hysteria and Allied Vaso-Motor Conditions* (London, 1909), p. 16.

103. Charles H. Hughes, "Psychiatry and Neuriatry in the Medical Press," *Alienist and Neurologist*, 26 (1906), pp. 452–460; quote from p. 455.

104. Karl Petrén, "Über die Verbreitung der Neurasthenie unter verschiedenen Bevölkerungsclassen," *Deutsche Zeitschrift für Nervenheilkunde*, 17 (1900), pp. 397–412; data from p. 399.

105. Paul Leubuscher and Wenzeslaus Bibrowitz, "Die Neurasthenie in Arbeiterkreisen," *DMW*, 21 (May 25, 1905), pp. 820–824; quote from p. 822. For further social data on neurasthenia see Franz Koelsch, "Arbeit bezw. Beruf in ihrem Einfluss auf Krankheit und Sterblichkeit," in Max Mosse and Gustav Tugendreich, eds., *Krankheit und soziale Lage* (Munich, 1913), p. 161.

106. Raymond Belbèze, *La Neurasthénie rurale* (Paris, 1911), pp. 24, 108–109.

107. The whole question of somatoform symptoms as a result of depression is so important that a chapter is devoted to it in volume 2 of this work. Accordingly depression will not be further discussed here.

108. Paul Hartenberg, *Traitement des neurasthéniques* (Paris, 1912), pp. 228–233.

109. Henri Feuillade, *Conseils aux nerveux et à leur entourage* (Paris, 1924), p. 26. Writing mainly for an audience of family doctors, he said he was reflecting the teachings of Charcot.

110. Edward A. Weiss, "A Consideration of Neurasthenia in its Relation to Pelvic Symptoms in Women," *AJO*, 57 (1908), pp. 230–235; quote from p. 231.

111. John L. Garvey, "Neuroses in Women—the Neurologist's Point of View," in Carl Henry Davis, *Gynecology and Obstetrics*, 3 vols. (New York, 1935), vol. 3, p. 5 (each chapter is paginated separately).

112. Joseph-Marie-Alfred Beni-Barde, *La Neurasthénie: les vrais et les faux neurasthéniques* (Paris, 1908), p. 370.

113. Levillain, *Neurasthénie* (1891), p. 17.

114. Of Hösslin's 828 private-clinic patients with neurasthenia, only 35 percent had positive family histories. Hösslin, though favorable to explanations involving heredity, said: "Neurasthenia in the absence of a neuropathic disposition may be acquired, if demands are placed on the organism which exceed one's physiological limits." *Neurasthenie* (1893), p. 68. One of the major German authorities, Rudolf Arndt, considered that neurasthenia could be either inherited or acquired: Patients with a positive family history would probably become symptomatic earlier in life. *Die Neurasthenie (Nervenschwäche): Ihr Wesen, ihre Bedeutung und Behandlung* (Vienna, 1885), pp. 107–109.

115. Joseph Collins, *Letters to a Neurologist* (New York, 1908), pp. 20–21.

116. Wilkie Collins, *The Woman in White* (1859); (reprint, Harmondsworth, England: Penguin, 1974), pp. 66–70.

117. Joseph Amann, *Über den Einfluss der weiblichen Geschlechtskrankheiten auf das Nervensystem* (Erlangen, 1868), pp. 1–2.

118. Berthold Stiller, *Die asthenische Konstitutionskrankheit (Asthenia universalis congenita, Morbus asthenicus)* (Stuttgart, 1907), p. 6.

119. Levillain, *Neurasthénie* (1891), p. 8.

120. Alfred Boettiger, "Über Neurasthenie und Hysterie und die Beziehungen beider Krankheiten zu einander," *MMW*, 44 (May 25, 1897), pp. 554–558; quote from p. 555.

121. Oswald Bumke, "Die Revision der Neurosenfrage," *MMW*, 72 (October 23, 1925), pp. 1815–1819; quotes from p. 1816.

122. Feuillade, *Conseils nerveux* (1924), p. 28.

123. Emil Kraepelin, *Psychiatrie. Ein kurzes Lehrbuch für Studierende und Aerzte*, 4th ed. (Leipzig, 1893). See "Dementia praecox," pp. 435–445.

124. Carl Lange, "Über die Ausflockung von Goldsol durch Liquor cerebrospinalis," *BKW*, 49 (May 6, 1912), pp. 897–901; also "Die Ausflockung kolloidalen Goldes durch Zerebrospinalflüssigkeit bei luetischen Affektionen des Zentralnervensystems," *Zeitschrift für Chemotherapie*, 1 (1912–13), pp. 44–78.

125. Sigmund Freud, "Über die Berechtigung, von der Neurasthenie einen bestimmen Symptomenkomplex als 'Angstneurose' abzutrennen," reprinted in *Gesammelte Werke*, vol. 1 (Frankfurt am Main: Fischer, 1952), pp. 315–342.

126. Pierre Janet, *Les Obsessions et la psychasthénie*, 2 vols. (Paris, 1903; vol. 2 was coauthored by Fulgence Raymond). For a critique of "psychasthenia" as a catchall, see Smith Ely Jelliffe, "Nervous and Mental Disease Dispensary Work," *Post-Graduate*, 27 (1912), pp. 593–607, especially p. 594 ("an artificial group, made up in large part, according to the Kraepelian [*sic*] conceptions, of dementia precox, manic depressives, alcoholic psychoses, hysteria, neurasthenia, and other disorders.")

127. Angelo Louis Marie Hesnard, *Les Syndromes névropathiques* (Paris, 1927), p. 202.

128. John C. Chatel and Roger Peele, "A Centennial Review of Neurasthenia," *AJP*, 126 (1970), pp. 1404–1413; quote from p. 1405.

129. Simon Wessely makes this point: "Once neurasthenia was viewed as psychiatric, a principal social function was lost." "Old Wine in New Bottles: Neurasthenia and 'ME,'" *Psychological Medicine*, 20 (1990), pp. 35–53; quote from p. 47. "ME" means "myalgic encephalomyelitis," an organic-sounding synonym for chronic fatigue.

CHAPTER 9

Doctors, Patients, and the Psychological Paradigm

1. Robert Whytt, *Observations on the Nature, Causes, and Cure of those Disor-*

ders Which Have Been Commonly Called Nervous, Hypochondriac, or Hysteric (Edinburgh, 1765), pp. 234–235.

2. William Rowley, *A Treatise on Female . . . Diseases* (London, 1788), pp. 63, 119.

3. See Edward L. Margetts, "The Early History of the Word 'Psychosomatic,'" *Canadian Medical Association Journal,* 63 (1950), pp. 402–404; Z. J. Lipowski, "What Does the Word 'Psychosomatic' Really Mean?" *Psychosomatic Medicine,* 46 (1984), pp. 153–171.

4. John Haygarth, *Of the Imagination as a Cause and as a Cure of Disorders of the Body, Exemplified by Fictitious Tractors* (London, 1800), pp. 2–4, 28. On the background see Roger Rolls, *The Hospital of the Nation: The Story of Spa Medicine and the Mineral Water Hospital at Bath* (Bath: Bird Publications, 1988), pp. 101, 164–165.

5. Edward James Seymour, "Clinical Lecture . . . Hysteria," *Lancet,* ii (May 5, 1832), pp. 134–136.

6. William Sudlow Roots, "Hysterical Paralysis," *St. Thomas's Hospital Reports,* 1 (1836), pp. 248–260; case from p. 260.

7. Robert Brudenell Carter, *On the Pathology and Treatment of Hysteria* (London, 1853), pp. 4–6.

8. Frederic Carpenter Skey, *Hysteria* (London, 1867), pp. 41, 60–61.

9. Dennis De Berdt Hovell, *On Pain and Other Symptoms Connected with the Disease Called Hysteria* (London, 1867), pp. 22–24. Leopold Löwenfeld believed Hovell among the first to recognize hysteria as a "psychische Erkrankung." *Pathologie und Therapie der Neurasthenie und Hysterie* (Wiesbaden, 1894), p. 4 n.

10. John Russell Reynolds, "Remarks on Paralysis, and Other Disorders of Motion and Sensation, Dependent on Idea," *BMJ,* ii (November 6, 1869), pp. 483–485; case from p. 483.

11. Joseph Skoda, "Geschichte einer durch mehrere Monate anhaltenden Katalepsis," *Zeitschrift der kais.[erlichen] kön.[iglichen] Gesellschaft der Ärzte zu Wien,* 8 (2) (1852), pp. 404–419; quote from p. 418. Skoda disagreed, thinking catalepsy a "reflex phenomenon."

12. Moritz Benedikt, "Über Hysterie," *WMW,* 18 (January 22, 1868), pp. 105–108; quotes from p. 105.

13. Carl von Liebermeister, "Über Hysterie und deren Behandlung," *(Volkmann) Sammlung klinischer Vorträge,* no. 236 (*Innere Medicin 82*) (n.d. [about 1884]), pp. 2139–2158; quotes from pp. 2140, 2142, 2147. Löwenfeld called Liebermeister the first German writer to recognize hysteria as a psychological disease (*Pathologie* [1894], p. 5). See also Löwenfeld, "Hysterie und Suggestion," *MMW,* 41 (February 13, 1894), pp. 117–119, contrasting the whole "psychological" school of Liebermeister, Paul Julius Möbius, and Adolf Strümpell to the "reizbare Schwäche"-style organicists.

14. Summary of paper by George Beard on "The Influence of Mind in the

Causation and Cure of Disease—The Potency of Definite Expectation," *JNMD*, 3 (1876), pp. 429–431; discussion on pp. 431–434. Beard borrowed the concept of "definite expectation" from Daniel Hack Tuke's book, *Illustrations of the Influence of the Mind Upon the Body in Health and Disease* (London, 1872), pp. 367f. There is no acknowledgment of Tuke's work in the summary of Beard's paper. According to Charles Dana, Beard "discovered psychotherapeutics" one day when his battery failed. "He continued his applications with the dead electrodes" and apparently the patient improved anyway. Charles L. Dana, "George M. Beard: A Sketch of His Life and Character . . . ," *Archives of Neurology and Psychiatry*, 10 (1923), pp. 427–435, especially p. 429.

15. On Möbius's life see Elisabeth Katharina Waldeck-Semadeni, *Paul Julius Möbius, 1853–1907: Leben und Werk* (Berne: med. diss., 1980), pp. 8–11 on these years.

16. Paul Julius Möbius, *Über den physiologischen Schwachsinn des Weibes* (Halle, Germany, 1900); the book had reached a ninth edition by 1908.

17. Adolf Strümpell, *Aus dem Leben eines deutschen Klinikers* (Leipzig, 1925), p. 141 for both anecdotes. Francis Schiller places Möbius in context in *A Möbius Strip: Fin-de-siècle Neuropsychiatry and Paul Möbius* (Berkeley: University of California Press, 1982).

18. Paul Julius Möbius, "Über den Begriff der Hysterie," *Zentralblatt für Nervenheilkunde*, 11 (1888), pp. 66–71.

19. Paul Julius Möbius, "Über die Behandlung von Nervenkranken und die Errichtung von Nervenheilstätten" (1896), reprinted in Möbius, *Vermischte Aufsätze* (Leipzig, 1898), quote from pp. 40–41.

20. See Möbius's obituary of Charcot, *MMW*, 40 (September 19, 1893), pp. 712–714.

21. Hannah Decker considerably underestimates the healthiness of this psychological paradigm in pre-Freudian Europe when she writes, "German psychiatrists' suspicion of or hostility to anything that was unmaterialistic partly explains their repugnance for the psychotherapies and hypnotic techniques in style in much of Europe." Further: "The scientist was supposed to be concerned with diseased organs, symptoms and syndromes, and the courses of diseases—not with individual patients." *Freud in Germany: Revolution and Reaction in Science, 1893–1907* (New York: International Universities Press, 1977), pp. 66, 68. In a previous article she attributed the slowness of German psychiatrists and neurologists to accept Freud's wisdom to "the overwhelming belief . . . in the organic etiology of mental illness." "The Medical Reception of Psychoanalysis in Germany, 1894–1907: Three Brief Studies," *Bulletin of the History of Medicine*, 45 (1971), pp. 461–481; quote from p. 475.

22. These facts come from biographical monographs available in standard reference works. For a retrospective view putting these individuals in the larger context of psychological theories, a context rejecting the brain para-

digm, see Oswald Bumke, "Fünfzig Jahre Psychiatrie," *Archiv für Psychiatrie und Nervenkrankheiten,* 76 (1926), pp. 58–67.

23. Adolf Strümpell, "Über die Entstehung und die Heilung von Krankheiten durch Vorstellungen," *BKW,* 30 (January 2, 1893), pp. 22–25; quote from p. 23. Hermann Determann, a society nerve doctor who ran a private clinic in the Black Forest, attributed to Strümpell the "psychogene Theorie" of neurasthenia. "Über Wirkung und Anwendung der Hydrotherapie bei der Neurasthenie," *Zeitschrift für diätetische und physikalische Therapie,* 3 (1899–1900), pp. 211–220; quote from p. 216.

24. Josef Breuer and Sigmund Freud, *Studies in Hysteria* (1895), Eng. trans. 1955 (Harmondsworth, England: Penguin, 1974), p. 58 n. 2.

25. Robert Sommer, *Diagnostik der Geisteskrankheiten* (Vienna, 1894), pp. 127–128. *Vorstellung* might also be translated as "representation" or "idea."

26. Hans H. Walser, ed., *August Forel, Briefe/Correspondance: 1864–1927* (Berne: Hans Huber, 1968), pp. 158–160, 167, 298.

27. Emil Kraepelin, *Psychiatrie: ein Lehrbuch für Studierende und Ärzte,* 5th ed. (Leipzig, 1896), p. 728.

28. J. Zutt et al., eds., *Karl Bonhoeffer Zum Hundertsten Geburtstag* (Berlin: Springer, 1969), "Lebenserinnerungen von Karl Bonhoeffer, geschrieben für die Familie" (about 1940), pp. 8–107; anecdote from p. 67.

29. The story is told in Ernst Kretschmer, *Gestalten und Gedanken,* 2nd ed. (Stuttgart: Thieme, 1971; 1st ed. 1963), p. 65.

30. Kurt Kolle himself relates this anecdote, in Kolle, ed., *Grosse Nervenärzte,* 2nd ed., vol. 1 (Stuttgart: Thieme, 1970), p. 175.

31. Hans W. Gruhle, "Kraepelins Bedeutung für die Psychologie," *Archiv für Psychiatrie,* 87 (1929), pp. 43–49; quote from p. 45.

32. For example, Alfred Hoche had trained in Heidelberg and was in 1902 at thirty-seven, senior lecturer (ausserordentlicher Professor) in psychiatry in Strasbourg. He said in that year, apropos the differential diagnosis between hysteria and epilepsy, "Die reine Hysterie ist functioneller Natur in dem Sinne, dass sie eine pathologische Anatomie weder besitzt noch jemals besitzen wird." Summary of his paper on "Differentialdiagnose zwischen Epilepsie und Hysterie," in *NCB,* 21 (July 1, 1902), p. 626. My comments about conceding the psychogenic to psychiatry apply only to the scientific elite of Central Europe, centered especially around Heidelberg and Leipzig. In France, Austria, England, and the United States a great turf war between psychiatry and neurology over hysteria and the other psychoneuroses was waged in the first half of the twentieth century. There is not enough space here to consider this contest in detail, but see the exchange between neurologist Jules-Joseph Dejerine and psychiatrist Gilbert Ballet in the *Presse médicale:* Dejerine, "Clinique des maladies du système nerveux, leçon inaugurale," (April 1, 1911), pp. 253–259; Ballet, "Le Domaine de la psychiatrie" (May 10, 1911), pp. 377–380; and Dejerine's rebuttal, "Le Domaine de la psychiatrie" (May 24, 1911), pp. 425–426.

33. Bumke, "Fünfzig Jahre" (1926), p. 62.

34. Antoine Le Camus, *Médecine de l'esprit* (Paris, 1753), cited in Jean Camus and Philippe Pagniez, *Isolement et psychothérapie* (Paris, 1904), brief summary p. 74. Camus and Pagniez give an excellent résumé of the vicissitudes of psychotherapy up to the 1890s, pp. 74–82.

35. Roy Porter, "Was There a Moral Therapy in Eighteenth Century Psychiatry?" *Lynchnos: Lärdomshistoriska Samfundets Årsbok 1981-1982*, pp. 12–26. On Tuke see Anne Digby, *Madness, Morality and Medicine: A Study of the York Retreat, 1796-1914* (Cambridge, England: Cambridge University Press, 1985). Reil is commonly seen as the founder of psychotherapy in Germany. See Martin Schrenk, *Über den Umgang mit Geisteskranken* (Heidelberg: Springer, 1973), pp. 61–79. His seminal text was *Rhapsodien über die Anwendung der psychischen Curmethode auf Geisteszerrütung* (Halle, 1803).

36. See for example François Leuret, "Des indications à suivre dans le traitement moral de la folie," *Gazette médicale de Paris* (January 10, 1846), pp. 26–31. Some private asylums did, however, implement moral therapy. See for example, Bruno Goergen, *Privat-Heilanstalt für Gemüthskranke* (Vienna, 1820), on "das sogenannte psychische Verfahren (moralische Behandlung)," pp. 9–10. His conception amounted to entertaining and distracting these wealthy private patients, simultaneously encouraging them in civilized behavior.

37. Daniel Hack Tuke, *Illustrations of the Influence of the Mind Upon the Body* (Philadelphia, 1873 [London, 1872]), pp. 361, 393.

38. Möbius, "Hysterie" (1888), pp. 69–70.

39. See Bernheim's *De la suggestion dans l'état hypnotique et dans l'état de veille* (Paris, 1884). Actually, Ambroise-Auguste Liébeault had begun using non-hypnotic suggestion as early as 1866, but was not widely recognized for having done so. See his "Confession d'un médecin hypnotiseur," *Revue de l'hypnotisme*, 1 (1886), pp. 105–110, 143–148. "Il y a plus de vingt ans ... que, par simple affirmation verbale, j'ai fait disparaître des symptômes morbides sur des malades non endormis et qui n'avaient jamais été hypnotisés" (p. 144).

40. See the report of Frederik van Eeden's 1889 talk on "La Psychothérapie suggestive" to the Dutch Psychiatric Society reprinted in *Revue de l'hypnotisme*, 4 (1890), pp. 370–377; and Frederik van Eeden and Albert Willem van Renterghem, *Psychothérapie* (Paris, 1894). For details on the outpatient psychotherapy clinic that Van Renterghem and Van Eeden opened in 1887 in Amsterdam, see Renterghem's "Liébeault et son école," *Zeitschrift für Hypnotismus*, 6 (1897), pp. 11–44, especially pp. 11–15. Van Eeden terminated his association with the clinic in 1893.

41. Frederik van Eeden, "Les Principes de la psychothérapie," *Revue de l'hypnotisme*, 7 (1893), pp. 97–120; quote from pp. 105–107. Arie de Jong, a psychiatrist in The Hague who was able to compare statistics on the suc-

cess of hypnotism in his public clinic and in a private practice, found working-class patients easier to hypnotize than middle-class patients, because the former were more accustomed to carrying out orders. "Quelques observations sur la valeur médicale de la psychothérapie," ibid., 6 (1891), pp. 78–86, especially pp. 79–80.

42. George M. Robertson, "Psycho-Therapeutics," *Lancet,* ii (September 17, 1892), pp. 657–658.

43. Joseph Babinski, "Définition de l'hystérie," *Revue neurologique,* 9 (1901), pp. 1074–1080.

44. John C. Burnham, *Jelliffe: American Psychoanalyst and Physician. His Correspondence with Sigmund Freud and C. G. Jung* (Chicago: University of Chicago Press, 1983), p. 49.

45. Paul Dubois, *The Psychic Treatment of Nervous Disorders (The Psychoneuroses and their Moral Treatment)* (1904), Eng. trans. (New York, 1905), pp. 226, 242–243, 388.

46. Ibid., p. 376.

47. Ibid., pp. 229–230.

48. These quotes from Jules Dejerine and Ernest Gauckler, *Les Manifestations fonctionnelles des psychonévroses: leur traitement par la psychothérapie* (Paris, 1911), p. viii. Dejerine began constructing his system in connection with a clinic for "isolation" therapy he had introduced at the Salpêtrière; see his, "Le Traitement des psycho-névroses à l'hôpital par la méthode de l'isolement," *Revue neurologique,* 10 (1902), pp. 1145–1148. Probably the best exposition of Dejerine's views appears in the work of his students Camus and Pagniez, *Isolement* (1904), pp. 24–26.

49. "Psychotherapy" appeared in the index of the *Index Medicus,* the main annual bibliography of medical literature, for the first time in 1895–96 ("Psycho-therapy"); "Psycho-therapeutics" made its appearance in the index, however, in 1893. "Psychotherapy" was used for the first time as a subject heading in 1906 (ser. 2, vol. 4, p. 639).

50. Angelo Hesnard, *Les Syndromes névropathiques* (Paris, 1927), p. 231.

51. David Drummond, "The Mental Origin of Neurasthenia . . .", *BMJ,* ii (December 28, 1907), pp. 1813–1816; quote from p. 1815.

52. Edwin Bramwell, "A Lecture on Psychotherapy in General Practice," *Edinburgh Medical Journal,* N.S., 30 (1923), pp. 37–59; quotes from pp. 44, 59.

53. Thomas Arthur Ross, "Observations on the Diagnosis and Treatment of Functional Nervous Disorder," *BMJ,* ii (December 7, 1929), pp. 1041–1044; quote from p. 1043.

54. Smith Ely Jelliffe, in a discussion of E. W. Taylor's, "The Attitude of the Medical Profession Toward the Psychotherapeutic Movement," *JNMD,* 35 (1908), p. 408.

55. Joseph Collins, "The General Practitioner and the Functional Nervous Diseases," JAMA, 52 (January 9, 1909), pp. 87–92; quote from p. 91.

56. Wilhelm Olivier Leube, "Über nervöse Dyspepsie," *Archiv für klinische Medizin*, 23 (1879), pp. 98–114. On Nothnagel see Erna Lesky, *Die Wiener medizinische Schule im 19. Jahrhundert* (Graz: Böhlau, 1978), p. 322.

57. On Rosenbach's life see F. C. R. Eschle, "Ottomar Rosenbach als Begründer der Psychotherapie," *Zeitschrift für Psychotherapie und medizinische Psychologie*, 2 (1910), pp. 50–62. Although Rosenbach was an important figure, the claim that he "founded" psychotherapy is ridiculous.

58. Ottomar Rosenbach's last major work on the subject was *Nervöse Zustände und ihre psychische Behandlung* (Berlin, 1897).

59. Ottomar Rosenbach, "Über psychische Therapie innerer Krankheiten," *Berliner Klinik*, 25 (1890), pp. 1–33; quote from p. 18; reprinted in Rosenbach, *Nervöse Zustände und ihre psychische Behandlung* (Berlin, 1897), pp. 65–95.

60. For an illustration see George M. Beard and Alphonso D. Rockwell, *A Practical Treatise on the Medical and Surgical Uses of Electricity*, 6th ed. (New York, 1888), p. 325.

61. Ibid., p. 87. For a summary of Rosenbach's ideas, see H. Temmen, "Ottomar Rosenbach (1851–1907) und sein Beitrag zur Psychotherapie," *Acta psychotherapeutica*, 12 (1964), pp. 10–20, especially pp. 14–15. Although Rosenbach often criticized hypnotism, he was in fact a founding member of the editorial committee of the *Zeitschrift für Hypnotismus*, the first issue of which appeared in 1892.

62. Ottomar Rosenbach, "Die Emotionsdyspepsie," *BKW*, 34 (February 1, 1897), pp. 97–101; quotes from pp. 99–100.

63. I follow here the summary of H. J. Weitbrecht, "Kurt Schneider 80 Jahre—80 Jahre Psychopathologie," *Fortschritte der Neurologie und Psychiatrie*, 35 (1967), pp. 497–515, especially p. 503.

64. Felix Gattel, *Über die sexuellen Ursachen der Neurasthenie und Angstneurose* (Berlin, 1898), pp. 52–57. Although Freud had initially been pleased to greet Gattel, and even took him along in September 1897 on the family vacation, the young man turned out something of a millstone around Freud's neck, and Freud was embarrassed by the publication in 1898 of Gattel's book. See Freud's complaints to Wilhelm Fliess, in letters from May 16, 1897, to April 3, 1898, in Jeffrey Moussaieff Masson, *The Complete Letters of Sigmund Freud to Wilhelm Fliess, 1887–1904* (Cambridge, Mass.: Harvard University Press, 1985), p. 244 ff. On February 15, 1901, Freud said, apropos collecting notes on neurotic patients: "I am doing roughly the same thing Gattel did at the time he made himself so unpopular in Vienna" (p. 436).

65. Leonard Seif, "Casuistische Beiträge zur Psychotherapie," *Zeitschrift für Hypnotismus*, 9 (1900), pp. 371–373; Franz Riklin, "Analytische Untersuchungen der Symptome und Assoziationen eines Falles von Hysterie (Lina H.), " *PNW*, 6 (February 11, 1905), pp. 449–452, and following issues.

66. Jakob Kläsi, "Über psychiatrisch-poliklinische Behandlungsmethoden," *Zeitschrift für die gesamte Neurologie und Psychiatrie*, 36 (1917), pp. 431–450; quote from p. 432, n.2.

67. Alfred T. Schofield, *The Management of a Nerve Patient* (London, 1906), p. 150.

68. Hermann Weber, summary of paper, "Die Behandlung der Nervosität" (given to a meeting of physicians in Dresden), *MMW*, 60 (April 15, 1913), p. 837. Although Weber had been born in Germany and maintained life-long ties to that part of Europe, he had qualified in medicine in 1855 in England.

69. William Henry Stoddart, "Hysteria and its Relation to Mental Diseases," *Clinical Journal*, 40 (July 31, 1912), pp. 257–261; quote from p. 259. He referred to second states as "systematised anaesthesia." On the reception of psychoanalysis by the British public in general see Dean Rapp, "The Early Discovery of Freud by the British General Educated Public, 1912–1919," *Social History of Medicine*, 3 (1990), pp. 217–243.

70. Robert T. Edes, "The Present Relations of Psychotherapy," *JAMA*, 52 (January 9, 1909), pp. 92–96; quotes from p. 96.

71. George M. Parker, "Hysteria under Psychoanalysis," *Medical Record*, 78 (August 6, 1910), pp. 219–226; case from pp. 221–222.

72. Edward E. Mayer, "The Present Status of the Psychoneuroses and of Psychotherapy," *New York Medical Journal*, 92 (December 10, 1910), pp. 1168–1176; quotes from 1170, 1171.

73. Among the many accounts of these events, compact and reliable is Henri Ellenberger, *The Discovery of the Unconscious* (New York: Basic Books, 1970).

74. Hilda C. Abraham and Ernst L. Freud, eds., *Sigmund Freud/Karl Abraham: Briefe, 1907–1926*, 2nd ed. (Frankfurt am Main: Fischer, 1980), pp. 65–66.

75. Johannes Heinrich Schultz, *Lebensbilderbuch eines Nervenarztes* (Stuttgart: Thieme, 1964), pp. 70–71.

76. Schultz, "Zur Technik der Suggestiv-Behandlung, besonders bei gebildeten Patienten," *Klinische Wochenschrift*, 9 (February 26, 1923), pp. 402–403. "In Deutschland, Österreich und der Schweiz das Hauptinteresse psychotherapeutischen Arbeitens in mehr oder weniger offener Weise auf psycho-analytische Fragen gerichtet ist" (p. 402). See also Schultz's résumé "Psychoanalyse: die Breuer-Freudschen Lehren, ihre Entwicklung und Aufnahme," *Zeitschrift für angewandte Psychologie*, no. 2 (1909), pp. 440–497.

77. Hans Prinzhorn, "Der Psychiater und die Psychoanalyse," *Zeitschrift für die gesamte Neurologie und Psychiatrie*, 80 (1923), pp. 1–9; quote from p. 8.

78. On this transformation see Mark Micale, "Hysteria and its Historiography: A Review of Past and Present Writings," *History of Science*, 27 (1989), pp. 223–261, 319–351, especially pp. 246–249.

79. Some authorities consider Alfred Adler's *Studie über Minderwertigkeit von Organen* (Berlin, 1907) as an influential forerunner in the interpretation of the unconscious roots of somatoform symptoms. I feel this claim is unfounded as the book has little of the authority conferred by clinical experience, thus gravely conflating organic and psychogenic, and is moreover largely an exercise in pseudoneurophysiology. Laying a more legitimate claim is Charles Creighton's *Illustrations of Unconscious Memory in Disease* (London, 1886).

80. Max Eitingon, *Bericht über die Berliner Psychoanalytische Poliklinik* (Leipzig, 1923), p. 8.

81. Martin Grotjahn, "Franz Alexander," in Franz Alexander et al., eds., *Psychoanalytic Pioneers* (New York: Basic Books, 1966), p. 386.

82. On the history of the clinic see U. Schultz and L. M. Hermanns, "Das Sanatorium Schloss Tegel Ernst Simmels—Zur Geschichte und Konzeption der ersten Psychoanalytischen Klinik," *Psychotherapie, medizinische Psychologie*, 37 (1987), pp. 58–67.

83. Advertisement in *PNW*, 30 (August 11, 1928), p. 354.

84. Ernst Simmel, "Die psychoanalytische Behandlung in der Klinik," *Internationale Zeitschrift für Psychoanalyse*, 14 (1928), pp. 352–370; quote from p. 357.

85. Wilhelm Stekel, "Eine interessante Somatisation," *Psychoanalytische Praxis*, 2 (1932), p. 148. For Stekel's use in 1924, see his "Der epileptische Symptomenkomplex und seine analytische Bedeutung," *Fortschritte der Sexualwissenschaft und Psychanalyse*, 1 (1924), pp. 17–57; for example, "Aus Somatisation dieser Gefühllosigkeit zeigt der Kranke eine vollkommene Anästhesie der beiden Arme" (p. 39). From 1922 on, Felix Deutsch became an influential propagandist among internists for psychoanalytic techniques in the treatment of psychosomatic disorders. See, for example, his "Psychoanalyse und innere Medizin," in Wladimir Eliasberg, ed., *Bericht über den II. allgemeinen ärztlichen Kongress für Psychotherapie in Bad Nauheim* (Leipzig, 1927), pp. 53–59.

86. Sigmund Freud, "Bruchstücke einer Hysterie-Analyse" (1905), *Gesammelte Werke*, vol. 5 ([London, 1942] Frankfurt am Main: Fischer), p. 277; Freud spoke of "das 'somatische Entgegenkommen.'" This phrase has been rendered in English as "somatic compliance." The subsequent theoretical vicissitudes within psychoanalysis of Freud's hysteria concept are too complex to be gone into here. Freud's own thinking underwent a major change in 1926 when he began to see conversion symptoms as a consequence of anxiety. "Hemmung, Symptom und Angst" (1926), in *Gesammelte Werke*, vol. 14, pp. 162–205. "Die Angst ist also ein besonderer Unlustzustand mit Abfuhraktionen auf bestimmte Bahnen." Some of these "Bahnen," or pathways, take the form of conversion symptoms. Later psychoanalytic thought would interpret conversion symptoms as a way of blotting up, or binding, anxiety.

87. Although other writers used the term after Stekel, it was really Z. J. Lipowski who gave "somatization" its current psychiatric meaning. See his "Review of Consultation Psychiatry and Psychosomatic Medicine," *Psychosomatic Medicine*, 30 (1968), pp. 395–422, especially pp. 412–414. Lipowski, "Somatization: The Concept and Its Clinical Application," *AJP*, 145 (1988), pp. 1358–1368.

88. Franz Alexander, "Functional Disturbances of Psychogenic Nature," *JAMA*, 100 (February 18, 1933), pp. 469–473; also "The Influence of Psychologic Factors Upon Gastro-Intestinal Disturbances: A Symposium. I. General Principles . . . ," *Psychoanalytic Quarterly*, 3 (1934), p. 501–539.

89. Franz Alexander, "Fundamental Concepts of Psychosomatic Research: Psychogenesis, Conversion, Specificity," *Psychosomatic Medicine*, 5 (1943), pp. 205–210; quote from p. 209. The summation of Alexander's work was *Psychosomatic Medicine: Its Principles and Applications* (New York: Norton, 1950).

90. Helen Flanders Dunbar, *Emotions and Bodily Changes: A Survey of Literature on Psychosomatic Interrelationships* (New York, 1935). On Dunbar and Alexander, see Robert C. Powell's reflective article, "Helen Flanders Dunbar (1902–1959) and a Holistic Approach to Psychosomatic Problems," *Psychiatric Quarterly*, 49 (1977), pp. 133–152.

91. Research findings from this sample of ninety-two patients in Shorter, et al., "A Study of Patients With Persistent Somatization on an Inpatient Unit for Psychosomatic Medicine," forthcoming in *Psychosomatics*.

92. Geoffrey G. Lloyd, "Psychiatric Syndromes with a Somatic Presentation," *Journal of Psychosomatic Research*, 30 (1986), pp. 113–120; quote from p. 113.

93. Anton Theobald Brück, *Das Bad Driburg in seinen Heilwirkungen dargestellt* (Osnabrück, 1844), p. 87.

94. See advertisements, unpaginated, in the *PNW*, 26 (December 27, 1924); 28 (October 9, 1926).

95. Benjamin Travers, *A Further Inquiry Concerning Constitutional Irritation and the Pathology of the Nervous System* (London, 1835), p. 444.

96. Rudolf Schindler, "Die Psychotherapie des Organspezialisten," *MMW*, 72 (September 4, 1925), pp. 1517–1518; quote from p. 1517.

97. Malcolm A. Bliss, "Psychotherapy," *JAMA*, 51 (July 4, 1908), p. 37.

98. Herbert Berger, "Management of Neuroses by the Internist and General Practitioner," *New York State Journal of Medicine*, 56 (June 1, 1956), pp. 1783–1788; quotes from p. 1784.

99. Daniel Webster Cathell, *The Physician Himself and What He Should Add to the Strictly Scientific* (Baltimore, 1882), p. 146.

100. Schofield, *Management* (1906), pp. 90–91.

101. Axel Munthe, *The Story of San Michele* (London, 1929), pp. 32–34.

CHAPTER 10
The Patients' Paradigm Changes

1. Samuel Alexander Kinnier Wilson, "The Approach to the Study of Hysteria," *Journal of Neurology and Psychopathology,* 11 (1931), pp. 193–206; quote from pp. 194–195.

2. Aldo Zalla, "Sulla Sintomatologia Attuale dell'lsterismo," *Rassegna di Studi Psichiatria,* 38 (1949), pp. 39–74, especially p. 45.

3. J. Frei, "Contribution à l'étude de l'hystérie: Problèmes de définition et évolution de la symptomatologie," *Archives Suisses de Neurologie, Neurochirurgie et de Psychiatrie,* 134 (1984), pp. 93–129, especially pp. 116–117. There were fifty-three hysteria patients in 1910–29, and fifty-five in 1970–80.

4. Walter von Baeyer, "Zur Statistik und Form der abnormen Erlebnisreaktionen in der Gegenwart," *Nervenarzt,* 19 (1948), pp. 402–408; quotes from p. 405.

5. Patria Asher, "A Case of Rapidly Cured Hysterical Paralysis," *BMJ,* i (March 9, 1946), p. 355.

6. James L. Halliday, *Psychosocial Medicine: A Study of the Sick Society* (New York: Norton, 1948), p. 61.

7. Angelo Hesnard, *Les Syndromes névropathiques* (Paris, 1927), pp. 134, 142. He felt that hysteria had "taken refuge in military circles and in work accidents" (p. 134).

8. See Lynn Payer, *Medicine and Culture: Varieties of Treatment in the United States, England, West Germany, and France* (New York: Henry Holt, 1988), pp. 62–64.

9. Israel S. Wechsler, *The Neuroses* (Philadelphia, 1929), pp. 185, 187.

10. Paul Chodoff, "A Re-examination of Some Aspects of Conversion Hysteria," *Psychiatry,* 17 (1954), pp. 75–81; quote from p. 76.

11. Henry P. Laughlin, *The Neuroses in Clinical Practice* (Philadelphia: Saunders, 1956), pp. 252–253.

12. François Sirois, *Epidemic Hysteria* (Copenhagen: Munksgaard, 1974), p. 15.

13. Headline and story, "The Toll Workers' Illness: Was It All in Their Minds?" *New York Times,* March 12, 1990, p. A16.

14. Oswald Bumke, *Erinnerungen und Betrachtungen: Der Weg eines deutschen Psychiaters* (Munich: Pflaum, 1953), p. 182. "Man braucht nicht zu zittern, man lässt sich lieber versprengen." In 1916 the German Society for Psychiatry and Neurology met in Munich, where Hermann Oppenheim, oriented toward central-nervous explanations of shell shock, confronted adherents of the psychological paradigm. The latter were considered to have carried the day. See the proceedings of the "Achte Jahresversammlung der Gesellschaft Deutscher Nervenärzte in München am 22. und 23. September 1916," *Deutsche Zeitschrift für Nervenheilkunde,* 56 (1917), pp. 1–214.

15. Hans Bürger-Prinz, *Ein Psychiater berichtet* (Hamburg: Hoffmann und Campe, 1971), p. 102.

16. P. Lefebvre and S. Barbas, "L'Hystérie de guerre: étude comparative de ses manifestations au cours des deux derniers conflits mondiaux," *Annales médico-psychologiques*, 142 (1984), pp. 262–266. "Le glissement de l'hystérie de conversion vers la pathologie somatique" (p. 265).

17. For an overview see H. Merskey, "Shellshock," in G. E. Berrios and H. L. Freeman, eds., *1841–1991: 150 Years of British Psychiatry* (London: Royal College of Psychiatrists, 1991).

18. Oswald Bumke, *Lehrbuch der Geisteskrankheiten*, 2nd ed. (Munich, 1924; 1st ed. 1919), p. 258.

19. Giovanni Mingazzini, "Die Modifikationen der klinischen Symptome, die einige Psychosen in den letzten Jahrzehnten erfahren haben," *PNW*, 28 (February 6, 1926), pp. 68–72; quote from p. 71.

20. Stephen Taylor, *Good General Practice* (London: Oxford U.P., 1954), p. 417.

21. The identity of the correspondent was not revealed. "Paris," *Lancet*, ii (November 15, 1890), pp. 1060–1061; quote from p. 1060.

22. Alfred T. Schofield, *The Management of a Nerve Patient* (London, 1906), p. 106.

23. Parkes Weber and his father had written one of the standard "balneological" guides. Hermann Weber and Frederick Parkes Weber, *The Mineral Waters and Health Resorts of Europe* (London, 1898).

24. In the Contemporary Medical Archives Centre of the Wellcome Institute for the History of Medicine in London; charts in a series of bound volumes beginning "1894–1900" and ending "1913–."

25. Parkes Weber, "1913–" vol.; case begins p. 198. The charts of several long-standing patients continued past 1909.

26. Ibid., vol. for 1907–9; note of July 18, 1929.

27. Ibid., vol. for 1906–7; case begins p. 142.

28. Ibid., vol. for 1906–7; case begins p. 337.

29. Ibid., vol. for 1903–6; case begins with the letters attached to p. 152.

30. Dennis De Berdt Hovell, *On Pain and Other Symptoms Connected with the Disease Called Hysteria* (London, 1867), pp. 19–20, 24–25.

31. Joseph Amann, *Über den Einfluss der weiblichen Geschlechtskrankheiten aus das Nervensystem* (Erlangen, 1868), pp. 29–30.

32. See Shorter, "The First Great Increase in Anorexia Nervosa," *Journal of Social History*, 21 (1987), pp. 69–96.

33. Silas Weir Mitchell, "Rest in Nervous Disease: Its Use and Abuse," in Edward C. Seguin, *A Series of American Clinical Lectures*, vol. 1 (April 1875) (New York, 1876), pp. 83–102; quote from p. 96.

34. Josef Schreiber, "Zur Behandlung gewisser Formen von Neurasthenie und Hysterie durch die Weir Mitchell-Cur," *BKW*, 25 (December 31, 1888), pp. 1070–1072; case from pp. 1070–1071.

35. August Diehl, "Erfahrungen über einige Arzneimittel in der Hand des Nervenarztes," *Monatsschrift für Psychiatrie*, 29 (1911), pp. 450–471; details from pp. 457–458.

36. Semi Meyer, "Hysterie-Typen," *PNW*, 13 (April 8, 1911), pp. 21–24; quote from p. 23.
37. Fernand Levillain, *La Neurasthénie: maladie de Beard* (Paris, 1891), pp. 91–92.
38. Paul Hartenberg, *Traitement des neurasthéniques* (Paris, 1912), p. 15.
39. Charles-Albert Fiessinger, *La Médecine du praticien* (Paris, 1942), pp. 437–438.
40. Raymond Pujol, "Reflexions sur la fatigue et ses aspects psychologiques," *Annales médico-psychologiques*, 125 (1967), pp. 23–35; quotes from pp. 26–27.
41. Augustus Hoppin, *A Fashionable Sufferer, or Chapters from Life's Comedy* (Boston, 1883), pp. 12–15, 19–25, 54, 67.
42. Robert T. Edes, "The New England Invalid," *BMSJ*, 133 (August 1, 1895), pp. 101–107; quote from p. 102.
43. Philip Knapp, in the discussion at a meeting of the Boston Society of Psychiatry and Neurology, January 19, 1906, *JNMD*, 33 (1906), p. 464.
44. L. Gibbons Smart, "Management and Treatment of Functional Nervous Conditions," *New York Medical Journal*, 97 (June 28, 1913), pp. 1345–47; case from p. 1346.
45. C. W. Dowden and W. O. Johnson, "Exhaustion States," *JAMA*, 93 (November 30, 1929), pp. 1702–1706. The series contained patients with hypothyroid disease, anemia and depression. The 110 exhaustion patients on whom data by apparent cause were available seem to cover the period 1910–28.
46. See for example John Madison Taylor, "Management of Exhaustion States in Men," *International Clinics*, 17th ser., 2 (1907), pp. 36–50.
47. Abraham Myerson, *The Nervous Housewife* (Boston, 1926), pp. 2–3.
48. Joseph De Lee, "Obstetrics versus Midwifery," *JAMA*, 103 (August 4, 1934), pp. 307–311; quote from p. 310.
49. Horace K. Richardson, "Psychopathy and the General Practitioner," *NEJM*, 213 (October 24, 1935), pp. 787–795; case from pp. 792–793.
50. Frank N. Allan, "The Differential Diagnosis of Weakness and Fatigue," ibid., 231 (September 21, 1944), pp. 414–18. Two hundred thirty-five patients with a diagnosis of "chronic nervous exhaustion" were reexamined at the Mayo Clinic an average of six years after the diagnosis was first made. Two hundred of them did not have organic disease, either then or later. Seventy-eight percent of this group were women. Twenty-one patients did have some organic disease, which however was not considered responsible for their symptoms. In most cases the disease found at follow-up, such as a cervical cancer, was unlikely to have been present at the original examination, which occurred an average of seven years previously for this particular group. Fourteen patients turned out to have an organic disease which explained the original fatigue: three with "chronic encephalitis," two with hypertension, three with tuberculosis, and six miscellaneous. The percent-

age of women in these latter two groups was unstated. John W. Macy and Edgar V. Allen, " A Justification of the Diagnosis of Chronic Nervous Exhaustion," *Annals of Internal Medicine*, 7 (1934), pp. 861–867.

51. William P. D. Logan and A. A. Cushion, General Register Office [England], *Morbidity Statistics from General Practice*, vol. 1 (London: HMSO, 1958), p. 86. Such obvious physical causes of fatigue as iron-deficiency anemia were reported elsewhere in these statistics.

52. This will be discussed in the second volume of this work.

53. Ivan Illich, *Limits to Medicine. Medical Nemesis: The Expropriation of Health* (London: Boyars, 1976 [Penguin Books, 1977]), p. 141. See also Horacio Fabrega, Jr., "Language, Culture and the Neurobiology of Pain: a Theoretical Explanation," *Behavioural Neurology*, 2 (1989), pp. 235–259.

54. See Shorter, *A History of Women's Bodies* (New York: Basic Books, 1982), chaps. 5 and 7.

55. Paul Joire, "Contribution à l'étude de la contagion hystérique ou des crises par imitation," *Bulletin médical du Nord*, 31 (1892), pp. 505–517; case from pp. 512–514.

56. Silas Weir Mitchell, *Lectures on Diseases of the Nervous System, Especially in Women* (London, 1881), pp. 87–88.

57. Armand Hückel, "Über psychische Lähmungen und ihre Behandlung," *MMW*, 36 (March 26, 1889), pp. 213–217; quote from p. 214.

58. John Conolly, "Hysteria," in John Forbes et al., eds., *Cyclopaedia of Practical Medicine*, 5 vols. (1833–59), vol. 2 (London, 1833), pp. 557–586; quote from p. 561.

59. Hector Landouzy, *Traité complet de l'hystérie* (Paris, 1846), pp. 95, 98.

60. Frederic C. Skey, *Hysteria* (London, 1867), p. 66. The lectures had been delivered in 1866. Dennis De Berdt Hovell, astride both central-nervous and psychological paradigms, considered the term *hysterical pain* a misnomer unless the pain actually arose from the uterus. Such pain was, he said, really "centric neuralgia," caused by "depressed nerve power." *On Pain* (1867), p. 18.

61. John Russell Reynolds, "Hysteria," in Reynolds, ed., *A System of Medicine*, 5 vols. (1866–79), vol. 2 (London, 1872), p. 91.

62. On the usefulness of "la belle indifférence" as a diagnostic sign, see the discussion in Harold Merskey, *The Analysis of Hysteria* (London: Ballière Tindall, 1979), pp. 148–150.

63. Joseph Breuer and Sigmund Freud, *Studies in Hysteria* (1895), Eng. trans. 1955 (Harmondsworth, England: Pelican, 1974), pp. 203–204.

64. Charles A. Stimson, "The Psychic Treatment of Nervous Disorders," *Journal of the Michigan State Medical Society*, 7 (1908), pp. 281–285; quote from p. 283.

65. Walter C. Alvarez, *Nervousness, Indigestion and Pain* (New York, 1943), pp. 197, 208.

66. Otto Binswanger, *Die Hysterie* (Vienna, 1904), p. 123. "Man wird für diese

Schmerzen deshalb die weitere Bezeichnung des psychogenen Schmerzes vorziehen."

67. William Victor Johnston, *Before the Age of Miracles: Memoirs of a Country Doctor* (Toronto: Fitzhenry and Whiteside, 1972), pp. 78–79.

68. Schofield, *Management* (1906), p. 147.

69. William Morse Graily Hewitt, *The Diagnosis and Treatment of Diseases of Women* (London, 1863), p. 488.

70. Mary Putnam Jacobi, *Essays on Hysteria, Brain-Tumor and Some Other Cases of Nervous Disease* (New York, 1888), p. 35.

71. Semi Meyer, "Was charakterisiert die Hysterie," *Medizinische Klinik*, 5 (September 26, 1909), pp. 1471–1475; quote from p. 1473.

72. Felix Preissner, "Die Abteilung für Nervenkranke des Krankenhauses der Landesversicherungsanstalt Schlesien in Breslau," *PNW*, 27 (December 19, 1925), pp. 523–527; quote from p. 525.

73. H. Merskey, "Headache and Hysteria," *Cephalalgia*, 1 (1981), pp. 109–119.

74. Logan, *Morbidity Statistics* (1958), pp. 72, 86.

75. Henri Schaeffer, "Conceptions nouvelles sur l'hystérie," *Presse médicale* (February 20, 1929), pp. 237–239; quote from p. 239.

76. Kristine von Soden and Maruta Schmidt, eds., *Neue Frauen, die zwanziger Jahre: Bilder Lesebuch* (Berlin: Elefanten Press, 1988), cover photograph.

77. See some of the evidence from my earlier work on the history of the family, Shorter, *The Making of the Modern Family* (New York: Basic Books, 1975). See also Philippe Ariès's analysis of the distinctively dramatic nineteenth-century style of confronting death. *L'Homme devant la mort* (Paris: Seuil, 1977), p. 389 ff.

CHAPTER 11

Somatization at the End of the Twentieth Century

1. Donna E. Stewart, "The Changing Faces of Somatization," *Psychosomatics*, 31 (1990), pp. 153–158; quotes p. 157.

2. Shorter, *Bedside Manners: The Troubled History of Doctors and Patients* (New York: Simon & Schuster, 1985), p. 213.

3. Arthur J. Barsky, "The Paradox of Health," *NEJM*, 318 (February 18, 1988), pp. 414–418; quote from p. 415. See also his *Worried Sick: Our Troubled Quest for Wellness* (Boston: Little Brown, 1988).

4. Theodore Diller, "A Study of Three Thousand Cases Seen in Private Neurologic Practice," *International Clinics*, 23rd ser., ii (1913), pp. 180–189; data from p. 188.

5. Robert Wood Johnson Foundation, *Medical Practice in the United States* (Princeton: R. W. Johnson Foundation, n.d. [1982]), p. 68.

6. Karen Dunnell and Ann Cartwright, *Medicine Takers, Prescribers and Hoarders* (London, Routledge, 1972), p. 16, table 7.

7. Martha S. Linet et al., "An Epidemiologic Study of Headache Among Adolescents and Young Adults," *JAMA*, 261 (April 21, 1989), pp. 2211–

2216. Emphasis supplied. Within the month before the interview, "3.0 percent of the males and 7.4 percent of the females had suffered from a *migraine* headache." Some further statistics on the frequency of headache: Of sixteen hundred individuals polled in the early 1970s in a county in north Florida, 9 percent had headaches regularly and 38 percent had them "occasionally" (John J. Schwab et al., "The Epidemiology of Psychosomatic Disorders," *Psychosomatics*, 15 [1974], pp. 88–93; data from p. 89). Twenty-four percent of the women interviewed randomly in 1976 in a community in Scotland experienced headaches, 13 percent of the men. (J. G. Ingham and P. McC. Miller, "Symptom Prevalence and Severity in a General Practice Population," *Journal of Epidemiology and Community Health*, 33 [1979], pp. 191–198; data from p. 193. The respondents reported here were "controls" for a study of patients seen by physicians.) When pain has a clear psychogenic component, it tends to center in the head. Of 430 cases of "psychogenic regional pain" seen in the practice of neurologist Allan Walters between 1950 and 1960, 43 percent concerned the "head and neck" (Allan Walters, "Psychogenic Regional Pain Alias Hysterical Pain," *Brain*, 84 [1961], pp. 1–18; data from p. 5.)

8. K. B. Thomas, "The Consultation and the Therapeutic Illusion," *BMJ*, ii (May 20, 1978), pp. 1327–1328. Those who were given a symptomatic diagnosis and treated did no better than those who were told they had no disease and not treated.

9. Charles G. Watson and Cheryl Buranen, "The Frequencies of Conversion Reaction Symptoms," *Journal of Abnormal Psychology*, 88 (1979), pp. 209–211.

10. Wayne Katon et al., "The Prevalence of Somatization in Primary Care," *Comprehensive Psychiatry*, 25 (1984), pp. 208–215; quote from p. 209.

11. Within psychiatric settings, one-half to two-thirds of all patients report chronic pain. See, for example, Harold Merskey, "Headache and Hysteria," *Cephalalgia*, 1 (1981), pp. 109–119; summarizing other studies, p. 116. For example, among 134 patients seen for psychogenic symptoms ("conversion reactions") at the Johns Hopkins Hospital between 1956 and 1960, pain was the primary complaint in 56 percent (Frederick J. Ziegler et al., "Contemporary Conversion Reactions: A Clinical Study," *AJP*, 116 [1960], pp. 901–910; data from p. 902.) "Pain was by far the commonest symptom in a series of patients referred for evaluation of unexplained symptoms to an Edinburgh psychiatric clinic," in the early 1980s (Geoffrey G. Lloyd, "Psychiatric Syndromes with a Somatic Presentation," *Journal of Psychosomatic Research*, 30 [1986], pp. 113–120; quote from p. 114).

12. Stanley Lesse, "Atypical Facial Pain Syndromes of Psychogenic Origin: Complications of Their Misdiagnosis," *JNMD*, 24 (1956), pp. 346–351; both cases from p. 346.

13. J. J. Gayford, "Atypical Facial Pain," *Practitioner*, 202 (1969), pp. 657–660.

14. The patients at the clinic are described in Shorter et al., "The Inpatient Treatment of Persistent Somatization," forthcoming in *Psychosomatics*.
15. Marcus Reidenberg and David T. Lowenthal, "Adverse Nondrug Reactions," *NEJM*, 279 (September 26, 1968), pp. 678–679.
16. Martin K. Chen, "The Epidemiology of Self-Perceived Fatigue among Adults," *Preventive Medicine*, 15 (1986), pp. 74–81; data from p. 76.
17. D. R. Hannay, "Symptom Prevalence in the Community," *Journal of the Royal College of General Practitioners*, 28 (1978), pp. 492–499; data from p. 493.
18. Simon Wessely et al., "Symptoms of Low Blood Pressure: A Population Study," *BMJ*, 301 (August 18, 1990), pp. 362–365; data from p. 363.
19. Rachel Jenkins, *Sex Differences in Minor Psychiatric Morbidity* (Cambridge, England: Cambridge University Press, 1985; Psychological Medicine, monograph supplement no. 7), p. 30.
20. Michael Shepherd et al., *Psychiatric Illness in General Practice*, 2nd ed. (Oxford: Oxford University Press, 1981), p. 114.
21. Simon Wessely and P. K. Thomas, "The Chronic Fatigue Syndrome—Myalgic Encephalomyelitis or Postviral Fatigue," in C. Kennard, ed., *Recent Advances in Neurology*, vol. 6 (Edinburgh: Churchill Livingstone, 1990), pp. 85–132; data from p. 88. G. Lewis and Simon Wessely provide a comprehensive list of community studies and primary-care studies of fatigue in, "The Epidemiology of Fatigue: Many Questions but Few Answers," forthcoming, table 1.
22. Sixty-six percent of the older women (over thirty-six) who presented in primary care in a Scottish town in the mid-1970s reported "tiredness," 34 percent of the older male patients. Of the younger patients, fully 43 percent of the women and 26 percent of the men were tired. (Ingham, "Symptom Prevalence" [1979], p. 193.) In one medical practice, 21 percent of five hundred "unselected" patients were identified as suffering from the kind of fatigue that these particular doctors (highly sympathetic to the diagnosis) and their patients attributed to "chronic Epstein-Barr virus" (Dedra Buchwald et al., "Frequency of 'Chronic Active Epstein-Barr Virus Infection' in a General Medical Practice," *JAMA*, 257 [May 1, 1987], pp. 2303–2307).
23. Kurt Kroenke et al., "Chronic Fatigue in Primary Care," *JAMA*, 260 (August 19, 1988), pp. 929–934.
24. Leone Risdale, "Chronic Fatigue in Family Practice," *Journal of Family Practice*, 29 (1989), pp. 486–488; data from p. 486.
25. Chauncey Warring Dowden and William Oscar Johnson, "Exhaustion States," *JAMA*, 93 (November 30, 1929), pp. 1702–1706. Statistics today usually exclude patients whose fatigue is owing to an organic illness, whereas those of Dowden and Johnson did not.
26. Landes-Irren-Anstalt Kierling-Gugging, chart no. 246 in Abgangjahr 1905.

27. E. Steinebrunner and Ch. Scharfetter, "Wahn im Wandel der Geschichte," *Archiv für Psychiatrie und Nervenkrankheiten*, 222 (1976), pp. 47–60; data from p. 52. From 3 percent of all delusional patients in 1912–16 to 12 percent in 1973.

28. Stewart, "Changing Faces of Somatization" (1990), p. 154.

29. P. W. Bassett-Smith, "Duration of Mediterranean Fever," *BMJ*, ii (December 19, 1903), p. 1589.

30. Alice C. Evans, "Chronic Brucellosis," *JAMA*, 103 (September 1, 1934), pp. 665–667. She wrote a major overview of the disease in "Brucellosis in the United States," *American Journal of Public Health*, 37 (1947), pp. 139–151.

31. Robert W. Trever et al., "Brucellosis: I. Laboratory-Acquired Infection," *Archives of Internal Medicine*, 103 (1959), pp. 381–397; Leighton E. Cluff et al., "Brucellosis: II. Medical Aspects of Delayed Convalescence," ibid., pp. 398–405; John B. Imboden et al., "Brucellosis: III. Psychologic Aspects of Delayed Convalescence," ibid., pp. 406–414. The phrase about "psychologic factors" appeared in Cluff, p. 405. The authors found no evidence of infection in these chronic patients (who had once suffered a real infection) and maintained that the profile of depression, fatigue, and so forth seen in chronic brucellosis resembled that of "psychoneurosis" (p. 404).

32. Hugh Fudenberg, in discussion, "Piercing the Smoke Screen View of CFIDS," *CFIDS Chronicle* (Spring/Summer 1990), p. 4.

33. *Newsweek*, November 12, 1990, p. 62.

34. See "Coming to Terms with a Wheel-Chair," *Myalgic Encephalomyelitis* [ME] *Association Newsletter* (Summer 1988), p. 14. On disability, see for example, Gary Boyd, "Claims under Policies of Disability Insurance," *ME Canada*, 1 (March–April, 1989), p. 4.

35. *ME Association Newsletter* (Summer 1988), p. 29.

36. A. G. Gilliam, *Epidemiological Study of an Epidemic, Diagnosed as Poliomyelitis, Occurring among the Personnel of the Los Angeles County General Hospital during the Summer of 1934* (Washington, D.C., 1938; Public Health Bulletin No. 240); quote from p. 69.

37. Alexis Shelokov et al., "Epidemic Neuromyasthenia: An Outbreak of Poliomyelitislike Illness in Student Nurses," *NEJM*, 257 (August 22, 1957), pp. 345–355; and David C. Poskanzer et al., "Epidemic Neuromyasthenia: An Outbreak in Punta Gorda, Florida," ibid., pp. 356–364.

38. Donald A. Henderson and Alexis Shelokov, "Epidemic Neuromyasthenia—Clinical Syndrome," ibid., 260 (1959), pp. 757–764.

39. See Irving E. Salit, "Sporadic Postinfectious Neuromyasthenia," *Canadian Medical Association Journal*, 133 (1985), pp. 659–663.

40. Michael A. Epstein and Y. M. Barr, "Cultivation in Vitro of Human Lymphoblasts from Burkitt's Malignant Lymphoma," *Lancet*, i (February 1, 1964), pp. 252–253. Gertrude Henle et al., "Relation of Burkitt's Tu-

mor-Associated Herpes-Type Virus to Infectious Mononucleosis," *Proceedings of the National Academy of Sciences* (Wash.), 59 (1968), pp. 94–101.

41. Raphael Isaacs, "Chronic Infectious Mononucleosis," *Blood*, 3 (1948), pp. 858–861.

42. On the significance of the "Lake Tahoe epidemic" in the iconography of the fatigue movement, see Byron Hyde, "The Cambridge Symposium on Myalgic Encephalomyelitis (ME)," in *The Nightingale* (newsletter of the Nightingale Research Foundation, a prominent sufferers' support organization), 1 (Spring 1990), pp. 1–4, especially p. 1.

43. Among the principle boosters of the EBV explanation were James F. Jones et al., "Evidence for Active Epstein-Barr Virus Infection in Patients with Persistent, Unexplained Illnesses: Elevated Anti-Early Antigen Antibodies," *Annals of Internal Medicine*, 102 (1985), pp. 1–7.

44. Gary P. Holmes et al., "Chronic Fatigue Syndrome: A Working Case Definition," ibid., 108 (1988), pp. 387–389. A further nail in the coffin of EBV was Deborah Gold et al., "Chronic Fatigue: A Prospective Clinical and Virologic Study," *JAMA*, 264 (July 4, 1990), pp. 48–53. Scare articles in such magazines as *Redbook* caused the Centers for Disease Control in Atlanta, Georgia, to attempt to monitor CFS in selected places. See the interview which the director of one sufferers' organization conducted with Holmes in the spring of 1988. *Chronic Fatigue Syndrome Society Reporter*, 2 (May 10, 1988), pp. 1–4.

45. The *National CEBV [chronic Epstein-Barr virus Reporter]*, which launched its first issue on May 15, 1987, changed its name with the issue of February 29, 1988, to *CFSS [chronic fatigue syndrome society] Reporter*, and then again with the issue of November/December 1988 to *CFIDS [chronic fatigue immune dysfunction syndrome] Society Reporter*.

46. Donna B. Greenberg, "Neurasthenia in the 1980s: Chronic Mononucleosis, Chronic Fatigue Syndrome, and Anxiety and Depressive Disorders," *Psychosomatics*, 31 (1990), pp. 129–137; quote from p. 135.

47. The Medical Staff of the Royal Free Hospital, "An Outbreak of Encephalomyelitis in the Royal Free Hospital Group, London, in 1955," *BMJ*, ii (October 19, 1957), pp. 895–904. A. Melvin Ramsay, a physician in the hospital, provided a true-believer's account in, *Myalgic Encephalomyelitis and Postviral Fatigue States: The Saga of Royal Free Disease*, 2nd ed. (London: Gower, 1988). Colin P. McEvedy and A. W. Beard rendered a setback to the organic interpretation of the epidemic with the judgment that some portion of the victims, especially the young nurses, were "pathological hysterics." "A Controlled Follow-Up of Cases Involved in an Epidemic of 'Benign Myalgic Encephalomyelitis,'" *BJP*, 122 (1973), pp. 141–150; quote from p. 149.

48. Editorial, "A New Clinical Entity," *Lancet*, i (May 26, 1956), pp. 789–790. This remarkably uncritical editorial compared the discovery of "benign myalgic encephalomyelitis" to the discovery by Viennese neurologist

Constantin von Economo in 1917 of encephalitis lethargica, a major organic (apparently viral) disease in which a fifth of the cases ended fatally!

49. Simon Wessely, "Chronic Fatigue Syndrome," in Kennard (1990), p. 85.

50. Charles-Humbert-Antoine Despine, *Observations de médecine pratique faites aux bains d'Aix-en-Savoie* (Annecy, 1838), p. 279.

51. W. R. Gowers, "Lumbago: Its Lessons and Analogues," *BMJ*, i (January 16, 1904), pp. 117–121. "I think we need a designation for inflammation of the fibrous tissue which has not [produced the same kind of inflammation as cellulitis], and yet we cannot doubt is of this nature. We may conveniently follow the analogy of 'cellulitis,' and term it 'fibrositis'" (p. 118).

52. Frederick Parkes Weber papers, Contemporary Medical Archives Centre, Wellcome Institute for the History of Medicine, London. Casebook 1907–9; case begins p. 58.

53. On the history of the diagnosis of fibrositis, see Nortin M. Hadler, "A Critical Reappraisal of the Fibrositis Concept," *American Journal of Medicine*, 81 (Suppl. 3A) (1986), pp. 26–30. A more credulous account is offered by Michael D. Reynolds, "The Development of the Concept of Fibrositis," *Journal of the History of Medicine*, 38 (1983), pp. 5–35. For an account by one of the principal figures in fibrositis's rebirth, see Hugh Smythe, "Fibrositis Syndrome: A Historical Perspective," *Journal of Rheumatology*, 16 (Suppl. 19) (1989), pp. 2–6.

54. Eugene F. Traut, "Fibrositis," *Journal of the American Geriatrics Society*, 16 (1968), pp. 531–538.

55. In the United States, Don L. Goldenberg of the Boston University School of Medicine became one of the main publicists of the disease. See for example his, "Research in Fibromyalgia: Past, Present and Future," *Journal of Rheumatology*, 15 (1988), pp. 992–996. A special issue of this journal in 1989 featured no fewer than three articles by Goldenberg. Ibid., 16 (Suppl. 19) (1989), pp. 12–14, 91–93, and 127–130.

56. Muhammad B. Yunus, "Fibromyalgia Syndrome: New Research on an Old Malady," *BMJ*, ii98 (February 25, 1989), pp. 474–475. Yunus was a rheumatology professor in Peoria, Illinois.

57. Thomas Bohr, letter, *JAMA*, 258 (September 18, 1987), p. 1476.

58. Simon Wessely, "Chronic Fatigue and Myalgia Syndromes," in Norman Sartorius et al., eds., *Psychological Disorders in General Medical Settings* (Berne: Hogrefe and Huber, 1990), pp. 82–97; quote from p. 86.

59. S. Alfici et al., "Primary Fibromyalgia Syndrome—a Variant of Depressive Disorder?" *Psychotherapy and Psychosomatics*, 51 (1989), pp. 156–161. Also James I. Hudson and Harrison G. Pope, Jr., "Fibromyalgia and Psychopathology: Is Fibromyalgia a Form of 'Affective Spectrum Disorders?'" *Journal of Rheumatology*, 16 (Suppl. 19) (1989), pp. 15–22.

60. See several contributions in the above-mentioned special number of the *Journal of Rheumatology* in 1989.

61. Byron M. Hyde, "Myalgic Encephalomyelitis," *CFIDS Chronicle* (Summer/Fall, 1989), pp. 37–40; quote from p. 37.

62. Summary of "COFA National Fibromyalgia Seminar," ibid., (Spring/Summer 1990), pp. 21–23. For an example of a medical enthusiast conflating the two diagnoses in a medical forum, see Charles Pritchard, letter, *Annals of Internal Medicine*, 106 (1988), p. 906. "In reality, is not the chronic fatigue syndrome just another name for fibrositis possibly secondary to a chronic viral infection?" he asked.

63. "Chronic Fatigue Syndrome: A Modern Medical Mystery," *Newsweek*, November 12, 1990, pp. 62–70.

64. Hillary Johnson, "Journey into Fear," *Rolling Stone*, July 16 and August 13, 1987.

65. Sue Finlay, "An Illness Doctors Don't Recognize," *Observer*, June 1, 1986, p. 43. The response was mentioned in Simon Wessely, "It's not *all* ME," ibid., May 21, 1989.

66. *ME Association Newsletter* (Summer 1988), p. 5.

67. *New York Times*, September 7, 1989, p. B18.

68. "M.E. Newsbrief," *Keeping in Touch. CFS/ME Newsletter*, no. 1 (March/April 1990), p. 9.

69. *CFIDS Chronicle* (Summer/Fall 1989), p. 112.

70. Dennis Jackson, "So I Really Have Something Real," ibid., pp. 108–111.

71. Elisabeth Keiffer, "The Illness You Can't Sleep Off," *Woman's Day*, March 1, 1990, pp. 26–32.

72. Stephen E. Straus, "Persisting Illness and Fatigue in Adults with Evidence of Epstein-Barr Virus Infection," *Annals of Internal Medicine*, 102 (1985), pp. 7–16; Straus, "The Chronic Mononucleosis Syndrome," *Journal of Infectious Diseases*, 157 (1988), pp. 405–412.

73. *CFIDS Chronicle* (Spring/Summer 1990), p. 98.

74. *Keeping in Touch*, no. 3 (July/September, 1990), p. 5.

75. Wessely, in Kennard (1990), p. 102.

76. Byron Hyde, reporting on the CIBA Symposium of October 11, 1988, in London. *The Nightingale*, 1 (Fall 1989), p. 6.

77. See for example Stephanie Woodcock, "Research Roundup," *ME Newsletter* (Autumn 1989), p. 10. "I was encouraged . . ."

78. *CFIDS Reporter*, no. 14 (1990), p. 5. The author was fighting both EBV and Candida.

79. *ME Newsletter* (Summer 1988), p. 38.

80. Ibid., p. 24. Nystatin is the generic term for an antifungal drug, large oral doses of which will themselves produce symptoms.

81. Ibid., (Autumn 1989), p. 51.

82. *Keeping in Touch*, no. 4 (October/November, 1990), p. 7.

83. Ibid., p. 30.

84. These examples all are taken from patients' newsletters, individual issues cited above.

85. See the *MEssenger*, 2 (Spring 1990), p. 1.

86. Stewart, "Changing Faces of Somatization" (1990), pp. 155–157.

87. Maggie Christensen, "Smart Consumers Present a Marketing Challenge," *Hospitals,* 63 (August 20, 1989), pp. 42–47; quote from p. 44.
88. Ibid., p. 42.
89. Gallup poll commissioned by the American Medical Association, quoted in *New York Times,* February 18, 1990, p. A21. These data represent a continuation of trends that had begun at least as soon as the early 1980s. See George D. Lundberg, "Medicine—A Profession in Trouble?" *JAMA,* 253 (May 17, 1985), pp. 2879–2880, on survey data for the years 1982–85 showing declines in the percent of the public who believe that "physicians explain things well," and that "physicians' fees are reasonable."
90. Shorter, *The Making of the Modern Family* (New York: Basic Books, 1975). For an updating of this analysis see Shorter, "Einige demographische Auswirkungen des postmodernen Familienlebens," *Zeitschrift für Bevölkerungswissenschaft,* 15 (1989), pp. 221–233. Also Shorter, "Recent Changes in Family Life and New Challenges in Primary Care," *Canadian Family Physician,* forthcoming.
91. Research note, "Age at First Marriage Continues to Rise; More U.S. Couples Cohabiting," *Family Planning Perspectives,* 18 (1986), p. 91.
92. Paul C. Glick, "A Demographer Looks Again at American Families," *Journal of Family Issues,* 8 (1987), pp. 437–439; quote from p. 438.
93. For social data see A. Thornton, "The Changing American Family," *Population Bulletin,* 38 (4), 1983; Paul Glick, "American Household Structure in Transition," *Family Planning Perspectives,* 16 (1984), pp. 205–211.
94. Michel Dahlin, "Perspectives on the Family Life of the Elderly in 1900," *Gerontologist,* 20 (1980), pp. 99–107, especially tab. 1, p. 100.
95. Donald A. West et al., "The Effects of Loneliness: A Review of the Literature," *Comprehensive Psychiatry,* 27 (1986), pp. 351–363; quote from p. 358.
96. J. N. Westhead, "Frequent Attenders in General Practice: Medical, Psychological and Social Characteristics," *Journal of the Royal College of General Practitioners,* 35 (1985), pp. 337–340.
97. Michael Brennan and Amy Noce, "A Study of Patients with Psychosocial Problems in a Family Practice," *Journal of Family Practice,* 13 (1981), pp. 837–843; quote from p. 837.
98. Maura C. Ryan and Joanne Patterson, "Loneliness in the Elderly," *Journal of Gerontological Nursing,* 13 (1987), pp. 6–12; quote from p. 9.
99. Salit, *Canadian Medical Association Journal* (1985), p. 660.
100. Carroll M. Brodsky, "'Allergic to Everything': A Medical Subculture," *Psychosomatics,* 24 (1983), pp. 731–742; data from p. 732.
101. Donna E. Stewart and Joel Raskin, "Psychiatric Assessment of Patients with '20th-Century Disease' ('Total Allergy Syndrome')," *Canadian Medical Association Journal,* 133 (November 15, 1985), pp. 1001–1006 for the report. Personal communication for the social data.

Index

Abend, Ludwig, 217
Abercrombie, John, 26–27, 106
Abernathy, John, 105
Abraham, Karl, 257–58
Adair, James Makittrick, 24
Addiction to surgery, 91
Adler, Alfred, 47
Aitken, John, 17
Alexander, Franz, 259–61
Allan, Frank, 284
Allbutt, Clifford, 58–59, 205–6
Alvarez, Walter, 86, 290
Amann, Joseph, 57, 97, 229, 278
Amputations of "paralyzed" limbs,
    126–27
Andree, John, 14
Anesthesias, 7–8
Animal magnetism, 129, 134–65. See also
    Hypnosis
Animals, attribution of internal sensation
    to, 52–55
Armand, Marquis de Puységur, 135
Asher, Patria, 269
Astasia-abasia, 108, 111–12
Autonomic symptoms, 4, 8–10. See also
    Internal sensation
Axenfeld, August, 35
Azam, Étienne Eugène, 145, 162

Babinski, Joseph, 175, 197–99, 241, 247,
    256
Backhaus, Carl, 87
Baeyer, Walter von, 269
Barker, Fordyce, 74
Barker, Lewellys Franklin, 282
Barr, Y. M., 309
Barsky, Arthur, 296
Baruk, Henri, 146
Bastian, Charlton, 192
Battey, Robert, 75–76

Battey's operation, 75–81
Baynard, Edward, 15
Beard, George, 221, 230, 239, 277, 281
Beauchêne, Edme-Pierre Cauvot de,
    17–18
Beecher, Henry Ward, 214
Belbèze, Raymond, 59–60, 225
Belhoome, Jacques-Etienne, 136
Benedikt, Moritz, 13, 33, 81, 99–100,
    127, 153, 191
Beni-Barde, Joseph-Marie-Alfred, 228
Bennett, Alice, 80
Berger, Herbert, 263–64
Berger, Oskar, 152–53
Berger, Paul, 214
Bernheim, Hippolyte, 246, 247
Berthier, Pierre, 49
Bichat, Marie François Xavier, 18
Billings, Frank, 77
Binswanger, Otto, 290
Bisoliére, Roget de la, 7
Blandin, Philippe-Frédéric, 136
Bleuler, Eugen, 257
Blocq, Paul, 111
Bödecker, Justus, 220
Boettiger, Alfred, 230
Bohr, Thomas, 313
Bonamaison, Léonce, 188–90
Bonhoeffer, Karl, 258
Bossi, Luigi Maria, 207
Bouchard, Charles, 175
Bourdin, Claude-Étienne, 145
Bournville, Desiré-Magloire, 179–80
Bowel disorders, 8–9, 25, 69
Braid, James, 135
Brain disease theories: see Central nervous
    theories
"Brain mythology," era of, 210
Bramwell, Byron, 126
Bramwell, Edwin, 250

Breuer, Josef, 68, 196, 242, 253
Brierre de Boismont, Alexandre, 144
Briquet, Pierre, 97–98, 116–18, 212
Brissaud, Edouard, 195–96
Brodie, Benjamin, 31–32, 42, 56, 110–11, 126–27, 212, 272
Brosius, Caspar Max, 211
Broussais, François Joseph Victor, 21, 69
Brown, Isaac Baker, 83, 85
Brown, John, 21
Brown, Thomas, 27
Brown-Séquard, Charles-Édouard, 45–46
Brucellosis, chronic, 305–6
Brück, Anton, 262
Brücke, Ernst Wilhelm von, 238
Bryant, Joseph, 92
Bumke, Oswald, 210, 230–31, 244, 271, 272
Bürger-Prinz, Hans, 271
Burns, John, 22
Burq, Victor Jean-Marie, 181
Busch, Dietrich, 52–53, 82, 213

Cabanis, Pierre Jean Georges, 18
Campe, Joachim Heinrich, 213
Carter, Robert Brudenell, 56, 73, 202, 236
Cassedy, James, 213–14
Castration
    of men, 93
    oophorectomy, 74–81
Catalepsy
    Charcot's hysteria and, 182–83
    decline of, 164, 165
    diagnosis of, 133
    hypnotic, 136–46
    symptoms of, 130–33
Catatonia, 145
Cathartic method, 253–56
Cathell, Daniel Webster, 63, 264
Cauterization of clitoris, 85
Central nervous theories, 201, 208–32, 277
    fatigue, 226–27, 277–85
    nerve doctors, 213–20
    neurasthenia, 220–32, 277–80
    pain, 285–89
    rise of, 208–13
Cerise, Laurent, 144
Charcot, Jean-Martin, 35, 42, 43, 79, 118, 120, 151, 166–86, 191, 193–200, 221, 227, 239
    biography of, 167–73

    personality of, 173–75
Charcot's hysteria, 166–200
    diffusion of, 186–93
    disappearance of, 196–200
    doctrine of, 175–81
    hypnosis and, 176, 181–85, 194
    metallotherapy and, 181
    "psychological" theories and, 193–96
Chéron, Jules, 214
Chevallier, Jean-Baptiste, 104, 117
Chevallier, Paul, 90–91
Chodoff, Paul, 270
Chronic fatigue immune deficiency syndrome (CFIDS), 306–7, 310
Chronic fatigue syndrome (CFS), 304–18
Church, Archibald, 93
Churchill, Fleetwood, 50
Circumcision, 93–94
Claretie, Jules, 174, 187
Clark, Andrew, 223
Claude, Henry, 146
Cleaves, Margaret, 80, 102–3
Cleckley, Hervey M., 164
Clegg, James, 5–6
Clemens, Theodor, 113
Clitoridectomy, 81–86
Cohen, Mandel, 91
Cohn, Hermann, 152
Colitis, 9, 265
Collins, Joseph, 163–64, 228, 251
Collins, Wilkie, 228–29
Coma, hysterical, 130–34
Conolly, John, 70, 110, 131, 288
Cullen, William, 19, 215
Culturally determined templates of illness, 2–3, 96, 266, 285, 314–19

Daudet, Alphonse, 171
Daudet, Léon, 166–67, 174–75, 183
Davis, Albert, 124
Davis, David, 212
Dejerine, Jules-Joseph, 175, 186, 197–98, 241, 247, 249
Dejerine-Klumpke, Augusta, 175
Delboeuf, Joseph, 182
De Lee, Joseph, 283
Dercum, Clara, 202
Despine, Charles, 105, 139–43, 149–50, 160–61, 312
Determann, Hermann, 37
Dewey, Richard, 93
Diehl, August, 279
Digestive tract, as master organ, 18

Dissociation, 129–65
    catalepsy: *see* Catalepsy
    defined, 129
    hypnosis and: *see* Hypnosis
    multiple personality disorder, 155,
        159–65
    "permanently benumbed" state,
        155–59
    somnambulism: *see* Somnambulism
Disturbing encounters, hysterical paraly-
    sis from, 113
Doctor–patient relationship, 56, 126–28,
    165, 249–50, 295
Drummond, David, 223, 249–50
Dubois, Paul, 185, 221, 247–49
Dunbar, Helen Flanders, 261
Dupotet, Jules, 144–45

Edes, Robert, 77, 108, 256, 282
Edinger, Ludwig, 242
Edis, Arthur, 50
Eeden, Frederik van, 246
Eger, Sänitatsrat, 152
Eitingon, Max, 259
Electrotherapy, 104
Ellenberger, Henri, 160
Emmett, Thomas, 99
Engelmann, George, 77
Environmental hypersensitivity, 318–19
Epidemic hysteria, 270–71, 305
Epstein, Michael, 309
Epstein-Barr virus infection, 285, 303,
    309–10, 312, 313, 317
Erb, Wilhelm, 35, 216–17, 241–42
Étiolles, Raoul LeRoy d', 82
Eulenberg, Albert, 219
Ewald, Karl Anton, 154
Expectation of disease presentation, 14

Facial pain, chronic, 297–98
Family
    Charcot's hysteria and, 186–87
    motor hysteria and, 120–25
    paradigm shift and, 294
    somatization in postmodern life and,
        320–23
Family tragedies, hysterical paralysis
    from, 113–14
Fatigue, chronic, 277–85, 304–18
    Epstein-Barr virus infection, 285, 303,
        309–10, 312, 313, 317
    fibrositis (fibromyalgia), 311–13, 316

incidence at end of 20th century, 300–
        301, 306–7
    mass media and, 314–18
    myalgic encephalomyelitis, 285, 311–
        13, 315–16
    neurasthenia and, 226–27, 277–80
    neuromyasthenia, 307–10
Feedback loops, 322
Fellner, Leopold, 61
Féré, Charles, 196
Feuillade, Henri, 227, 231
Fibrositis (fibromyalgia), 311–13, 316
Fiessinger, Charles, 280
Fischer, F., 162
Fits, hysterical, 5–6, 25, 95–102, 107–8
    in Charcot's hysteria, 175–80, 187, 189,
        190
    clitoridectomies to arrest, 82–83
    vs. epileptic fits, 96–97
    main variations of, 96
    precipitating symptoms of, 98
    predominance of, 96
    secondary gain element of, 98–99
    social class and, 101–2
    typical course of, 97–98
    unsympathetic assessments of, 99–100
Fixed illness attribution, 301–7, 319–20
Flaccid paralysis, 108–10
Flaconer, William, 234–35
Flechsig, Paul, 80, 210, 241–42
Fliess, Wilhelm, 67–68
Folk culture, 319
Forel, August, 210–11, 215–16
Förster, Richard, 49
Foster, Edward, 17
Fräkel, Ernst, 152
Francis, Henry A., 66
Franque, Arnold von, 107
Frederick, Carlton C., 87
Freud, Sigmund, 67–68, 121, 169, 191,
        196, 210, 218, 219, 222, 231, 242,
        253–54, 256, 259, 289
Freund, Hermann Wolfgang, 49
Friedreich, Johannes, 15, 208

Gamgee, Arthur, 182
Garvey, John, 227
Gattel, Felix, 254–56
Gaupp, Robert, 244
Genital irritation, 92–93, 117–18
Georget, Étienne-Jean, 202
Giffard, William, 20
Glick, Thomas, 320

413

Globus hystericus, 6
Gmelin, Eberhard, 161–62
Goltz, Friedrich, 203
Goncourt, Edmond de, 174, 188
Goodell, William, 77
Gowers, William, 312
Griesinger, Wilhelm, 69, 208–10, 215, 219
Gudden, Bernhard von, 210–11
Gull, William, 109
Gynecological surgery, 69–94
  clitoridectomy, 81–86
  to cure nervous and mental illness, 73–81
  decline of use of, 202–8
  desire for, as psychosomatic symptom, 86–92
  pelvic organs as supposed cause of insanity, 69–73

Hack, Wilhelm, 65
Hall, Marshall, 41–42
Haller, Albrecht von, 20–21, 24
Halliday, James, 269
Hammond, William Alexander, 34, 239
Hansen, Carl, 151–53
Harling, Robert, 85
Hartenberg, Paul, 226, 280
Hartmann, Arthur, 64
Harvey, William, 16
Haygarth, John, 234–35
Headaches, 290–91, 296–97
Hecker, Ewald, 211, 219
Hegar, Alfred, 75, 76
Heidenhain, Rudolf, 153
Heinroth, Johann Christian August, 234
Hemiplegias, 108–9
Hesnard, Angelo, 231–32, 269
Hewitt, Graily, 291
Hinds, Frank, 276
Hoffmann, Friedrich, 19
Hohnstock, G. L. V., 8–9
Holmes, Gary, 310
Holmes, Oliver Wendell, Sr., 32
Holst, Valentin von, 121–22, 190–91
Hooper, J. M., 48
Hoppin, August, 281–82
Hösslin, Rudolph von, 224
Houston, William R., 77
Hovell, Dennis de Berdt, 114, 236–37, 278, 288
Hovell, Thomas, 66
Hubertus, Kurhaus, 220

Huchard, Henri, 188
Hückel, Armand, 287
Hughes, Charles H., 224
Humoral theory, 14–15
Hyde, Byron, 313
Hypnosis, 129–65
  Charcot's hysteria and, 176, 181–85, 194
  first wave, 134–50
  hypnotic catalepsy, 136–46
  induced somnambulism, 135–36, 146–50
  multiple personality disorder, 155, 159–65
  "permanently benumbed" state and, 155–59
  second wave, 150–55, 246
  sensory symptoms and, 150–51
Hypochondria, 9, 12
Hysteria
  as central nervous disease, 212–13, 215, 220, 223–24
  Charcot's: *see* Charcot's hysteria
  epidemic, 270–71, 305
  Freud and, 259
  motor: *see* Motor hysteria
  psychological view of, 234–44, 293
"Hystero-epilepsy," 176, 177, 179

Illich, Ivan, 285
Immunologists, 314–15
Internal sensation, 4, 51–64
  attributed to live animals, 52–55
  medicalizing of, 55
  ovary, fixation on, 60–63
  uterus, fixation on, 56–60, 63–64
Intimate relationships, 294, 320–21
Irritable bowel syndrome, 9
Irritable weakness, 209–10, 220
Irritation, 20–22. *See also* Reflex theory
  genital, 92–93, 117–18
  vs. inflammation, 21, 22, 28
  in males, 117–18
  spinal, 25–39, 73
Isaacs, Raphael, 309
Isenflamm, Jacob Friedrich, 18, 24, 117
Israel, James, 202–3

Jaccoud, Sigismond, 111
Jacob, John, 130
Jacobi, Mary Putnam, 50–51, 80, 223–24, 291
Janet, Pierre, 53, 162–63, 195, 231

Jelliffe, Smith Ely, 250–51
Joal, Joseph, 66
Johnson, J. Taber, 77
Johnson, Walter, 30–31
Johnston, Victor, 290–91
Joint pain, 108, 110–11
Joire, Paul, 286
Jolly, Friedrich, 216–17, 219
Jones, Ernest, 68, 218
Juliusburger, Otto, 220

Kalhbaum, Karl, 211–12, 219
Kalischer, Siegfried, 220
Kaltenbach, Rudolf, 206
Katon, Wayne, 297
Keetley, Charles Bell, 204
Kehrer, Erwin, 46–47
Kerner, Justinus, 147–49
Kläsi, Jakob, 256
Klotz, Hermann, 78
Kluge, Carl, 135
Knapp, Philip C., 57, 282
Koömer, Richard, 93
Kopiopia hysterica, 49
Kraepelin, Emil, 154, 231, 241–44
Krafft-Ebing, Richard von, 13, 35, 72, 154, 215
Krecke, Albert, 90
Krishaber, Maurice, 119
Kroner, Traugott, 152
Krönig, Bernhard, 81, 206
Kühner, August, 222

Laehr, Heinrich, 74, 213
Landouzy, Hector, 53, 107–8, 118, 288
Laughlin, Henry, 270
Laycock, Thomas, 43–44, 53
Le Camus, Antoine, 245
Lesse, Stanley, 298
Leube, Wilhelm Olivier, 217, 251
Levillain, Fernand, 228, 280
Leyden, Ernst von, 121
Lhéritier, Sébastien-Disier, 36–37
Lièbeault, Ambroise-Auguste, 246
Liebermeister, Carl von, 238–39
Lisfranc, Jacques, 82–83, 107
Lockhart-Mummery, John Percy, 61–62
Loneliness, 321–23
Louyer-Villermay, Jean-Baptiste, 18, 82, 98–99
Löwenfeld, Leopold, 66, 214
Luys, Jules-Bernard, 172, 182

Maass, Martin, 220
Macario, Maurice, 105, 150
Macartney, William, 33
Mackenzie, John Noland, 65
Mackenzie, Sir Morell, 222
Macnaughton-Jones, Henry, 50, 71, 72, 85
Magendie, François, 23
Magnan, Valentin, 213
"Magnetizers," 129, 134–65. See also Hypnosis
Males
  motor hysteria in, 117–20
  sexual surgery for, 92–94
Mankiewitz, Samuel, 220
Mannerism, hysterical paralysis as kind of, 115–17
Manning, Henry, 101
Manton, Walter P., 80
Marie, Pierre, 168, 176
Mass media, 314–17, 319–20
Master organs, theory of, 16–18
Maubray, John, 131
Maudsley, Henry, 71
Maupassant, Guy de, 186–87
Mayer, August, 207
Mayer, Edward, 257
Mayer, Louis, 70–71
Medical authority, loss of, 314–20
Medical encounters, hysterical paralysis from, 115
Medicalization, 203–4
Mendel, Emanuel, 218–19
Menninger, Karl, 91
Mental illness
  gynecological surgery to cure, 69–81
  pelvic organs as supposed cause of, 69–73
Mesmer, Franz Anton, 134–36
Mesmerism, 135. See also Hypnosis; Somnambulism
Mesnet, Ernest, 111
Meyer, Semi, 112, 279, 291
Meynert, Theodor, 210
Mezler, Franz Xaver, 131–32
Michell, Jan Petersen, 24
Miles, Francis, 239
Mingazzini, Giovanni, 272
Möbius, Paul Julius, 154, 239–41, 244, 246
Moll, Albert, 154
Monakow, Constantin von, 222
Mononucleosis, infectious, 309

Monoplegias, 108–9
Morel, Benedict-Augstin, 213
Morestin, Hippolyte, 268
Morgagni, Giovanni Battista, 19
Motor hysteria, 4, 95–128
  catalepsy: *see* Catalepsy
  decline of, 267–73
  diagnosis of, 12–14
  fits: *see* Fits, hysterical
  internal sensation and: *see* Internal sensation
  in males, 117–20
  paralysis: *see* Paralysis, hysterical
  reflex theory and, 95
  somnambulism: *see* Somnambulism
  uterus and, 17–18
  vapors, 6, 11, 17–19, 24
Motor symptoms, 3–7, 95–96
Müller, Johannes, 70
Multiple personality disorder, 155, 159–65
Munchausen's syndrome, 91–92
Mundé, Paul, 88–90
Munthe, Alex, 185, 264–65
Murray, William, 84
Musil, Robert, 3, 214
Myalgic encephalomyelitis (ME), 285, 311–13, 315–16
Myerson, Abraham, 127, 282

Nancy school, 154–55, 196, 246
Nasal-reflex theory, 64–68
Nerve doctors, 213–20
Nervous system
  autonomic, 4, 8–10
  central nervous theories: *see* Central nervous theories
  irritation doctrine, 20–22
  reflex theory: *see* Reflex theory
  somatosensory, 3–4
  spinal irritation, 25–39
  theories stressing role of, 18–23
Neurasthenia, 220–32, 277–80
Neuromyasthenia, 307–10
Neuroses, central nervous theory and, 215–16
Nissl, Franz, 244
Nothnagel, Hermann, 251
Nymphomania, treatment of, 81–86

Obersteiner, Heinrich, 153–54
Ogle, John, 119
Ohr, C. H., 51

Oppenheim, Hermann, 217–19
Organ-falling theory, 47
"Organic brain" theories, 210
Osler, William, 125, 166, 224
Ovaries
  Charcot's hysteria and, 178–81
  preoccupation with, 60–63
  reflex theory doctrine and, 43–44, 49, 202, 203
  removal to cure nervous and mental illness, 74–81, 202, 203

Pain, psychogenic, 1, 4, 8, 12, 277, 285–93
  central nervous theory and, 285–89
  culture and, 285
  current hypersensitivity to, 295–99
  from fibrositis (fibromyalgia), 311–13, 316
  gender differences in incidence of, 292–93
  joint, 108, 110–11
  from myalgic encephalomyelitis, 285, 311–13, 315–16
  psychological paradigm and, 289–92
  reality of sensation of, 287–88
Pallen, Montrose, 119
Palmer, Chauncey, 58
Pan-nervousness, 223
Paradigm shift, 1–2, 267–94
Paralysis, hysterical, 4, 7, 95, 102–17, 294
  doctors' dislike of, 125–28
  family psychodrama and, 120–25
  forms of, 108–12
  physical trauma as trigger for, 114–15
  reflex theory and, 45, 46, 95
  rise of, 102–8
  shock as trigger for, 112–14
Paraplegias, 108–9
Parker, George, 257
Parker, Harry, 125–26
Parkes Weber, Frederick, 60–62, 66, 204–5, 273–77, 312
Parrish, Isaac, 28–29
Pathoplasticity, 266, 305, 318–19
Pelvic organs: *see* Ovaries; Uterus
Penis, reflex theory and, 51
Peretti, Josef, 78, 207
Peripheral localization theory, 18
"Permanently benumbed" state, 155–59
Petetin, Jacques-Henri-Désiré, 137–39
Petrén, Karl, 225

Peyer, Alexander, 51
Physical trauma, hysterical paralysis from, 114–15
Pierce, Robert, 7, 8
Piorry, Pierre-Adolphe, 97, 105, 136
Pitres, Jean-Albert, 190
Placebo operation, 202–3
Player, R. R., 26
Pomme, Pierre, 24, 131
Preissner, Felix, 55, 101–2, 292
Priestly, William, 87
Prinzhorn, Hans, 258
Proschaska, Georg, 23
Pseudoepilepsy: see Fits, hysterical
Psychoanalysis, 253–61, 289
Psychological paradigm, 201, 233–66
  forerunners of, 233–39
  pain and, 289–92
  patients' rejection of, 261–66
  psychoanalysis, 253–61, 289
  psychotherapy, 245–53
  rejection by chronic fatigue patients, 317
  rise of, 239–45
Psychoneuroses, 215, 222
Psychoses, central nervous theory and, 215–16
Psychotherapy, 245–53
Pujol, Raymond, 280
Purcell, John, 6, 213

"Railway spine," 114
Raspe, Rudolf Erich, 91
Rayer, Pierre, 167, 168
Raymond, Fulgence, 197, 248
Receptionists' syndrome, 280, 284
Reflex neurosis, 43, 73–74, 93
Reflex theory, 14, 40–68, 201
  brain and, 69–70
  clitoridectomy and, 81–86
  defined, 40
  destruction of, 202–8
  evolution of, 42–44
  founding of, 41–42
  genital irritation, 92–93
  medicalizing of internal sensation and, 55
  motor hysteria and: see Motor hysteria
  nasal, 64–68
  ovarian, 43–44, 49, 74–81, 202, 203
  pelvic organs as supposed cause of insanity, 69–73
  pelvic preoccupation and, 56–60, 63–64

reflex arc concept, 20, 22–23, 41, 95
  sexual surgery on males and, 93–94
  total-body, 45–48
  uterine, 40–43, 49–51, 70, 72–74, 202–8
Renterghem, Albert Willem van, 246
Reynolds, Russell, 205, 237–38, 288–89
Rheinstädter, August, 63
Riadore, Evans, 29, 42
Richardson, Horace, 283–84
Rieger, Conrad, 222, 242
Riklin, Franz, 255–56
Rivet, Maria, 123
Robertson, George, 246–47
Rockwell, Alphonso, 221
Rohé, George, 79–80
Romberg, Moritz, 35, 38, 42–44, 118
Roots, William, 17, 235–36
Rosenbach, Ottomar, 251–53
Rosenthal, Moritz, 64, 85
Ross, Sheila M., 71–72
Ross, Thomas Arthur, 250
Rowley, William, 234
"Royal Free epidemic," 310–11

Sadler, John, 16
Sandras, Clause-Marie-Stanislas, 82, 221
Sarradon, Jean, 50
Savage, George, 62, 223
Savill, Thomas Dixon, 192
Sayre, Lewis Albert, 94
Schaeffer, Henri, 293
Schindler, Rudolf, 263
Schizophrenia, 231
Schlesinger, Wilhelm, 144–45
Schoder, Johann, 136–37
Schofield, Alfred Taylor, 256, 272–73, 291
Schreiber, Joseph, 278–79
Schröder, Karl, 76, 81, 89
Schultz, Johann, 258
Schultze, Bernhard, 207
Schütz, Eduard Robert, 217
Schützenberger, Charles, 44
Seif, Leonard, 255–56
Sensory symptoms, 3–4, 7–8, 12, 150–51, 177, 285
Seymour, Edward, 235
Shap, Jane, 16
Shaw, George Bernard, 89–90
Shell shock, 271
Shepherd, Michael, 300–301
Shock, hysterical paralysis from, 112–14

417

Siemerling, Ernst, 207
Simmel, Ernst, 259
Simon, Clément, 197
Simpson, Alexander Russell, 76
Simpson, Frederick, 96
Simpson, John, 30
Singer, Charles, 21
Sirois, François, 270
Skey, Frederic, 32, 127, 236, 288
Skoda, Joseph, 137, 238
Smart, Gibbons, 282
Smart, T. N., 28
Smith, Heywood, 76
Smith, Tyler, 83–84
Social isolation, 321–23
Sollier, Paul, 157–59
Somatogenic symptoms, 2
Somatosensory nervous system, 3–4
Sommer, Robert, 17, 242, 244
Somnambulism, 134, 154
    Charcot's hysteria and, 183
    decline of, 165
    induced, 135–36, 146–50
    symptoms of, 130
Souques, Alexandre, 199
Spas
    hysterical paralysis cures and, 104
    spinal irritation cures and, 35–37
Spastic contracture, 108, 109
Spinal cord, reflex arc theory and, 22–23
Spinal irritation, 25–39, 73
Stekel, Wilhelm, 68, 198, 216, 259–60
Stewart, Donna, 305, 322
Steyerthal, Armin, 199–200
Stiebel, Salomon, 149
Stiller, Berthold, 230
Stilling, Benedict, 35
Stimson, Charles, 289
Stoddart, William, 256
Straus, Stephen, 317
Stromeyer, Louis, 115–16, 118–19, 127
Strümpell, Adolf, 241, 242, 244
Subculture of illness, 304
Suckling, Cornelius, 192
Surgery
    desire for, 86–92
    gynecological: see Gynecological surgery
    hysterical paralysis from, 115
    sexual, on males, 92–94
Sutleffe, Edward, 107
Sympathy, doctrine of, 20

Symptoms, psychogenic, 1–12
    autonomic, 4, 8–10
    catalepsy: see Catalepsy
    categories of, 3–4
    central nervous theories: see Central nervous theories
    Charcot's hysteria: see Charcot's hysteria
    defined, 2
    desire for surgery as, 86–92
    18th-century census of, 10–12
    fatigue: see Fatigue, chronic
    fits: see Fits, hysterical
    hysterical paralysis: see Paralysis, hysterical
    internal sensations of women, 51–64
    motor, 3–7, 95–96
    multiple personality disorder, 155, 159–65
    neurasthenia, 220–32, 277–80
    ovary, fixation on, 60–63
    pain: see Pain, psychogenic
    permanently benumbed" state, 155–59
    pool of, 2–3, 5–10
    psychological paradigm of: see Psychological paradigm
    sensory, 3–4, 7–8, 12, 150–51, 177, 285
    "shaping" of, 1–2, 4, 13, 24, 25, 63, 129, 136, 166, 266, 293, 307–20
    somnambulism: see Somnambulism
    spinal irritation, 30–33
    uterus, fixation on, 56–60

Tanner, Thomas, 84–85
Taylor, Stephen, 272
Teale, Thomas Pridgin, 27–28
Theilhaber, Adolph, 206–7
Thigpen, Corbett H., 164
Thomas, Robert, 82
Todd, Robert Bentley, 29, 212
Total-body-reflex theories, 45–48
Tourette, Georges Gilles de la, 79
"Traumatic neurosis," 114–15
Traut, Eugene, 312
Travers, Benjamin, 26, 42, 110, 117, 263
Tuke, Hack, 245–46
Tuke, Samuel, 245

Underwood, E. Ashworth, 21
Uterus
    as master organ, 16–18
    preoccupation with, 56–60, 63–64

reflex theory doctrine and, 40–43, 49–
    51, 70, 72–74, 202–8
as supposed cause of insanity, 70–72
surgery to cure nervous and mental ill-
    ness, 73–74
viewed as live animal, 52, 53

Vance, Ap Morgan, 34, 59, 127–28
Vapors, 6, 11, 17–19, 24
Vaughan, Peter, 316
Verhaeghe, Louis, 36, 104
Villar, François, 79
Virchow, Rudolph, 191
Voisin, Auguste-Félix, 72, 172, 182
Volkmann, Alfred Wilhelm, 70
Voltolini, Friedrich, 64
Vulpian, Félix, 170

Wagner-Jauregg, Julius, 13
Wanke, George, 262
Weber, Sir Hermann, 256

Wechsler, Israel, 102, 269–70
Wegelin, Adrian, 101
Weil, Julius, 220
Weir Mitchell, Silas, 111, 126, 127, 132–
    33, 278, 287
Weiss, Edward A., 57–58, 227
Wessely, Simon, 311, 313
Westphal, Karl Friedrich, 43, 80–81, 219
Whytt, Robert, 22–23, 234
Wiederhold, Moritz, 94
Wilks, Samuel, 192–93
Williams, Leonard, 48
Wilson, Kinnier, 193, 268
Windscheid, Franz, 207
Winternitz, Wilhelm, 37, 66, 216
Wollenberg, Robert, 100–101
Wundt, William, 241

Yeast infections, 318–19

Zola, Emile, 186